Foundations of Anthroposophical Medicine

You may also be interested in...

Anthroposophical Care for the Elderly
Annegret Camps, Brigitte Hagenhoff & Ada van der Star

Anthroposophical Therapeutic Speech
Barabara Denjean-von Stryk & Dietrich von Bonin

Biographical Work
The Anthroposophical Basis

Gudrun Burkhard

Compresses and other Therapeutic Applications
A Handbook from the Ita Wegman Clinic

Monika Fingado

Foundations of Curative Eurythmy
Dr Margarete Kirchner-Bockholt

The Physiology of Eurythmy Therapy
Hans-Broder and Elke E. von Laue

Rhythmic Einreibung
A Handbook from the Ita Wegman Clinic

Monika Fingado

Foundations of Anthroposophical Medicine

Edited by
Guus van der Bie & Machteld Huber

Floris Books

Translation from Dutch by Jan Kees Saltet

First published in Dutch as *Opleiding Antroposofische Geneeskunde*

First published in English by Floris Books in 2003
Fourth printing 2014

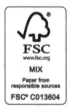

FSC
www.fsc.org
MIX
Paper from
responsible sources
FSC® C013604

British Library CIP Data available
ISBN 978-086315-417-1

Printed in Great Britain
by CPI Group (UK) Ltd, Croydon

Contents

Introduction

This manual was originally written in Dutch under the aegis of the teaching committee of the Dutch Anthroposophical Doctors Association. The authors are medical doctors and a medical biologist, all active in the medical profession and/or in teaching anthroposophical medicine. All authors have had an education in anthroposophical medicine in some form. They are familiar with the current literature and practice in this field.

Excellent basic literature on anthroposophical medicine is available, albeit mostly in German.

In this manual, which is part of the Dutch training course for doctors an attempt is made to come to a new way of teaching. On the one hand there is the content of the manual which contains elements which can build bridges between conventional medicine and anthroposophical medicine. For example, anthroposophical medicine is set in its historic and philosophical context. Then, extensive attention is given to the way sense perception and the assimilating process of thinking connected with it, can lead to new insights and also place hitherto unrelated aspects into a common context.

Examples of this are worked out in biological and medical themes.

Subsequently, nature is observed in such a way that its 'elements' can be recognized, both in the surrounding natural world and in ourselves, and related to one aspect of the anthroposophical image of the human being: the four bodily members.

Inevitably, if we study anthroposophy, we need to study the works of its founder, Rudolf Steiner. A method for the study of Steiner's works which may prove fruitful to the reader is described. Finally the path of inner development for the physician is discussed. It is an essential aspect of becoming an anthroposophical doctor. All these topics together constitute the first steps of an extension of medicine; they are not yet the actual practice of anthroposophical medicine.

On the other hand the form in which this content is offered, is new. The text contains many assignments and exercises that the reader can apply in daily practice. Through this the manual can lead the reader to new experiences and new skills. However, anthroposophical medicine cannot be learned merely from a book. It becomes a living reality in the way each individual doctor lives and works with it. That is why, in the Dutch doctors' training, the study of this manual is used in the context of frequent contact with a personal tutor, an experienced anthroposophical doctor. And after this an extended program is offered in which anthroposophical medicine is introduced in a more practical way.

The intention of this manual is to present a diversity of themes, to give doctors with different interests and inclinations the opportunity to recognize subjects that connect to their specific interest. It is inevitable that not all chapters will have the same appeal to each reader. However, this diversity can enrich, when those working together strive for communication and mutual understanding. Some physicians, by their natures, tend more towards reflection, others towards action; for still others, their empathy with the patient is primary. The different styles of the authors have been kept to add to the variety.

We would like to make a special comment about how to begin to use this manual. We recommend that the reader review Chapter 10, before starting with Chapter 1. Through this the reader will best be able to keep clearly in mind the thread that runs all through this manual.

A comment about gender usage: when 'he' or 'she' is written, both sexes are meant.

With the translation into English the attempt was made to stay as close as possible to the intentions and way of thinking of the authors. We thank translator Jan Kees Saltet for his great concern and preciseness. Next to him we owe great gratitude to Dr Alicia Landman-Reiner from the U.S.A. and Dr Frank Mulder from the U.K., both experienced anthroposophical doctors, who meticulously edited the text for language, content and translation from their professional perspective. We think they all did a great job!

This translation has been made possible by gifts from the Physicians' Association for Anthroposophical Medicine in the U.S. via the Seward Fund, the New Zealand Association of Anthroposophical Doctors, The Hermes Trust in the U.K. and the Dutch Iona Stichting. We are very grateful to them all.

Guus van der Bie and Machteld Huber
on behalf of the authors

CHAPTER 1

The Art and Science of Medicine

Anthroposophical Medicine and its Place in the History of Medicine

ANTON DEKKERS

1.1 Introduction

In 1920 Rudolf Steiner held the first cycle of lectures for physicians *Geisteswissenschaft und Medizin,* in English: *Spiritual Science and Medicine,* now commonly called the *First Medical Course.**

Before that he had touched on medical subjects in individual lectures and also in one small lecture cycle given in 1911, for a general audience, *Occult Physiology* [*Eine okkulte Physiologie*]. In the *First Medical Course,* however, lectures specifically given to physicians, a broad foundation for anthroposophical medicine was laid for the first time. In the first of twenty lectures Steiner starts off by giving a sketch of the history of medicine. He did this primarily, he says, to demonstrate that people had ideas about health and illness in the past which differ very much from the notion which prevails today, which is that illness is a deviation from the norm and that healing is a return to the norm. In the course of the lecture it becomes clear that this changing view of health and illness is bound up with the *evolution of human consciousness* in the course of time, and is therefore connected with the way in which we perceive and think, for example. In addition to this, he *introduces the notion of the ether body — Archaeus,* and discusses the importance of *the intuitive attitude of the physician.*

It is recommended at this point to read the first part of the first lecture of the First Medical Course, *in the Appendix.*

---

* A list of current English translations of Steiner's medical works is given in the Bibliography.

1.2 Two principal streams in the history of medicine

This chapter, loosely connected to the first lecture of the *First Medical Course,* deals with the different streams in medical thinking and the physicians representing these streams.

In this historical survey, the main focus will be on those elements which we often encounter in anthroposophical medicine. At the conclusion of the chapter a brief sketch will be given of the relationship of anthroposophical medicine to these streams.

It is important for physicians to enter into the history of medicine for several reasons. These are:

1) In medical school we are educated from one specific viewpoint, which looks at things on a cellular-molecular level. We're so much immersed in this viewpoint, that we are in danger of no longer seeing its relativity. The history of medicine teaches us that there are also other viewpoints concerning health, illness and healing. This can lead us to rethink our present viewpoints and we can also experience whether and how our own ideas sometimes link up with those of physicians of former times. We thus gain a clearer idea of our own position.

2) This can call forth *enthusiasm,* and kindle the will to further penetrate the riddles posed by health and illness in our daily work as physicians.

3) We learn to think in terms of *developmental processes.* The importance of this will become more obvious in the ensuing chapters. Every process of development has its own specific traits, its individual signature. If we look at the way in which Steiner describes history in the lecture, it turns out that he specifically focuses on the changing consciousness of humanity. He makes clear that our internal changes manifest in external changes, resulting in, for example, discoveries.

Assignment 1
Suppose you visit a patient with pneumonia. What are your thoughts, what have you been taught? What do you do? Are there other concepts about pneumonia that come to mind? If so, what other aspects do you consider?
Look at these questions again after working through this entire chapter.

The three aspects mentioned above usually receive little attention in books dealing with the history of medicine. The development of medicine is usually represented somewhat as follows:

> People used to have limited knowledge, and this was compensated for by substituting magical thinking. In the time of Hippocrates (fifth to fourth century BC) people began for the first time to observe more clearly and to reflect on those observations. This way of observing and thinking gradually developed and more and more was discovered as time went on: how the body functions, what causes diseases etc. This led to insight into the cellular and molecular basis of disease, and engendered the hope that answers will be found to everything that is still a riddle today.

The history of medicine, however, can be viewed differently, and when we do this we immediately come to the first point which Steiner makes: Hippocrates not only marks the beginning of medicine as we know it today, but at the same time marks the end of an old atavistic medicine, i.e. a medicine which was rooted in a clairvoyance characteristic of human consciousness in the past. After the time of Hippocrates, increasingly poorly understood traces of this old form of medicine remain trickling down until the middle of the nineteenth century.

Thomas Kuhn's thoughts on paradigms (also see Chapter 2), namely that every worldview is based in pre-scientific ideas (states of consciousness), did have a certain amount of influence, but the majority of physicians have rarely, if ever, taken notice of these ideas. If this were the case, a new light could be shed on many medical problems we are wrestling with in our time.

We can thus distinguish roughly speaking two principal streams: the first, powerful in its origins, dates from before Hippocrates and gradually wanes after his time until it ceases to exist around 1850; in the lecture Steiner describes this cessation as being linked to the controversy between Rokitansky and Virchow. In this chapter we will mark the cessation by connecting it to Hufeland. The other stream, which starts in the time of Hippocrates with a budding ability to observe concretely with the senses and to digest these impressions with thinking, becomes ever stronger after 1500 and ends up by dominating the first stream after 1850. In the second half of the nineteenth century we then come to the time in which therapeutic nihilism prevails in the practice of medicine. All older forms of advice are thrown overboard and the question becomes: what really does work? Are we actually able to help a sick person, or are we reduced to stand by and only improve the surrounding circumstances a bit in the hope that the patient heals by herself?

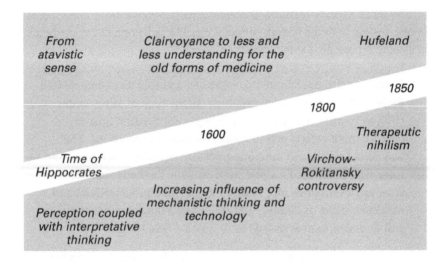

We will elaborate on this classification in Section 1.4.3.

1.2.1 A metaphor

In order to elucidate the development of these two streams further, we can use the metaphor of child and adult. A grown-up can all too easily forget how it was to be a child, being completely absorbed in adult consciousness. Childhood can then be felt as a stage we have grown out of. We have 'made progress.'

However, we can also view childhood as a phase which we have lost, to which we no longer have access. This can lead to the realization that we have grown more limited in one sense. We can look back to our childhood with nostalgia, when our consciousness used to be much less differentiated and narrowed down into a specific track. If we follow through with this, and continue going in reverse direction, back into the time of being a baby and an embryo, we finally come to the fertilized ovum. This cell is tiny in terms of matter, but huge in potential. Thinking back this far we can come to the realization that we have developed very little of the total potential present at that time, and this in turn can lead to a feeling of nostalgia in adulthood.

If we apply this to history and think in a similar vein, we might be inclined to give more credit to the state of consciousness people had in the past. Earlier humanity still had faculties which we no longer possess, and vice versa.

The consciousness of pre-Hippocratic man is characterized by a gradually waning clairvoyance, not only *quantitatively* but also *qualitatively.* In both respects we can imagine that old clairvoyance was no longer reliable and became prone to error. This atavistic, clairvoyant consciousness slowly died out (traces were still to be found in the Middle Ages), and the kind of consciousness that began to develop is the one we still have today. In its initial stages it was slumbering, but began to unfold fully from 1500 onwards.

This comparison of history to the development of child into adult can open further perspectives. In the eighteenth century the German author Lessing (1729–81) was the first to introduce in writing the concept of reincarnation, i.e. the thought of repeated earth lives, into modern Western thinking. He describes how there are successive historical epochs in which the human being returns again and again to earth and in which new and different things can be learned each time. Lessing focuses specifically on moral development, stating that human beings are led at first by laws imposed from the outside (Old Testament). This corresponds to childhood. By way of love (New Testament) the human being develops towards (future) freedom, which corresponds to the state of mature adulthood. And Lessing interprets this as follows: just as the individual human being undergoes many changes throughout life, yet remains the same entity, development in history only *makes sense* if an individuality is able to experience every successive phase.

And that is only possible when this individuality is born again and again in successive phases, absorbs what can be learned during life in that phase, and dies again. Steiner connects to this later in a much more concrete way on the basis of his own spiritual-scientific research.

We can put it as follows: the deeper meaning of history only reveals itself when we take the concept of reincarnation into account. The concept of reincarnation enables us to look at former times with a totally different feeling. Applied to ourselves this means that we may have lived repeatedly in Greece, Egypt, Mexico, China etc., with a different kind of consciousness and a different relationship to nature, to our fellow human beings and to the cosmos.

When we review all this, it becomes more understandable why Steiner considers it an enormous mistake not to see Hippocrates also as standing at the end of an old clairvoyant medical tradition.

Assignment 2

This is, in a certain sense, a somewhat optimistic view of historical development. What are your thoughts about it? Supposing you adopt this viewpoint, how would you look at the enormous technical possibilities of our time?

1.3 The time before Hippocrates

We have to build a picture of the pre-Hippocratic era in order to imagine what medicine was like in that time. This of course can only be done in a limited way. After all, we simply look and think differently today, so it already is quite an accomplishment when we gain a very general idea of those times. To the same degree that our orthodox medicine is rooted in our present-day state of consciousness, medicine back then had its roots in the Greek consciousness. From 850 BC onward, in the Greek period, several nuanced stages can be indicated, which demonstrate that the consciousness of humanity underwent very gradual changes.

1.3.1 Historical phases before Hippocrates

1. Homer *(c. eighth century BC)*

In Homer the relationship between gods and human beings is very close. Right at the beginning of the *Odyssey*, Homer calls on the muses to tell him about the life of Odysseus, so that he can pass on the story. When Pallas Athena whispers something to Odysseus, which others can neither see nor hear, this process can be compared to what we do when we are deliberating with ourselves. Such interactions can be found on nearly every page of Homer's work. We can see from this that the process of thinking which we experience inside ourselves as our own, was experienced by the Homeric heroes at least partly as something which came from the outside, as in the example given above of the muses and of Pallas Athena. Similarly, the relationship between nature and the gods is experienced as a very close one. The goddess Thetys, mother of Achilles, manifests herself in the waves of the water and then proceeds to have a conversation with Achilles *(Iliad,* Book 1). In general, what happens in nature is often described as the manifestation of a god or goddess.

We can also put this in different words: the separation between the human being and nature is not yet very strong. The human being experiences the unity intensely because the divine manifests both within the human being, as well as in nature. And this manifestation of the divine in nature and the human being was experienced pictorially. That is to say, not as an abstract thought, but as an image. We find such images in all ancient myths. From this it becomes understandable that the gods also played an important role in sickness and health. This becomes clear right at the beginning of the *Iliad.* A plague-like illness rages around Troy, caused by the arrows of Apollo, who will only stop when the daughter of the priest of Apollo has been returned. This girl was Agamemnon's war prize. The girl is returned, accompanied by sacrifices to Apollo and after that the plague ends. So we are obviously not dealing with abstract thinking at this time. Similarly, the concepts for body, life, soul, and spirit were not used in a delineated abstractly differentiated way. Experience of sense impressions are closely interwoven with supersensory experiences. Feelings are direct and elemental in the *Iliad.* Such a perspective throws a totally new light on the *Iliad,* and read in this way it becomes palpable how people lived in a completely different state of consciousness back then.

2. The early pre-Socratics

We now go on to the next phase, that of the pre-Socratics. These were the philosophers who lived before Socrates (d. 399 BC). Examples are Pythagoras, Heraclitus, Empedocles, and Thales. Steiner describes one philosopher of this phase in his book *The Riddles of Philosophy* [*Die Rätsel der Philosphie*]. He chose Pherekydes of Syros as being illustrative of this time. On the one hand this philosopher still has a pictorial, clairvoyant consciousness, on the other hand he also has the first sparks of abstract thinking. Pherekydes gives a picture of the earth as a winged oak tree, around which Zeus drapes the land and the sea. But he also speaks of the three primeval principles such as Kronos, Zeus and 'Chthoon' (Greek for earth), which we could translate into modern terms of time, space and matter. Out of these three the world of the phenomena comes into being. However, we must realize at the same time that Pherekydes had a different notion of these abstract concepts of time, space and matter than we have nowadays. His ideas were still richer and more saturated, they tended to have more the character of images. In *The Riddles of Philosophy,* Steiner indicates how we can try to understand this way of thinking. The god Kronos can be experienced in the activity of fire, when we think of fire as something which consumes and digests. In expanding vapours, cloud formation, lives what expands radiantly: that is what Zeus is. In the *Iliad* he gets the epithet 'cloud-gatherer.' And finally, when we come to Chthoon, we can experience the various relationships between fluid and solid.

We can summarize this as follows:

Fire	—	*Kronos*
Between Water and Air	—	*Zeus*
Between Fluid and Solid	—	*Chthoon*

3. The later pre-Socratics

After Pherekydes the later pre-Socratic philosophers worked out the abstract conceptual side more and more, each in his own way. Great efforts were made to transform the old pictures into concepts. As indicated before, pictures came from the outside as it were, concepts were experienced more as inner possessions. It is extremely refreshing to experience the vigour with which people were practising philosophy in those days. A frequent topic, for example, was the various primal states. For Heraclitus it was fire; for Anaximenes it was air; for Thales water; for Democrites it was the smallest solid particles, the 'atoms.' For these philosophers, the primal states did not arise purely out of speculation. We cannot overestimate how nuanced the transition from pictures to concepts actually was. With Socrates we find the real start of truly conceptual thinking, but just before that, with these later pre-Socratics, a certain personal constitutional one-sidedness still plays a strong role. It decidedly colours the conceptual content. Thus we can imagine when Heraclitus chooses fire as the primal principle that this was determined by a fiery side in his constitution, something which is confirmed by the oral traditions handed down about the philosopher.

1.3.2 Medicine in the mystery temples before Hippocrates

Up to the time of Plato and less so in the time after that, the mysteries were the source of all cultural renewal. These were places where initiates, hierophants, maintained contact with the higher spiritual world. In these places one could be apprenticed and ultimately after years of discipline and meditation be initiated. This training was one aspect of the mysteries. Another aspect was that this initiation imbued one with the notion that the whole of society had to reflect the spiritual world in its structure and organization. We still find many vestiges of this in Plato's dialogues. To a much greater extent than would be possible today, people used to be convinced of the reality of the spiritual worlds and knew that initiates were conversant with this. Therefore they put much more trust in advice which was as it were handed down 'from above' and passed on for the well-being of society. In that sense the mysteries were the source of all manifestations of culture. Pupils at the mystery centres were sworn to secrecy. Even in the mysteries of Eleusis, where in later days, when it was much more open, thousands of people were still initiated, but the essential teachings remained a strictly guarded secret. This is also the reason why very little information has come down to us, because little or nothing was written down.

Another reason is that writing things down only became necessary when abstract thinking began to develop. This coincided with the gradual decline of the mysteries. The principle of self-reliance which is part and parcel of conceptual thinking, is incompatible with the strict authoritarian principle which governed the mysteries.

Another important task of the mysteries was temple medicine. Ancient Greek medicine had two sides: temple medicine and secular medicine, the latter developing in close relationship to the nascent pre-Socratic philosophy. We know a little more about temple medicine because Plutarch, amongst others, makes mention of it.

W.J. Stein (see bibliography) has summarized these and other sources: after a preparation of several days of fasting or dieting, bringing sacrifices and worshipping of the god Asclepius, the patient, lying on a lamb's skin, was brought into a sleeping state by the priest. In this process sleep was supervised by the priest-physician.

This temple sleep (incubation) brought the sick person into contact with Asclepius during the night, and on awakening the patient would either have a dream of the cure or an image of the disease. So these came in picture form. The priest had the ability to interpret these images.

The priests knew that there is a close connection between the world outside the human being and the inner world, between macrocosm and microcosm. This enabled insight into the specific connection between human illnesses and processes in outer nature, which could be applied for therapeutic purposes.

In his essay about Socrates' *Daimonion,* Plutarch speaks about our ability to have a meeting with our 'genius' or 'demon.' Nowadays we would speak of our higher self. In other words, the patient would contact his higher being. The temple sleep was as it were a lower form of experiencing the divine, the experience the patient had unconsciously while being asleep corresponding to the experience of initiation. At Eleusis this correspondence between conscious initiation and temple sleep also appears in that one day of the mystery celebrations was devoted to Asclepius.

Assignment 3
Can you recognize these different states of consciousness in your own life?

Very little of this ancient knowledge of the relationship between macrocosm and microcosm has trickled through. One finds a limited reflection of it in the *Corpus Hippocraticum,* the work which is ascribed to Hippocrates but actually contains contributions by various authors from several centuries. (See also excerpts in the Appendix).

We can wonder how people could heal in this way. Many eyewitness accounts of healings have come down to us. These remain incomprehensible to us until we realize that the Greek state of mind was fundamentally different and that the finer bodies were also structured differently in ancient Greece, which opened up distinctive possibilities. This goes especially for the life principle, which Paracelsus called *Archaeus,* and is called ether body in the lecture by Steiner. This life body was less firmly connected to the physical body and hence more accessible to nonmaterial healing forces.

1.4 Four schools of medical thought:

1.4.1 Hippocrates

It is not so easy to judge and comprehend the *Corpus Hippocraticum.* Although opinions vary, the general consensus is that the *Corpus* does give a reasonable impression of Greek medicine in the time of Hippocrates. Among other things the book contains:

— Sections which strike one as fresh and modern, in which observation has the upper hand.
— Sections which show strong influence from the pre-Socratics (specifically Empedocles, Pythagoras, Heraclitus).
— Sections which seem to originate more from the school of Knidos. Distinction is often made between the school of Kos, where Hippocrates was from, and the school of Knidos, which was situated very close to the isle of Kos on the coast of what is now the Turkish mainland. The school of Knidos had more clearly defined categories of illnesses and their treatments, handed down from previous times and adhered to fairly rigidly. This gave the whole school a more abstract and deductive character. The Kos approach, by contrast, was more individual and hence more inductive.
— Vestiges of mystery wisdom can be sensed behind much of what was written in the *Corpus.*

Little is known about Hippocrates himself. He lived from about 460 to 375 BC. He came from a line of physicians who traced their ancestry back all the way to Asclepius. He was born on Kos and died in Thessalia. Legend has it that he also visited Egypt, where he came into contact with the conservative teachings of Knidos. In later life he became a travelling physician. It is said that he strongly experienced the pain of losing the old mystery culture, while realizing the necessity of its descent. It is also said that a pamphlet published at the time accused him of betraying the secrets of the mysteries, but he was spared because of his fame. (Betraying the mysteries customarily resulted in the death penalty in those times.) Legend or fact, these stories clearly indicate that Hippocrates lived in a time of change. Steiner's summary of the work of Hippocrates in the lecture mentioned above is very brief:

The four elements around us correspond to the four humours within:

warmth	**air**	**water**	**earth**
yellow bile	sanguis	phlegma	black bile
	blood	slime	

— The right or wrong mixture is of the essence: *crasis* or *discrasis,* that is to say thinking in terms of *balance* is thought to be important (see also the excerpts in the Appendix)
— Early Greek medicine viewed black bile as the only one of the four humours which was not totally permeated by cosmic forces.

The following themes are dealt with by Hippocrates, but are not mentioned by Steiner:

— The *vis medicatrix naturae (healing force of nature):* 'nature' within the human being always works for the good by means of the internal warmth.
— The great importance of *atmospheric, geological* and sometimes also *astronomical* influences (see also the Appendix).
— The physician as *assistant* of 'nature' within the human being, summarized in the dictum *medicus curat, natura sanat (the physician treats, nature heals).*

These themes are dealt with extensively in the subsequent lectures in the *First Medical Course,* but without mentioning Hippocrates specifically.

Below follow some aphorisms from the *Corpus Hippocraticum.* It should be realized that a large part of these aphorisms used to be learned by rote by physicians in the past. The first one is the most famous, and reflects a spirit of acceptance, something which is quite characteristic for large parts of the *Corpus Hippocraticum.*

1.   Life is short, art is long, opportunity fleeting, experiment treacherous, judgment hard. The physician must not only be willing to do his duty, but also make sure that both patient and nurses are willing to cooperate, and must take pains to secure good care.
2.   Changes of season are especially likely to cause illnesses, and within the times of year the big fluctuations of cold and warm ...
3.   Older people stand up better to fasting than people of middle age, youngsters have a hard time with it, and most of all children, especially those whose vivaciousness is above average.
4.   Growing creatures have most natural warmth. Therefore they also need most food; if they do not get enough of it their bodies waste away. Old people have little natural warmth and therefore do not need much fuel; too much fuel makes the body expand. That is the reason why older people have less acute fevers than young people, because their bodies are cold.
5.   Pains above the diaphragm necessitate vomiting for a cure. Pains below the diaphragm call for a laxative.
6.   When a woman vomits blood, the onset of menstruation is her cure.
7.   Matter left over after the crisis of an illness is prone to cause the illness to reappear.

These seven aphorisms contain much wisdom. Medicine is indeed a difficult art. And it is true: the physician has to take good notice of changes in the atmosphere.

In the third and fourth aphorisms we find some observations concerning age. Age was strictly taken into account in all treatment. Aphorism No. 5 and 6 deal with the location of the illness. Above and below the diaphragm were considered different worlds, requiring totally different treatments. Much was done to promote elimination, which was based on the following thought: if there is less of the ailing substance, the life force gets more of an opportunity to regain control. In No. 6 the direction in which the blood flows is of great importance. The blood flowing upwards in the woman will be balanced out by menstruation, which is a movement down of the blood. This is also the principle behind the fact that in later times bloodletting out of the elbow was prescribed in the case of menorraghia, but in the case of an amenorrhea, bloodletting out of the ankle was prescribed. In the former case the big flow downward had to be balanced out by an upward flow. In the latter case the flow downward had to be set in motion to begin with.

Aphorism No. 7 indicates how important it is that the life forces regain control of everything. As long as ailing substance (later called *materia peccans,* sinful matter) remains in the body, these remnants will cause the illness to flare up again and again, as is the case with a splinter which is left in the wound: even if the pus around it is removed again and again, the process will continue.

Assignment 4

Read the section of Steiner's lecture from the First Medical Course *again in the Appendix. This time consider the following illnesses from the perspective of the four elements: pneumonia, kidney stone, glue ear, rickets. In the case of rickets, the enormous importance of light plays in too. Can you connect this, in a very rudimentary way, with what Steiner says in the lecture about the cosmic forces, which are at work in three of the four humors?*

1.4.2 Paracelsus and the decline of Hippocratic thinking

In the lecture Steiner deals with the time between Hippocrates and Paracelsus (1493–1541) very briefly, even though this comprises a time span of nearly two thousand years.

He says that few new things happened in that time period. Physicians still depended on the old work of the Greeks, but understand it less and less. In later lectures, Steiner dealt much more extensively with this time period, specifically with the way Greek knowledge was absorbed by the Arab world in the East and how Arab culture in turn influences Europe in the Middle Ages. (A well-known name connected with this is, for example, is Avicenna). When Steiner talks about Paracelsus, he stresses how Paracelsus was clairvoyant and could therefore put into words many things which his contemporaries no longer were able to perceive. As a result, Paracelsus became an opponent of the medicine of his time.

We strongly meet these two sides of Paracelsus, clairvoyant and polemic, when we study his work. His inner powers gave him enormous self-confidence, as is apparent from this quote:

Follow me, not the other way around, Avicenna, Rhases, Galen, Mesur. Follow me, and not the other way around, you from Paris,

you from Montpellier, you from Swabia, you from Meissen, you
from Cologne, you from Vienna and whatever other towns on the
Danube or the Rhine, you from the islands in the sea, you from
Italy, from Dalmatia, from Athens, you Greek, Arab, Israelite. You
should follow me and not the other way around, mine is the
kingdom.

Paracelsus had searched very much, and found even more.

Paracelsus grew up in Einsiedeln near Zurich, where his father's medical practice covered the whole area. His mother died when he was eight
and he moved with his father to the south of Austria; he started his study
of medicine early, amongst other places in Padua. Not satisfied with what
he had learned there, he travelled all over Europe learning everywhere and
from everybody, wherever he could. Later on in life he prided himself on
having learned much from simple peasants, traders in the marketplace,
etc., and preferred that living knowledge over the dead book-learning of
the universities. The distances he covered are astounding. After these travels he finally became town-physician in Basel, a post which he largely
owed to good contacts with several humanists in that town. He met with a
lot of misunderstanding and much unjust treatment, which makes it understandable that he often made short shrift with the practice of medicine of
his time, and he made many enemies in this way. Things came to such a
state that he finally had to flee in the middle of the night in order to save
himself.

Later on in life he also worked for a time as a lay preacher, and he built
up a considerable theological body of work in that period. This theological work is just as large as his medical-philosophical achievements; it consists largely of commentaries on the Psalms.

The age in which he lived was highly exciting. It was a time of explo-
rations and discoveries in many fields (1492 Columbus, 1543 Copernicus
and Vesalius), a time in which old assumptions were being questioned.
Individual exploration was in the air. In this, Paracelsus went the way of
many other innovators of his time and also had to suffer the same disbe-
lief and opposition that others met. In taking his strong stance, Paracelsus
was guided by a strong connection with forces deeply embedded in nature
and the human being, and always spoke out of this direct experience.
Many other innovators distanced themselves from the old and relied more
and more on sense perception, systematized by the intellect. This mode of
doing research formed the beginning of our natural science. A schism took
place here, which Paracelsus had already foreseen, as many passages in
his work show.

Reading Paracelsus is a special experience. It is best to read him out loud, because he often writes the way one speaks, and his discourses are punctuated with repetitions to make his points clear. His style is often polemic, and many passages seem naive. On closer scrutiny, however, one can gain the impression that he gives literal descriptions of both sense experiences and supersensory perceptions. He obviously has a very concrete way of approaching the occult, in a manner that I have only met in Steiner's work. No wonder Steiner often refers to him as someone from whom one can still learn a lot today. He refers to him repeatedly in the *Course for Young Doctors* [*Meditative Betrachtungen und Anleitungen zur Vertiefung der Heilkunst*] (given early in 1924). This was mainly because Paracelsus had such a profound relationship to the natural world.

As an introduction to his works, two pamphlets are very appropriate, which he wrote a few years before his death, *Sieben Defensiones* and *Labyrinthus*. I will describe them briefly, using a dramatic form, *adopting his stance as it were.*

Seven Defences *(Sieben Defensiones)*

Medicine, in the time of Hippocrates and before, used to be pure but has gradually sunk into a state of darkness. The practice of medicine is no longer imbued with the spirit of truth. There is endless talk and mindless imitation without proper insight. The universities have become rigid and are behind the times in the way they teach medicine.

Everything has to be looked at anew. The tendency to speak of incurable diseases is pernicious in medicine. As doctors, we have to start by admitting that we are powerless as individual persons. If we realize, however, that we have to keep searching and that God is the final ground of medicine, we shall find if only we continue to seek.

A good physician is shaped neither by his talent, nor by human teaching alone. In the final analysis, a physician is shaped by God.

My way of working meets with many prejudices, for example because I work with fasting and praying, especially when dealing with people who are possessed. But does the word not also heal? And when I give new names to diseases, is it not so that names for diseases differ from village to village? I look at the origin of diseases and determine their names in accordance with what I find. What do I have to do with books that were written two thousand years ago? Have earth and heaven, and with them the nature of illness, not changed radically in the bygone two thousand years?

I am also being condemned for prescribing poisons. But is poison not a great mystery in nature, also made by God? Are all things not poison in the final analysis? Does the dosage not determine whether a poison actually poisons? The way a remedy is prepared is of essential importance, after all. The good has to be separated from the bad, as taught by alchemy, and my recipes have been prepared strictly in accordance with the laws of nature! Personal speculation plays no role in their preparation.

People also reproach me for travelling much. Do they expect my teacher to be behind my stove at home? A medical doctor must be astronomer, cosmographer, philosopher and alchemist all in one. That necessitates travel. Other countries do not seek you out and neither do the mountains. You have to seek them out for yourself. A lover goes a long way to see a beautiful woman. Much more is needed to learn the beautiful art of medicine. Did the Queen of Sheba not come from all the way across the sea to Solomon, to absorb his wisdom? Those who seek the gifts of God, have to go to the place where they are to be found. Those who want to follow their stomachs should not follow me, they should follow those who walk in soft garments.

This also goes for the work of the physician. Egotism in medicine is pernicious, only medicine done out of love will bear fruit. So there are two kinds of doctors, those who act out of love and those who are after money. Egotism brings falsehood into medicine, and false appearance will stand out. Therefore a physician must sell all he has, so as to strengthen his healing capacities.

People reproach me for my rough nature, and say I'm full of wrath. No subtle strands have been woven into the fabric of my nature ... Where I come from, we were not fed with figs, nor with flour, nor with wheat bread, but with cheese, milk, and oat bread. That does not make you genteel, it stays with you all your life. Those who have grown up in soft clothes and women's chambers and we who have grown up under the pine trees, we do not mix well.

Then there are those who say that I give coarse answers. True, I will not call a merchant in the marketplace a squire, and I will not try to win somebody over with sweet words; my work should speak for itself.

People also say that I do not give an immediate judgment or prescribe medicine straightaway when I first see a patient. That is true. I gradually arrive at the truth. How can you immediately recognize hidden diseases the same way you see colours? When a colour is veiled, you also do not recognize it immediately, do you?

This gives a succinct impression of the kind of criticism Paracelsus levied at his colleagues.

Assignment 5

1. What are your thoughts on the way a medical doctor should be trained? Paracelsus names talent, human teaching and God. How does that tend to work in your own life?

2. What do you think of the contrast made in the passage above: those who act out of love and those who are after money. What is the role of money in your life as a doctor?

Labyrinthus (The Labyrinth)

In *Labyrinthus* Paracelsus describes the books a physician has to learn to read. A summary follows below.

1. Book of Wisdom

First seek the kingdom of God and all will follow from the wisdom which lies within that.

If we want to take it from the hand of God, the way is through prayer, seeking, and knocking at the door. Such is the way to school. Using force or theft does not bring us further. Those who constantly seek for wisdom in the old books, are seeking a treasure which is being consumed by rust. They do nothing but learn and learn and never arrive at the art of truth.

2. Book of the Firmament

This is a book which we have to learn to read in the full realization that it is a book with a message from further away. The book of the firmament is a book which deceives no one. The one who wrote it needed no paper to teach us. Books which have been written about it on paper often lead us away from the real book.

3. Book of the Elements

The four elements which are in the outside world are also to be found within. There is a strong correspondence between outer and inner. Within the human being lives the strength of thistles, of mercury, of gold pigment, for instance. By getting to know the creations, the sons and daughters of the elements, the physical body and the illnesses must be recognized, distinguished and judged.

4. Book of the Physical Body As a Microcosm
This entails amongst others that ordinary anatomy must be studied again in correspondence with the world. Paracelsus reiterates here that knowledge must grow out of a practical relationship of the human being to the world and not out of speculative thinking. Just as there are many kinds of wood, there are also many kinds of bone. Similarly, there are many winds, and many colics in people.

5. Book of Alchemy
All is unfulfilled seed. It is fulfilled by the fire of Vulcan. Wherever we look, in the kitchen, in the stove, in the smithy, in the pharmacy or in the human body, we find the *Archaeus*. When our eyes rest on the herb, we do not see the medicine, we only see the shell. The medicine lies within, hidden behind the shell. First you have to take away the shell. Only then can you reach the medicine. That is alchemy, and that is the task of Vulcan. This way all is in a process of transformation. Nature makes first matter until wheat is harvested. Harvest follows, and grinding, then baking. These are all alchemical processes that follow, resulting in middle matter. Then comes the microcosmic alchemy inside the human being; through mouth and stomach bread turns to flesh and blood, thus forming last matter. But there is another alchemy: weakness is the first matter, sickness the second, death the last.

6. Book of Experience
The work of the doctor must be grounded in knowledge, ground which can be likened to a tree bringing forth fruit. God bestowed this basic knowledge on the plants. We in turn have to learn it from the plants. If our experience is limited to what the eye can see, it does not count for Paracelsus. Everything in the cosmos can be brought to light, be it ever so hidden. A mighty alchemy must stand behind the tree's wisdom for it to carry through the whole process which in the end brings forth fruit. In a like manner, the human being contains the seed of knowledge, which needs cultivation in order for it to produce the ears and berries in the autumn.

7. The Book of Natural Pharmacies and Physicians
The natural world around us is a vast pharmacy. This natural pharmacy is far superior to the human pharmacy. A doctor and a pharmacy dwell in every human being. We are all born with a disposition towards illness

('man is born to fall over'), but this is constantly balanced by the inner doctor with a pharmacy, which restores again and again what the disposition to illness breaks down. The outer doctor is powerless without the inner doctor. If the inner doctor fails to maintain the balance, the outer doctor must intervene, using the cures contained in outer nature.

8. The Book of Medical Theory
Where are the remedies? Answer: in nature.
Where is the illness? Answer: in the patient.

These two lead to the following medical theory: the theory of the treatment and the theory of the cause, which two have to become *one!* The book must be read in the *light of nature*. This theory must shed light on the seed of all diseases (see Book 11).

9. The Book on How to Find the Art of Medicine
The art of medicine is found not by speculation, but by the certainty of revelation. When we follow the teachings of magic and of the cabala, we learn to see with the true vision of the seer how man and nature are related.

10. The Book of the Way of the Drug from First Matter to Last Matter
Everything changes shape, metamorphoses. The seed turns into the flowering plant and withers again. In the mother's belly the human being is a growing fruit, then the child is born, grows up and goes through all the stages of life until old age. All form, all physiognomy, both of plant and mineral, tells us something specific and points to the organ or the illness it can heal.

11. The Book of the Genesis of Diseases
The ancients taught that the cause of diseases was to be found in the humours. That is not so. The humours correspond to the elements, they represent the female part which has to be fructified by the seed of Vulcan, which is the male part. Likewise the apple does not go forth from the elements of the earth, but from the seed. Disease originates in the seed, not in the elements. Disease is to be understood in terms of the elements, as they were understood by the ancients, the same way that the apple can be described in terms of the elements, even though it originates in the apple-seed. There are thus two seeds of disease: *Iliastrum* and *Cagastrum*. *Iliastrum* is the origin of the more or less inborn weakness which gradually grows more pronounced and also brings forth the more chronic diseases. *Cagastrum* is the origin of the more infectious and febrile diseases.

This summary of the eleven books of the *Labyrinthus* was included here
not only because it brings us into closer acquaintance with Paracelsus, but
also because through it we meet many aspects of a form of practising medicine which we will meet again in anthroposophical medicine, albeit in a
metamorphosed form.

I would like to elaborate on two questions here. The first one is: What
is the 'light of nature' of which Paracelsus speaks in Book 8? The second
question is: How does Paracelsus' view of illness compare with the somewhat resigned attitude which we find in the *Corpus Hippocraticum*?

The 'light of nature' is definitely not meant to signify the ordinary
sense experience of the eye. It is much more to be seen as a form of higher
cognition such as we meet it in Goethe's 'seeing in beholding'
[*anschauende Urteilskraft*], or developed even further (see Section 2.3.3).
It goes towards a form of clairvoyance fused with precise observation similar to the way Steiner speaks of in the *Course for Young Doctors*.
Paracelsus speaks frequently of this 'light of nature' and it should most
probably be understood in this wider sense.

It will be clear from the above that Paracelsus was not complacent by
nature. On the one hand, he accepted illness as a given. But there was
another side to illness for him. *Illness enables the human being to come
closer to God.* Paracelsus already saw illness as being embedded within a
human biography, as finding its expression there. This was viewed within
the confines of his time, of course. Paracelsus speaks about this very concretely and therefore the profession of the doctor was so important to him,
because the doctor helps people to come closer to God.

So in Paracelsus we see a human being who stands at the threshold of
modern times, a man with very strong clairvoyant powers who could
therefore look much deeper than his contemporaries into the essence of
the human being and nature. Working out of this insight he put many
things into words which contain germinal thoughts that could be developed further even today. Paracelsus was a true innovator, but in such a
way that we can surmise that he still was endowed with a way of knowing such as doctors had before the time of Hippocrates. Hence his unstint-
ing admiration for Hippocrates.

Summary
In the lecture Steiner sketches the descent of Hippocratic thinking in
broad terms, taking as a last representative, if we can even call him that,
Rokitansky (1804–78). Aside from that he points to the rise of a totally
different stream represented by Morgagni (1682–1771), who was in a
sense the founder of modern pathology. Gradually the view that the
human being is permeated by cosmic forces disappears; life as such is

no longer understood. Illness and health can only be grasped in a dead form, i.e. by dissecting bodies. We are all familiar with the kind of medicine which resulted from this stream. We have grown up with it. And of course we should not forget that this stream also has very positive qualities.

At this point Steiner also points to *homeopathy* as an attempt with a strong orientation towards the future, which is of such importance that it cannot be dealt with adequately in an introduction. In his next lectures he speaks in a variety of ways about homeopathy, potentizing, and so on.

To sum up, we can distinguish four separate medical streams.

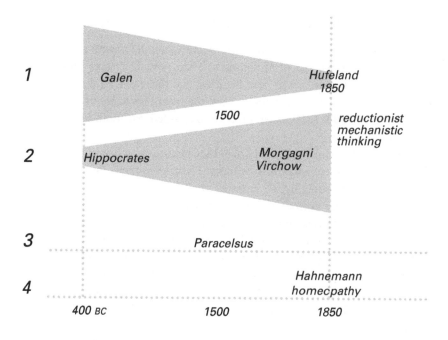

1. The first stream originates before Hippocrates and has its source in clairvoyant perception. It gradually declines and the last vestiges of it can be found as late as 1850; Steiner describes Rokitansky (a pathologist!) as a last representative. We will describe Hufeland in this chapter as a last well-known practising physician of this stream. An essential trait of this stream is a thinking in terms of equilibrium, which degenerates with time into a thinking in terms of opposites. We will encounter this latter type of thinking when we come to Hufeland.

2. The second stream begins with Hippocrates and is characterized by its emphasis on sense perception. This stream only comes into its own

around 1500 and from 1850 onwards it becomes cellular molecular thinking.

3. The third stream is represented by Paracelsus and his followers. Its hallmark is thinking in terms of development; it sees illness as meaningful.

4. Homeopathy represents the fourth stream (Hahnemann). Homeopathic thinking starts from the premise that 'like cures like.' We could call it a thinking in terms of similarities.

Of these four streams 1 and 2 are the most distinct.

1.4.3 Hufeland as a last representative of Hippocratic thinking

Even though Hippocratic thinking was declining, it did absorb new developments. Due to the ascent of natural science, new facts were brought to the surface that gave rise to new theories, and these placed the inherited wisdom in a new light. Therefore we see the rise of a variety of schools in the period of 1600–1850, often prone to one-sidedness, both in their theories and practices.

Christian Wilhelm Hufeland (1762–1836) indicates in his autobiographical sketch how these schools took turns. There were times that physicians only practised bloodletting, other times in which they only prescribed opiates, and yet other periods in which emetics or laxatives were the chief cures. Hufeland himself did not tend to follow the fashion of the times, his system was based on finding a balance between extremes, as was his own life. His father had a large practice as a physician near the town of Weimar, where Hufeland grew up with the strong values of both religion and classical antiquity of a Lutheran Grammar school. He was conscious specifically of absorbing the values of the Stoic Epictetus at an early age. At the age of twenty-one he took over the practice of his father, who had become practically blind. For four years he was under 'the true Hippocratic tutelage' of his father, who died in 1787. During ten years of practice, up to his thirty-first year, he began to study the theme of *life* in his spare time, and his considerations were later published under the title of *Makrobiotik* (1796).

Important characteristics of Hufeland emerged early on. All that he had absorbed in his youth in the way of Christian, classical and medical elements are digested and applied systematically in practice. He found his Christian values in Herder, to whose church he also belonged. His contacts with Goethe and Schiller brought him back in touch with his classical values; they were also his patients. He was systematic and conservative in a positive sense, a man who wanted to make everything he had learned *practical,* and wanted to reach out to a wide public.

We also meet this practical bent strongly in his *Makrobiotik*. The first part of the book contains thoughts which are typical of the time; we also find them for example in the work of Novalis and Schelling, but Hufeland goes further: he writes a second part in which he puts these thoughts into practice. In the first part he delineates the notion of *life*. He views this in a wide sense, describing how we meet life in seeds, plants, animals and human beings; how we have to see it in relation to light, warmth, air and water. He has gathered many observations. Even though he calls life 'a breath of divinity,' he does not define it but only names the conditions for its appearance. The duration of life is determined by the following factors.

1. the sum total of all life force
2. the condition of the organs
3. the process of consumption (of life force)
4. regeneration

The third especially, consumption, can be influenced, because it depends to a high degree on our behaviour. What he calls 'living too fast' is fatal. In general it is the *aurea mediocritas,* the middle ground between extremes, which promotes life.

In the second part, which deals with more practical aspects, he goes into concrete detail concerning conditions which shorten life.

1. education which weakens (too soft, too many impressions)
2. excessive sexual life
3. exaggerated emotions
4. illnesses
5. air pollution, city life
6. excessive eating and drinking
7. specific 'soul moods': agitation, boredom, fearfulness
8. poisons
9. old age

To give an impression of his writing style, a passage follows about fear.

Fear is a continuous cramp which constricts all the small vessels; the whole skin turns pale and cold, evaporation is completely blocked. The blood all collects inside the large vessels, the pulse falters, the heart fills to overflowing and cannot move freely. This way the most important work of circulation is disturbed. Digestion is also interrupted, cramping diarrhoeas ensue. All muscle strength is lamed, one wants to walk but cannot, an overall trembling arises, breathing is shallow.

Hufeland lists the following factors as contributing to a healthy life:

1. a good infancy, with specific indications for the care of the newborn and the growing baby
2. realistic educational measures, including the advice not to start schooling too early. He says amongst other things, 'It is possible to start too early when one chooses the time in which nature is still busy forming the bodily forces and organs and needs all its strength, and that is the time before the seventh year. If one induces children to sit too much and to learn, one deprives the body of the noblest parts of those forces, which are then consumed by thinking, which definitely causes retardation in growth ...'
3. an active youth
4. a happy marriage
5. healthy sleep
6. exercise
7. fresh air
8. moderate temperatures
9. country life
10. regular travel
11. hygiene and baths
12. temperance in eating and drinking
13. peace of mind
14. truthfulness

Goethe and Duke Karl August heard him in a public lecture and secured him a position as a professor at the University of Jena, where his classes were very popular. In 1795 he started editing a magazine called *Journal der praktische Medizin,* later known as *Hufeland's Journal.* Because of difficulties at the University of Jena, in 1801 he transferred to the University of Berlin, where he was also director of the hospital and held the post of court physician to the Royal House of Prussia. Between 1806 and 1810 he accompanied the royal couple to Königsberg where they hid from Napoleon, after which they resumed their normal lives again in Berlin. He continued to work and teach until 1831, when he turned sixty-nine. In spite of deteriorating eyesight, he still managed to write his last work, *Enchiridon Medicum,* which appeared a few weeks before his death in 1836.

All during his working life, and even in his career as a teacher, he did not really discover new things. New developments, such as the stethoscope and homeopathy, had little effect on him. He did take note of them and was not necessarily negatively disposed to them — he did not see much value in them, they remained marginal for him. He said himself in an autobiographical sketch how his whole life was focused on the general picture rather than on specific details. He did, however, always keep his eye on practical applicability. Always thoughtful and considerate, he was a man who kept an even keel in all he did, and in his final work as a medical scholar, the *Enchiridion Medicum,* he managed to encompass the sum total of the heritage of Hippocrates and Galen. Even so, he did not really fathom the deeper sides of man and nature. We have seen how he skirted around the concept of 'life' without penetrating to the heart of the matter. He did not go as far as seeing it as a strictly material phenomenon, but he did, among other things, resort to comparing it to electricity. In the *Enchiridion* he was not able to do more than summarize more or less all that had been thought for centuries without truly penetrating to deeper foundations in the way that Paracelsus was able to do. Incidentally, Hufeland wanted to have nothing to do with Paracelsus.

Space does not allow a discussion of this 600-page book. It is still eminently readable, especially because it contains descriptions of diseases which, in the western world, we only rarely observe in their full-blown form, such as tuberculosis and typhoid fever.

In typical late Hippocratic fashion the book contains a few pages with aphorisms, also a chapter on how to deal with patients and colleagues ('Never speak condescendingly about colleagues'). He also stresses how important it is to keep a journal at night and note down the most important points of patients' medical histories, and reflect on changes and developments once again. He even goes as far as saying that this is the most important way to become a truly competent doctor. Here are two examples of aphorisms which demonstrate the Hippocratic nature of his thinking.

1) Never forget that it is *nature* who accomplishes the healing, not you. Your role is to help and assist her work, and you have the option to either allow and enable her to gain access, or, sad to say, hinder her and even make her work impossible.
2) Always maintain the dignity of the art, both within yourself and for others, and do not debase or demean her out of low motives.

Apart from three hundred recipes (nearly all of which could still to be found in a 1950s formulary!) the last hundred pages contain a description of the three cardinal treatments of medicine: *bloodletting, emetics, and opium.* For Hufeland, these are the basic tools in his medical practice. Whoever masters these three holds the key to life and death; whoever does not master them: he shall spread death and destruction. He always focuses on the broader aspects of these interventions; his description of opium especially is a treat for the reader, and after that he goes on to describe concrete case histories which give a clear insight into the practical application.

Two things emerge clearly: First, these medicines serve to assist nature, for example in the case of a coated tongue, bloated stomach, and slight nausea, an emetic is to be recommended. Secondly, the above-mentioned thinking in terms of opposites appears in the principle that one should take away where there is too much, and add where there is too little. In principle, bloodletting is antiflogistic, so counteracts inflammation. The emetic is obviously *the* gastric remedy, and opium *the* stimulant!

When we practice bloodletting, we cause a weakening of life, and with that we diminish the excessive life tendency of the inflammation. Hence it is recommended at the onset of an inflammatory disease. However, it also has a weakening effect, it dissolves cramping. Thirdly, the quantity of blood is lessened, which is the aim when there is an excess of blood. To complete the picture: we can see bloodletting as a way to divert things; in the case of pleurisy on the right side, for example, bloodletting is done on the right side, whereby we divert out and away. All this obviously makes no sense whatsoever if we stay within our cellular molecular medical frame of mind.

Opium works in two ways. On the one hand conscious nervous activity is dampened, on the other hand the cardio-vascular system is strengthened, which, in cases of loss of strength, can result in restoring the pulse and can also easily give rise to local congestions, strengthening warmth of life. Lastly it promotes the *motus periphericus,* i.e. the movement from centripetal to centrifugal becomes stronger, resulting in sweating but also possibly bleeding of the skin. Opium is therefore the medicine of choice for Hufeland when patients suffer from nervous diseases like overexcitement or hypersensitivity, coupled with a lack of life forces as is the case in certain forms of typhoid fever, alcoholic delirium, conditions of severe loss of blood through being wounded, and advanced stages of whooping cough and diabetes ...

The emetic has a much wider application for Hufeland than just emptying the stomach. He sees its effect throughout the body; the gastrointestinal tract, the liver, the skin, the bronchi, the kidneys, even the nervous system is affected. It has an emptying effect, specifically in the gastrointestinal tract and the bronchi, it strongly relaxes cramps, and changes the mood. It should also be taken into account that many traditional cough syrups are emetics when given in higher doses, for example

Ipecacuanha. It was recommended in all cases in which the tongue is very clouded and there is nausea, furthermore for all diseases which originate in the stomach, which were many in Hufeland's days. Examples include pharyngitis and the beginning stages of tonsillitis. Emetics are also prescribed for mumps, diphtheria, pneumonia, facial erysipelas and bronchial asthma.

These medicines were not just given separately or prescribed without careful consideration of the circumstances. When for example opium was prescribed, but there was an excess of blood, there would be a danger of a CVA.

Preventive bloodletting would have to be performed first, after which opium could be given without danger. We can interpret all this as follows: we as physicians cannot cure, we can only assist nature. We do this by alleviating the weight of the physical body both in a quantitative as a quantitative sense, so that the life forces (what Paracelsus calls the *Archaeus* and what Hufeland calls the 'Life-force') can do their healing work better. The location of the pain or swelling, or whatever the symptoms are, is not without significance. The head is located high up on the trunk, it has a high position, whereas the feet have a low position and stand on the ground. When we find in one of the aphorisms of Hippocrates that purgation upwards (= vomiting) is necessary when the ailment is above the midriff, but that purgation downward (= laxation) when the ailment is below the midriff, we are at first inclined to see that as a naive and simplistic cure. The considerations above give us more of an understanding of how these thoughts were arrived at.

Assignment 6
How would you apply these three medicines in the following cases.
1) an attack of bronchial asthma
2) pneumonia
3) threatening gangrene in the foot (in the case of diabetes for
   example)
4) pseudo-croup attack in a four-year-old
5) hemorrhagic CVA, detected early
Try to approach this assignment not by guessing, but by logical reasoning within the parameters of this medical view.

With this description of Hufeland's life and work, we have characterized the time just before the transition from Rokitansky to Virchow, as described by Steiner in the lecture.

1.4.4 Hahnemann

Samuel Hahnemann lived from 1755 to 1843, and is known as the founder of homeopathy. He was almost a contemporary of Hufeland, and in a certain sense their lives were closely connected. Whereas Hufeland's life was harmonious and quiet in spite of the Napoleonic wars, Hahnemann's life by contrast was full of ups and downs. He was born in Meissen in Saxony, Germany and grew up in a family which held values such as discipline, hard work, obedience to parents, and especially unpretentiousness in high esteem. Many a household in Meissen depended on the porcelain industry for its income. There certainly was not always bread on the table, so that Samuel was often taken out of school to earn some extra money. A certain Master Johann Müller played a prominent role in his life. He recognized his intellectual gifts and promoted them; at the age of twelve Samuel was even allowed to teach the young children Greek.

Hahnemann struck out on his own quite early in life. For example, when he was sent to a grocer's after elementary school to earn some extra income, he was back in no time because he was so miserable. Just around this time Master Müller was appointed Rector at the royal Gymnasium* which enabled the boy to attend lectures as a guest. Müller was almost like a father to him, and he profited a lot from his tutelage, becoming particularly adept at languages.

At the age of twenty, he left for Leipzig to study medicine. This was also the beginning of decades of painful poverty. He earned money tutoring rich students and translating. Afterwards he studied in Vienna, which he preferred because of the opportunity it offered to do practical work. His chief teacher here was Dr Quarin, who was also the personal physician of the Empress Maria Theresa. He formed a strong connection to him also. They were so close that Hahnemann was the only one who was allowed to accompany him when he visited his private patients. After two years of practice in what is now Romania, where he also studied languages, botany and chemistry, Samuel got his degree in 1779, when he was twenty-four years old. This marked the end of the first phase of his life.

In the following period up to 1805 (aged fifty), he moved twenty times, married, had many children and no satisfaction whatsoever in his practice. He supported his family by writing books and translating books

---

*   The Kurfürstliches Gymnasium was the most elite form of secondary education in those days, providing comprehensive training based on the humanist tradition, including Latin, Greek, maths and science.

on chemistry. His work was generally held in high esteem and considered thorough. His own writing comprises the following areas:

1. the treatment of old wounds and chronic sores
2. a pharmaceutical Lexicon, which soon became a standard text for pharmacists
3. Characteristics of Purity and Impropriety of Drugs
4. The Friend of Health; A Book for the Layman

A number of characteristic traits of Hahnemann emerge from these works. In the first, for example, he shows that shepherds, blacksmiths and veterinary surgeons are actually much better at treating chronic wounds than physicians are. He registers his first dissatisfaction with the practice of bloodletting, purging and emetics. He demonstrates the importance of such things as fresh air, free exercise and healthy food. He is also concerned with the purity of remedies. He would have many a bone to pick about this with pharmacists later on. This is an important cause of the birth of homeopathy. So we see that Hahnemann during the first forty years of his life observed contemporary medicine very critically, questioned it all the time and even came to the realization that this form of medicine did more harm than good. This led him to seek alternatives.

In 1796 his *Study Concerning a New Principle to Determine the Medicinal Power of Drugs* appeared in Hufeland's Journal. In this article he describes how drugs must be taken singly by healthy subjects of experiment in order to determine from the symptoms that develop what effect the substances have, and also to gauge their medicinal potential. Mixtures will not do for this. A Hahnemann realized that one cannot tell the effect of medicines anymore when they're always mixed in concoctions containing many ingredients. How individual ingredients worked was not known very well, so this was the primary aim of his research. And how else can we find out if we do not use ourselves or healthy subjects for our experiments?

Thus the basic principle of homeopathy was born in 1796! It will be clear to what extent it stemmed from tremendous dissatisfaction, but also from a vast knowledge and erudition. Hahnemann was quite certainly one of the most erudite physicians of Germany at the time, something which was clearly acknowledged in reviews of his work. The basic principle now needed to be elaborated, which soon happened. As a corollary, he began to enjoy practising medicine again. After yet another move, he established himself in Torgau around 1805, where he quickly established a flowering practice and would stay for seven years. He was 50 years old, and he had discovered a totally new principle, which filled him with enthusiasm.

In 1805 test results of 26 medicines were published. The substances he had researched were the ordinary medicines prescribed at the time. 1810 saw the first printing of the famous *Organon der rationellen Heilkunde* [Organon of the Medical Art].

The book starts with a long introduction in which Hahnemann gives a thorough account of his objections to the medicine of his time. This medicine, so he says, can only see the material side of illness, hence the welter of physical treatments such as bloodletting. What a strange thing to have to believe that someone, who is still perfectly healthy on the first of June and has exactly the appropriate amount of blood, suddenly would have too much blood on the second of June when he has got a fever, and would therefore need a bloodletting! It would be total nonsense. Illness is a dynamic principle resulting in certain symptoms, 'dynamic disturbances of our spiritual life, affecting both our feeling and actions. Those definitely remain *nonmaterial disturbances* of our sense of well-being.' He lamented how his colleagues were blind to such views; 'they have debased the profession to a kind of janitorial service.'

So doctors called themselves assistants of nature. But what is it that this nature shows us? Helpless attempts, usually causing more suffering than healing. In this sense no help at all can be given. God gave man reason to do better than nature. The secretions and excretions which nature brings about in acute cases of illness are only chaotic attempts to relieve the body. Should we assist these primitive, chaotic attempts, or even strengthen them? A patient's condition after receiving medicines like Calomel, Digitalis, or quinine bark is invariably worse than it was before. Moreover, blending them seems to be almost obligatory, and with so many other medicines mixed in there is no way to tell any more what effect a substance actually has.

This introduction is followed by 291 chapters of varying length, the first 70 of which deal with theory, the rest with practice. The first two short chapters deal with this thesis: 'The sole and highest calling of the physician is making sick people better, which is termed curing or healing.' (Paragraph 1). Then follows this comment, which is quoted here verbatim.

> It is not his calling to cobble together hollow assertions and
> hypotheses into theoretical systems about the essence of the life
> processes or about the genesis of illnesses in the invisible realm
> within (so many doctors, hungry for fame, have wasted time and
> effort in this endeavour, and many keep trying up to this very day).
> It is not necessary to keep up these countless efforts to find an
> explanation for the symptoms of diseases and what causes them

and what not, *for these have always been elusive.* He does not have to wrap things up in incomprehensible terminology and a plethora of abstract terms, aimed to sound learned and to astound the ignorant lay-person, while sick people are desperate for help in the meantime. Such learned fantasies are officially called theoretical pharmacology, and university positions have even been created for them, but we have more than enough of them. It is high time that those who call themselves physicians at last make an end of deceiving people with such waffling. It is high time for doctors to *get down to business,* that is, to truly help and heal.

The highest ideal of healing is a *rapid, gentle and lasting* restoration of health, either through getting rid of the disease or destroying it in its totality, *in the shortest, most reliable and harmless way possible,* and in a way that is *readily comprehensible* (Paragraph 2).

Style and content of the first two paragraphs are sharp and to the point, as is the whole of the *Organon.* In the first paragraph we can detect a certain form of *agnostic thinking,* in that he denies the possibility of knowing the ultimate causes. At least, he presents it in this context as a futile pursuit, but a few lines later on he postulates an invisible life principle, which indicates that he is not completely closed to more nuanced and elaborate thoughts concerning this. He specifically pinpoints this life principle, the 'Dynamis' or 'Autocracy'; when this is out of harmony, the symptoms of the disease manifest themselves. In the first instance, this is a nonmaterial process. The totality of what meets the eye are the symptoms; together they make up the illness. That totality will have to lead us to the choice of the specific medicine. The principal requirement of a remedy is that it must carry in itself the ability to change the condition of the patient. The next question is: how do we find out which forces are present in which substances? Here Hahnemann says:

... this can in no way be discovered by pure thinking alone. Only when we see the actual effects in a patient, when we can see how the condition changes, only then do we have tangible evidence of the forces contained in a specific medicine, then we will be able to clearly see how it works (Paragraph 20).

This is how Hahnemann arrives at his testing procedures for medicines, which he described in 1796 in his first article. Two more steps are needed to complete the train of thought.

> The healing power of medicines depends on their symptoms, *which are similar to those of the illness* but exceed them *in strength.* Normal illnesses only come about in people who have a susceptibility, so they do not occur in many people. Symptoms of the illness, however, occur in each subject who takes the medicine that is being tested ... [That means that] pathogenic agents often have a minor and limited, often even *extremely limited power* to cause illness. In contrast to that, the forces which dwell in medicines have an absolute, unlimited and *much stronger power* to disturb the well-being of a human being (Paragraph 33).

And further down 'the first requirement for healing to occur is *the strongest possible similarity* between the disease the patient has naturally and one that is induced' (Paragraph 34), known as the 'Similia'-principle. The aim in therapy is therefore to give a very small quantity of the substance which causes very similar symptoms to those of the actual disease, but in a sense cancels out that disease by virtue of its stronger potency. The fleeting illness caused by the medicine which remains after that, can be easily restored by the Dynamis.

Homeopathic history-taking does take time, because the aim is to penetrate to the heart of the symptoms.

> The important thing here is to have an eye for the more striking, characteristic and unusual symptoms which typify the specific illness, almost exclusively so. Because it is especially those which have to correspond to the symptoms belonging to the chosen medicine ... (Paragraph 153).

Hahnemann made great progress in the preparation of medicines, which he called the 'dynamizing' or potentizing of homeopathic medicines. He indicates the procedure very exactly. In a footnote to paragraph 269 he says, 'Triturating of the substance or succussion of the solution (dynamizing, potentizing) enhances the medicinal power and develops the latent force within to an ever greater degree. Maybe one could say that this procedure spiritualizes matter.'

With this *all essential aspects of homeopathy* were outlined in 1810. They only found a lukewarm reception in the medical world.

Having gained a clear vision of these basic principles, he now wanted to spread the word, and so it is that we find Hahnemann teaching at the University of Leipzig from 1812 to 1820, where previously he had been a student for a year. He made a dignified start, but his lectures gradually deteriorated into a tirade against the medicine of his time. Only a small group of students remained. During all this time he kept working with a group of subjects, which included his wife and two of his daughters. And so it came about that the six volumes of *Materia Medica Pura* were written between 1811 and 1821, in which *all symptoms of 66 medicines* are described.

After losing a legal battle for the right to make his own medicines in 1820, a fight he waged against the local pharmacists, he departed to the town of Köthen, where the Duke was his patient and protector. From this time onwards he kept in the background in public discussions. In 1828 he finished his book *Die chronische Krankheiten* [Chronic Diseases], in which he tried to describe why they exist and how they can be treated homeopathically. In March 1830 his wife died. She had shared his fate, poverty, the almost yearly moves, and a family life which seemed doomed to disaster: two daughters were murdered, one child was stillborn, one died in the cradle after an accident with a carriage, three daughters had unhappy marriages, and one son was practically insane. In the town of Köthen it seemed as if Hahnemann could come to rest a little bit, in spite of the many squabbles connected with the directorship of a homeopathic hospital in Leipzig. Hahnemann was almost eighty years old. But a big change was in store for him. In October 1834, a thirty-year-old Parisian woman by the name of Melanie d'Hervilly came to consult him. People said that she seduced Hahnemann. Their marriage in 1835 caused quite a stir in Köthen and surroundings. The couple departed for Paris, where Hahnemann still spent eight happy years of married life, filled with much work, but also with pleasure. He went to concerts and operas, had access to the beau monde of Paris, and became one of the most celebrated physicians of Europe. He died in 1843, just after completing the sixth edition of the *Organon,* which only surfaced again in 1922 and was then published.

Reviewing Hahnemann's life we can notice a strange paradox. Even though he himself was one of the most thoroughly grounded physicians in the natural sciences, and especially in the field of chemistry, the close relationship between these natural sciences and homeopathy was broken later on. Some people already noticed this during his life. This was due in part to two factors. On the one hand, Hahnemann and his pupils were too busy with practical work (see the *Organon,* paragraph 1), on the other, Hahnemann's own belligerence against colleagues who did not agree with him was the reason why the group of homeopathic physicians did not become very large and why he met so much opposition. Yet this situation remained virtually the same even later when there were more homeopathic doctors (around 1900, for example, 25 percent of doctors in the United States worked according to homeopathic principles). No doubt this is also due to the agnostic tendency in his writing, which was pointed out earlier in this chapter.

We have seen how Hahnemann speaks about a nonmaterial life

principle, and nonmaterial forces in nature, and he even goes as far as calling potentizing *'spiritualizing matter.'* In medicine, these are each entirely novel thoughts.

Whereas in Hufeland's work there still is a last 'solid' vestige of Hippocratic knowledge, especially with regard to practical application, in Hahnemann's work there is the mention of a nonmaterial principle again (comparable to the *Archaeus* of Paracelsus), but the relationship with 'solid' natural science is severed. This has certainly coloured the image of homeopathic medicine up to the present day, especially when it comes to finding wider recognition in the academic world.

1.5 The place of anthroposophical medicine

All in all, we can distinguish four streams which Steiner either describes or only names in the lecture.

1. The Hippocratic stream

This one started before Hippocrates and is summarized in the *Corpus Hippocraticum.* Comprehension of its background declines from Galen (129–199) onwards, even though the heritage of this stream continues to work on into the nineteenth century. In origin, this medical science had a broad foundation based on a thinking in terms of balance, which gradually becomes a thinking in terms of opposites. We described Hufeland as one of the last representatives of this stream.

2. Paracelsus and his followers

A stream, which places the development of the human being in sickness and health at the centre. An occult Christian vision of man and nature lies at the basis of Paracelsus' method.

3. Hahnemann and homeopathy

This stream essentially thinks in terms of similarities. Even though we already find this principle in the *Corpus Hippocraticum,* and also in the work of Paracelsus, it is usually associated with the name of Hahnemann. He is the first to clearly put it into words.

4. Cellular-molecular medical science

The medical science which forms the basis of university education today. Beginning in the time of Hippocrates with an emphasis on *sense perception,* it only comes into its own around 1500, and begins to dominate the other streams after 1850.

Elements of all four streams are to be found in medical-anthroposophical literature. This includes Steiner's medical work. We also find the fourth stream represented, for example in the way it values natural science in general, and also in the fact that Steiner frequently urged scientists and doctors to put his pronouncements to the test. He welcomed this. He also went to great lengths to indicate where his findings were mentioned before in history. Examples are: the idea of reincarnation in Western history, or the idea that inner development can lead to true insight into the nature of the human being and the world around us. He never ceased to stress, however, that these concepts have to find a new foundation in modern times.

Likewise we find many aspects in the history of medicine, which are also to be found within anthroposophical medicine. The most important and relevant aspects are summed up below in aphoristic form, referring back to what has been discussed above.

1. **The physician's attitude and schooling**
    1. Be honest concerning what you can actually bring about (Hahnemann)
    2. The physician's schooling (Paracelsus)
    3. Difference between abstract knowledge and living experience (Paracelsus)
    4. Understanding out of the light of nature (Paracelsus)
    5. The importance of having an eye for geological and meteorological circumstances (Hippocrates)
    6. The moral aspects of being a doctor; the doctor as a servant of God (Paracelsus, Hufeland)

2. **Understanding the human being**
    1. The importance of age; changes in physiology in the course of a life (Hufeland)
    2. The first seven years in relation to intellectual learning (Hufeland)
    3. The big difference between above and below the diaphragm (Hufeland, *Corpus Hippocraticum)*
    4. Vix Medicatrix Naturae (Hippocrates)
    5. Archaeus (Paracelsus)
    6. Dynamis (Hahnemann)
    7. The perception that illness is anchored in a specific human physiology (Paracelsus)
    8. The four elements

3. **Health/illness**
    1. Sleep as an important healing factor *(Corpus Hippocraticum,* Hufeland)
    2. The great importance of taking psychological, spiritual, and environmental factors into account (housing, climate, poverty, war, etc.) (Hufeland)
    3. The importance of secretion, and the suppression of it *(Corpus Hippocraticum,* Hufeland, Hahnemann)
    4. Aurea Mediocritas (Hufeland)
    5. The perception that illness is anchored in a specific human physiology (Paracelsus)
    6. Illness as a physical manifestation of something spiritual (Hahnemann)
    7. The view that illness offers an opportunity for development (Paracelsus)
    8. The difference between acute and chronic illnesses (Paracelsus, Hahnemann)

4. **Healing, therapy**
    1. Potentizing (Hahnemann)
    2. How healing really works (Hahnemann)
    3. The alchemy of medicine-making (Paracelsus)
    4. The three cardinal interventions (Hufeland)
    5. The physician as assistant of nature *(Corpus Hippocraticum,* Hufeland)

5. **Deeper aspects**
    1. Mystery medicine; Temple sleep
    2. Threefold human being. Briefly indicated in this chapter in the discussion of Pherekydes with the triad of Kronos-Zeus-Chtoon. The metamorphoses of these concepts we meet again in Paracelsus, and in anthroposophical medicine as Sal–Mercur–Sulphur
    3. Correspondence of macrocosm and microcosm

In Steiner's medical work we meet these aspects in a variety of ways. The lecture cycle *Occult Physiology,* for example, elaborates on the correspondence of macrocosmic and microcosmic aspects which emerges when we study the human being. It deals, for example, with the fact that our organs have a very specific relationship to the planets. In Steiner's *First Medical Course,* basically all aspects which are listed above are touched upon. We can gain the impression that the streams of Hippocrates, Paracelsus, and Hahnemann (homeopathy), are forged into a new unity, with Steiner adopting viewpoints from the different streams at different points. Yet this should not be seen as rekindling traditional concepts. Present-day consciousness has undergone too much of a change to just accept traditional concepts without questioning them. The enormous development of natural science during the last century especially was for good reasons. That in itself is an expression of present-day consciousness.

The *First Medical Course* was given for physicians who were also acquainted with anthroposophy and were practised in inner schooling. Therefore Steiner could refer back to this acquaintance and experience when he said later in the cycle that true insight into the deeper causes of health and disease is only possible when our inner faculties of perception are renewed and transformed. Steiner mentions the meditative schooling on the side as it were, in a way that could almost be overlooked when one is immersed in the enormous depth of the perceptions offered in this cycle.

The meditative side of the medical work comes to the fore much more from January 1924 onwards, when Steiner gave the *Course for Young Doctors.*

The Dutch physician Ita Wegman was of great importance to Steiner in bringing this about. They worked together intensively. Ita Wegman cultivated a strong meditative life, intent on reconnecting with the old mystery knowledge. She was also a thoroughly practical woman so that her inner knowledge could become fruitful for her outer work in everyday life. As a result, the book, *Extending Practical Medicine (Fundamentals of Therapy)* [*Grundlegendes für eine Erweiterung der Heilkunst*] was written in close collaboration between Steiner and Wegman. Steiner referred to this book a few times as containing 'the seeds for a new mystery-medicine.'

During the last years of his life, Steiner frequently spoke about the old mystery streams, and how they could come to life again in anthroposophy. During one of these cycles of lectures Ita Wegman asked Steiner if it would be possible for modern medicine to reconnect with the old mystery knowledge. Steiner answered with a full 'yes.' We can distinguish three phases within the development of anthroposophy in reference to medical content given.

First phase
For a long time Steiner gave medical content in general anthroposophical lectures, not specifically in courses for doctors. Much is contained in *Occult Physiology;* many facts are to be found in various lectures.

Second phase

The *First Medical Course* and sequels to that were given in response to questions from physicians who were pupils of Steiner and wondered how anthroposophy could become fruitful for their medical work.

Third phase

The phase after the question posed by Ita Wegman. This phase resulted in the *Course for Young Doctors* mentioned above, which contains indications for young doctors concerning the meditative path, and the book, *Extending Practical Medicine.*

This book is written in an extremely compact style; one gets the impression that this content only reveals itself in meditation. This style is typical of the general anthroposophical writing of Steiner's last years. His *Anthroposophical Leading Thoughts* [*Leitsätze*] have a similar compactness.

In anthroposophical medicine after Steiner's death, we meet the following elements. On the one side present-day consciousness is totally accepted, including the technical aspects which result from it. However, our consciousness is recognized as being limited but definitely capable of expanding and developing. At the same time there is a renewed appreciation of medical ideas from the past. Anthroposophical thinking is able to interpret them anew. Lastly, spiritual scientific medicine contains seeds for a new mystery medicine.

CHAPTER 2

A Philosophical Foundation of Anthroposophical Medicine

ERIK BAARS

One does not usually find a philosophical orientation at the start of a practical medical training. There are two reasons for including one. First of all, we feel a responsibility towards our patients; they need to know where we stand. Morally speaking, the way we think about the human being and illness in general has its consequences. After all, what we do as physicians is a direct product of our medical approach and the way we look at the human being. Is the human being a chance conglomerate of cells or a spiritual entity manifesting in a physical body? This is an important question to consider, for the answer to this question determines medical ethics. Secondly, many people feel it as a real omission if there is no philosophical justification right at the start of an academic training. Just imagine how many medical students would react inwardly, if a professor were to declare right at the onset of years of university study that materialism would be the sole basis of the entire training, and that a scientific outlook as understood in this context would be the outlook of materialistic natural science, without any further discussion! Other forms of science are often condescendingly treated as non-scientific, even though the phenomenological approach has had many important proponents in recent times. To name but a few important scientists: Bolk, Buytendijk, Van den Berg, Blechschmidt, Portmann, Sax and Holdrege.

In medical science, many questions are waiting for answers, and there is a wealth of facts which are known but not understood in their context. The increase of ethical questions in medicine merely illustrates this point.

The authors of this training manual are of the opinion that present-day medical science needs a broader foundation and needs to do justice to our full humanity. The introductory philosophical remarks of this chapter form a beginning. We realize that these contributions are short and incomplete, but they are nevertheless offered in the hope that their intent will be clear to the reader.

2.1 What is science?

Those who presently study, or have studied medicine may question the relevance of this question. After all, science is being practised in every university setting, and there is unlimited access to scientific knowledge anywhere in the world; we have a wealth of up-to-date information at our fingertips through the widespread use of computer technology. In light of this, advice given to the Dutch Board of Health in a 1993 report is all the more remarkable. It states that:

> There is no comprehensive or generally accepted definition or delineation of the concept 'science.' But even the so-called 'delineation-criterion' is a point of contention. What distinguishes scientific from non-scientific, what is the difference between science and belief, myth, or just plain nonsense? With regard to criteria which could be used in order to make this distinction, (when there is talk of identification, confirmation, falsification, consensus within a scientific discipline, verification through statistics or testing, the question of what constitutes proof, reliability of predictions based on theories, etc. etc.), opinions vary.[1]

According to this report to the Dutch Board of Health, we find *that there is more than one opinion about the meaning of scientific and non-scientific.*

This finding justifies the aim of this chapter, which is to delineate the philosophical foundation of anthroposophy and its views regarding science, epistemology, and medicine. Section 2.2 gives an overview of philosophy in order to have a historical perspective as a basis for what follows. Rudolf Steiner's theory of knowledge, the philosophical underpinning of anthroposophy, is the subject of Section 2.3. This leads us to Section 2.4 where we deal with a fundamental philosophical question: are there boundaries to knowledge? In conclusion, we summarize where anthroposophy stands philosophically in a formal sense. Anthroposophy and anthroposophical medicine are based on a monistic, spiritual, and realist view of the human being and the cosmos. This is elaborated in Section 2.5.

2.2 An outline history of philosophy

2.2.1. Up to modern times

Socrates (469–399 BC) could probably be called the first true philosopher in the history of mankind. He grew up in Greek culture, where the mysteries, such as the oracle of Delphi, played a central role. In these mysteries oracles formed the link between gods and humans. Socrates was the first to no longer refer people to an oracle or point them to the old norms, but urged people to come to an independent judgment (Blommaard, 1995).

Then came Plato (427–347 BC), a pupil of Socrates, who first began to make a principal distinction between body and soul, between perception and thinking. Before him, thinking was described as a special form of perception, *coming towards the human being from the outside.* For Plato thinking is on the one hand a kind of perceiving, but it is all taking place in an invisible realm, separate from the body, and clearly distinguished from sense perception. Before birth, according to Plato, the human being lives in a world of ideas, a world which is subsequently forgotten after we are born. In earthly life sense perception leads us step by step to remembering this pre-birth experience of the world of ideas. It is this process which actually leads to knowledge. These two realms interpenetrate in the human mind.

A little later, Plato's most important pupil Aristotle takes another step. In order to acquire knowledge, we first need sense perception, secondly the ability to retain the acquired sense perceptions (memory), and thirdly the ability which can only develop on the basis of these two, namely thinking in concepts (knowing). About the latter Aristotle says, 'I know that these concepts make sense, because they stem from the spirit.' Aristotle is conscious of the spiritual origin of the concepts, but the spirit is no longer of importance for the actual process of knowing. The further course of the history of philosophy continues to move between these poles, stressing now the world of ideas more, then the world of sense perception. For example, the Hellenistic philosophical system known as Stoa, which started right after Aristotle, only recognized the direction arising from sense perception. Things were reversed a few centuries later by the Gnostics, for whom consciousness does not quite 'descend' into earthly life anymore.

This dynamic alteration persists until a thousand years later in the Middle Ages, where we see a similar polarity within Scholasticism. The scholastics speak about 'two types of truth,' the truth of the mind and the truth of revelation, each comprising totally different areas. Mental truth is acquired by the activity of the mind, which occupies itself with what enters the human being through the senses. This activity can be seen as the perfection of the train of thought which Aristotle, focusing totally on the sense perceptible world, set in motion. Truth through revelation on the other hand comprises a part of reality (for example the Trinity) which can only be known through revelation. This last standpoint emerges out of the Scholastic battle about what were called the 'Universals,' a philosophical debate between the 'Nominalists' and the 'Realists.' This debate centred around the question whether the general concepts (Universals) such as for example the concept of 'horse,' are only the general *names* for separate objects (in this case 'horse' would be the common name for all separate horses) (nominalism), or whether the horse in general, the idea horse, has real existence (realism). One can also formulate this question as follows: are ideas real?

The realists distinguished three 'levels of existence' within the Universals.

1. The *Universalia ante rem* (universals before the thing) are those ideas which exist within themselves, that is to say, *before (ante)* they have begun to work within a thing which has become visible. In other words before they have manifested in this sense world. So the word 'res' means a visible thing.
2. The *Universalia in re* are the ideas *working creatively* and manifesting *within* sense perceptible things of the world.
3. The *Universalia post rem* are those ideas which, *after (post)* having worked within visible nature, appear as inactive ideas within the thinking consciousness of a human being who has studied visible nature, and through that has gained insight and knowledge, regarding the universals.

Subsequent history shows how 'modern times' radically abolish any notion of knowledge through revelation (see Francis Bacon below). Knowledge begins with sense perception and 'ascends' to abstraction, shaped consciously by the human being in the act of knowing. Instead of the spiritual world of antiquity and the world of revelation of scholasticism, we see, metaphorically speaking, a closed off, individual 'head-formation' taking place. Thinking is new in two aspects. First of all, the human being begins to think without the help of higher orders of being, and takes individual responsibility, 'using his own head.' The second aspect is that thinking is experienced as a subjective activity. Metaphysical speculation takes the place of spiritual experience (further elaborated in Dietz 1986).

2.2.2 Modern times

At the beginning of the new age, two thinkers exerted a great influence which lasted for centuries. Those two were Bacon and Descartes.

Francis Bacon

Francis Bacon (1561–1626) is generally regarded as the founder of empiricism. This stream starts from the premise *that experience or sense perception forms the only source of knowledge about reality* and that what this experience gives us forms the foundation of knowledge. The basic thesis of this view is that everything which springs from human consciousness must be removed from the process of knowing, because it leads to subjectivity. *This goes especially for thinking.* We're thus left with 'objective' factors, that is to say everything that sense perception offers. Bacon's ideas have set the tone for many themes which are still with us today at the beginning of the twenty-first century: regarding sense perception, the experiment, the possibility for human error, and the whole way we approach nature. In order to flesh this out, we will now highlight these themes by giving Bacon's vision on them.

Sense perception and the experiment

> But by far the greatest impediment and aberration of the human understanding proceeds from the dullness, incompetency, and errors of the senses; since whatever strikes the senses preponderates over everything, however superior, which does not immediately strike them ... For the senses are weak and erring, nor can instruments be of great use in extending their sphere or acuteness. All the better interpretations of nature are worked out by instances,* and fit and apt experiments, where the senses only judge of the experiment, the experiment of nature and the thing itself. (*Novum Organum,* Aphorism 50, p. 111)

As a consequence, insight arises straight from the observations gathered in the experiment. Nothing new is added by thinking, after all!

---

* The 'instances' refer to interpretation through thinking.

Sources of error: the four Idols

The first source of error is the *Idola Specus* or the 'error of the personal standpoint.' Bacon writes about this:

> The idols of the den are those of each individual; for everybody (in addition to the errors common to the race of man) has his own individual den or cavern, which intercepts and corrupts the light of nature either from his own peculiar and singular disposition, or from his education and intercourse with others, or from his reading, and the authority acquired by those whom he reverences and admires or from the different impressions produced on the mind, ... and the like so that the spirit of man ... is variable, confused, and, as it were, actuated by chance. And Heraclitus said well that men search for knowledge in lesser worlds and not in the greater or common world *(Novum Organum,* Aphorism 42, p. 109).

The second source is the *Idola Tribus* or the 'distorted image stemming from human error'

> The idols of the tribe are inherent in human nature and the very tribe or race of man; for man's sense is falsely asserted to be the standard of things; on the contrary, all the perceptions both of the senses and the mind bear reference to man and not the universe, and the human mind resembles those uneven mirrors which impart their own properties to different objects, from which rays are emitted and distort and disfigure them (p. 109).

The third source is the *Idola Fori* or the 'errors of the marketplace.'

> There are also idols formed by the reciprocal intercourse and society of man with man, which we call idols of the market, from the commerce and association of men with each other; for men converse by means of language, but words are formed at the will of the generality, and there arises from a bad and unapt formation of words a wonderful obstruction to the mind (Aphorism 43, pp. 109f).

The last source of error is the *Idola Theatri.*

> Lastly, there are idols which have crept into men's minds from the various dogmas of peculiar systems of philosophy, and also from the perverted rules of demonstration, and these we denominate idols of the theatre: for we regard all the systems of philosophy

hitherto received or imagined, as so many plays brought out and performed, creating fictitious and theatrical worlds.

Approach to Nature

According to Bacon, the aim of natural science is progress, practical application and human control of nature. In order to achieve that the human being must get to know the laws of nature and 'put nature on the rack to force her secrets from her.' The experiment plays the role of the rack in this.

René Descartes

René Descartes (1596–1650) is generally regarded as the founder of modern philosophy. He himself claimed that he was the first since Plato and Aristotle who had something new to say. According to Descartes we *arrive at knowledge* by starting from first principles which are totally clear, beyond any doubt and irrefutable. From these first principles we can deduce other knowledge if we stick to rules which are totally clear and are valid beyond a doubt. Euclidean geometry is always given as a standard example for this form of knowing. There is no doubt about the first principles, which are the five postulates, nor about the rules of deduction. It would be desirable and possible if the same method would be applied to natural science, which is synonymous with mechanics for Descartes. (He looked upon mechanics as the dynamic principle behind reality, in the same way that geometry is the static principle behind reality.) Examples of Descartes' rationalism can be found even today in science and especially in the language we still use to *prove* something. The first principles and the rules of deduction are assumed to be needing no proof. With that, mathematical thinking has been elevated to the sole source of knowledge and the only valid method. According to those who see the only just foundation for science in a mathematical approach, *Cartesian doubt* forms the basis of modern theory of knowledge.

> When I doubt everything, sense perception is the first to go; after all, I could be dreaming or hallucinating. Mathematics gives more certain knowledge, because it is also valid in our dreams. But it remains possible to doubt, because God or a devil could make it so that this knowledge also is only an illusion. Only one thing remains that I can not have any doubts about, namely the fact that I doubt, therefore think, therefore exist. My body could be an illusion, but however erroneous my thoughts may be, it is necessary that the thinking ego must exist. *I think, therefore I am.*

Only when we come to the twentieth century does this rock-solid trust in science begin to show some cracks. Important contributions to this development are the paradigm theory of Kuhn, Popper's ideas about falsification and the scientific nihilism of Feyerabend. A few brief remarks about these three follow below.

Thomas Kuhn

Thomas Kuhn's central theme is the *'paradigm,'* which is the idea that science stands or falls with a historically determined, pre-scientific, philosophically and ideologically determined framework of thinking. This contains fundamental views concerning a part of reality which reflects what is alive in the *Zeitgeist;* only through this, things can be observed, interpreted, and be even comprehended, so that problems can be recognized. Typical examples are the Copernican worldview or the anatomy of Vesalius. Such frameworks of thinking arise more or less spontaneously in the course of history; their origin and genesis are at any rate highly unclear. In any case, the way paradigms come into being and the way a certain thinking framework is chosen by scientists to serve as a paradigm in their field are in many respects irrational processes.

Sociology, history, and other non-philosophical disciplines have remarkable things to say on the subject. This irrational character of the paradigm theory has been attacked by critics with the argument that it does away with the most important trait of science: progress. Kuhn has countered this with the argument of the 'good reasons,' meaning that scientists have always had definite good reasons in selecting the best possible paradigm choosing from all the possible prescientific views current in their time, and elevating that to *the* paradigm. But up to now nobody has been able to put together a precise and convincing argument as to what the grounds are for calling these reasons 'good.'

Yet Kuhn's ideas regarding paradigms have generally been well received. Such a paradigm makes it possible to distinguish between problems that can be solved and those that cannot, and are therefore of no interest or relevance to science. This may give a very static impression of science, but only on the outside; Kuhn's paradigm theory is highly dynamic. After all, paradigms do not last forever. They emerge, grow and flourish for a long or a short time, then fall into decay and are replaced again by another paradigm. An astute observer might even notice how a paradigm begins to grow obsolete before it goes under. That would be at the moment when all the problems which have become definable and solvable within the paradigm have actually been resolved. Another reason why an existing paradigm could be doomed, is that its right of existence has become questionable. This might happen in a case where people are faced with new problems which cannot be solved within the framework of the existing paradigm, but must find a solution nevertheless (further elaborated in Verbrugh).

Karl Popper

Karl R. Popper (1902–94) is generally regarded as the one who has brought about a real epistemological breakthrough in this century, with his *'logical positivism'* and theory of *'falsification.'* In his thinking, *there is no form of scientific knowledge, which we can be totally certain about in the end.* In this theory, scientific knowledge is not stated positively, but must be open to criticism and should be refutable. So the characteristic of Popper's scientific knowledge is that knowledge is in principle *falsifiable.* This principle promotes scientific progress, because the inherent weaknesses of established theories will become very apparent and can then be challenged, leading to a constant search for better alternatives. Popper also coined the concept *demarcation criterion,* which is the criterion which distinguishes between scientific and non-scientific.

Paul Feyerabend

In 1975 Paul Feyerabend draws the following conclusion from Popper's theory about science and Kuhn's approach of the history of science: neither science nor epistemology is capable of openly explaining the grounds and intention of scientific rationality. He recognizes that what former times considered scientific was always dubbed prescientific or unscientific in later times. Hence Feyerabend draws a conclusion, which *openly questions whether science is at all scientific.*

> Science [he says] is one of many forms of thinking developed by human beings, and not necessarily the best one. It is loud, shameless, and glaring. Only those consider her superior in principle, who have already chosen a specific ideology, or have accepted science without ever having considered her advantages and weaknesses ... Modern science has silenced her opponents, not convinced them. Science took the helm by force, not by reasoning (Kiene 1984).

By the end of the twentieth century, empiricism (see Bacon) has become outmoded. It has become clear that pure facts, unaffected by any theory, do not exist. Something very important has been said with this, because if empiricism held that everything which was not sense-perceptible was not real, and if we now hold that everything sense perceptible does not guarantee 'reality,' we find ourselves in a *total loss of reality.*

So what are we dealing with in science, if not with a form of reality? Since the sixties, a new theory of truth has emerged more and more, namely the *consensus theory.* What a group of competent individuals can agree on is considered true. This goes for *all* questions, including those posed in mathematics and geometry. For example, if the sum of the angles of a triangle cannot be proved in any way, but we reach consensus that it is 180°, then it is so, and if we do not reach consensus, it is not so. The consequence of this, however, is that a widespread feeling arises of losing all touch with reality. Since everything which our minds can grasp is questionable, our heads are effectively severed from the world, so to speak. We all have our different mental concepts, but they lead separate lives. There may be consensus, but individual conceptions may bear little relation to actuality. Therefore we no longer speak of 'objectivity,' but of 'intersubjectivity.'

Another stream which tries to solve the results of the criticism of empiricism, is called 'irrationalism.' Ever since Kuhn published his theories of paradigms, no one can quite shake the notion that science has been subject to very real irrational influences in the course of history. The latest development in this respect is called 'constructivism.' This is grounded in the notion that knowing the world comes down to creating the world (further elaborated in Dietz 1986).

2.2.3 Summary of the history of philosophy

From this overview we can conclude that a clear development has taken place in the history of philosophy. Here follows a summary of the main points in this development:

— The time before Socrates: norms were set by the mysteries, and oracles were consulted
— From Socrates onwards: beginning of individual judgement
— Plato: sense perception points to the world of ideas
— Aristotle: the sense perceptible world itself becomes the object of research
— Medieval scholasticism: two types of truth, through the mind or through revelation

The human capacity for judgement develops, at times more oriented towards the world of ideas, at other times more oriented to the world which can be grasped by the senses. At the end of this development the world of ideas is considered real, but inaccessible for human knowledge!

Leaping ahead to modern times:

— *Bacon* introduces empiricism and sense perception becomes the sole source of what is considered real and can be known. The world of ideas is seen as fanciful and subjective. Thinking is excluded from the process of knowing and nature's secrets are extorted from her: experiments will supply the necessary data.
— *Descartes* makes the mathematical approach the foundation of science.
— *Kuhn* introduces the paradigm-theory, the idea that science stands or falls with different philosophical and ideological frameworks which alternate through history, that paradigm precedes scientific theory.
— *Popper* maintains that science never leads to certainty.
— *Feyerabend* doubts whether science is scientific.

Further twentieth-century developments:

— Empiricism is superseded; sense perception is no longer taken to guarantee reality.
— The consensus theory gains ground; a group of competent individuals decides what can be agreed upon collectively.
— Irrationalism recognizes that influences beyond our control always play in.
— Constructivism holds that knowing the world is in reality creating the world.
— Even if there is such a thing as a world of ideas, this would be inaccessible to scientific inquiry.
— Sense perceptible data no longer guarantee reality, and with that empiricism is superseded.

All this adds up to a general sense that reality is inaccessible. Science can say nothing regarding the truth.

So far this general philosophical history. Now we come to the vision which Rudolf Steiner developed with regard to the theory of knowledge and reality.

2.3 Steiner's theory of knowledge

2.3.1 Rudolf Steiner

Rudolf Steiner (1861–1925) was a philosophical thinker who has remained relatively unknown in academic circles. To place his work in a proper context within the history of philosophy it is important to take three things into consideration.

1. The spiritual experiences which he had from early childhood on.
2. His experience of the reality of the ego.
3. His relationship to the work of Goethe.

> Rudolf Steiner relates how, at the age of twenty, he was able to perceive the spiritual individuality of a human being, and could follow the process of incarnation, how this individuality manifests in a human body and finds its way back into the spiritual world after death. The question regarding the relationship of the spirit to nature and science becomes crucial for him; it is *the* essential question which occupies him in the first half of his life. *How does thinking bridge the gap between natural science and the inner experience of the spirit, grasped clairvoyantly?* (Sijmons 1995).

In his autobiography, Steiner relates how as a young philosophy student, he comes to an experience of the *reality of the ego,* in the night between February 10 and 11, 1881:

> During the last year I endeavoured to research whether Schelling is right when he says, 'Deep inside we possess a hidden and miraculous capacity to withdraw out of the vicissitudes of time into an inner sanctum, and there, stripped of all externals, behold the eternal within ourselves in the guise of the immutable.' I believed and still believe I have discovered this most inward capacity very clearly within myself — I've had an inkling all along: my whole view of idealistic philosophy has essentially changed now.*

---

* See also 'Experiencing the reality of thinking,' p.64.

From 1882 until 1889, Steiner worked on the Kürschner edition of the works of Goethe. From 1889 until 1897 he worked at the Goethe and Schiller Archives in Weimar, where the complete works of Goethe were being edited and published. In order to understand Steiner properly, we will now give a short survey of Goethe's work relevant to this chapter.

2.3.2 Goethe

Johann Wolfgang von Goethe (1749–1832) lived in Germany and was not only a well-known author, poet, and politician, but also a very great natural scientist. For a long time he was director and lecturer at the anatomical Institute of Jena and conducted extensive botanical, zoological, geological and meteorological studies. He gained scientific recognition amongst other things with his discovery of the intermaxillary bone, his botanical studies *(The Metamorphosis of Plants),* and his *Colour Theory.* There are many quotations which characterize Goethe's scientific approach. Here are two of them. They speak of the role of the senses and our relationship to art.

> Our mind and judgment can mislead us, so we must be watchful there. But our senses themselves do not mislead us.

> In our scientific striving, we human beings have always tried to grasp the specific nature of living organisms, to understand the separate outwardly visible parts in their interconnectedness, and to see them as manifestations of their inner being. We have tried to penetrate to an all-encompassing vision and represent that; how strongly this striving is related to the innate human urge for artistic expression and imitation needs little elaboration.

2.3.3 Goethe's scientific method

The quotations above show that Goethe attached great value to sense perception, looking for connections, seeing the whole picture, and an artistic approach to the phenomena. These elements appear again when we focus on three essential phases which can be discovered in his scientific approach.

1. Exact sense perception combined with imagination
The whole process of observation needs to be schooled, and the first step is to strive for the most exact correlation possible between the memory of what was perceived and the actual perception. When the objects we

observe undergo a clear process of development in time, we need to *reconstruct this development exactly in our memory*. Examples of this are plant study and the study of the development of the human embryo.

2. Self-restraint

When one occupies oneself this way regularly with the same object, one notices that one *lives into* the object more and more. One also finds that all one knows about the object tends to stand in the way of truly getting to know it in the way indicated above. So in this phase preconceived notions about the object have to be overcome. *Restraining oneself and holding back preconceived notions* enhances the ability to inwardly imitate.

3. The language of gesture

Having practised phases 1 and 2, the memory (closely matching the percept) can now reveal something of what Goethe called the *Gebärdensprache*, which we could translate as 'language of gesture,' or simply the gesture. By working in the way indicated, Goethe learned to read this language, and this enabled him when he occupied himself intensively with plant growth to discover archetypal gestures in the morphology of plants. Thus he came to speak of an *Urpflanze*, or an archetypal plant, a form lying at the basis of the entire plant kingdom. One should not conceive of this 'archetypal plant' as something static, but rather as a plastic being, from which every manifestation in the plant world is derived (see Chapter 6).

Such a way of approaching nature study is entirely different from the method Bacon strove after, when he suggested putting nature on the rack.

2.3.4 Rudolf Steiner's philosophical works

Implicit in Goethe's work, Steiner found a practical application of the scientific method in which both the reality of the spiritual world (which Steiner had experienced directly since childhood) and the activity of the individual ego play a central role. In his own philosophical writings, Steiner builds on this work of Goethe. He takes Goethe's approach, builds it up further and gives it a philosophical foundation. He thus bridges the gap between natural science and the spiritual world (which was a reality for him). In so doing, he also laid a philosophical basis for anthroposophy. Steiner's approach was as follows: he always entered fully into the philosophical thoughts current in his time and commented on them, after which he arrived at his own conclusions with regard to philosophical aspects of the way we come to knowledge, and the question of freedom of action, observation and thinking.

His doctoral thesis, *Truth and Science* [*Wahrheit und Wissenschaft*], appeared in 1892 and was subsequently reworked into a book. In this work Steiner deals with the epistemology of Immanuel Kant, who was a contemporary of Goethe and lived from 1724 to 1804. The passages quoted below are relevant to many subsequent philosophical and episte-mological arguments, in that Kant's whole train of thought is based on a *preconceived notion,* and thus loses its very fundament. This preconceived notion consists of the idea that 'all we experience is our own conceptions' [*alle uns gegebenen Gegenstände unsere* Vorstellungen *seien*]. Of course it is not uncommon to 'catch' somebody else's prejudices, but that is not the reason why Steiner's book is quoted here. A good reason to cite this book, however, is that Steiner goes on to indicate that a judgment marks the end of an epistemological process (a process to come to know some-thing), which also goes for a prejudice.

The task of a theory of knowledge

In *Truth and Science,* Steiner writes, 'epistemology is the scientific study of what all other sciences presuppose without examining it: *cognition* itself.' So before I can actually work with 'knowing' (something in the world), I first have to know how I know, how that process works. Therefore a theory of knowledge must first come to an understanding of this process, before any judgment can be formed. For a judgment is the result of the activity of coming to know something and should therefore not be dealt with at the end of a theory of knowledge, but at the beginning. So this also goes for Kant's pronouncement in the (German) quote above.

Immediate experience of the world

Steiner takes the next logical step by asking what the world would look like before we actually come to know it. The starting point is what Steiner logically calls the *pre-cognitive starting point.* When we perceive the world around us and have not made any judgements yet or come to know it, we have what we could call an immediate experience of the world; immediate because nothing has intervened yet. From this point without prejudice where we have this immediate experience of the world, we per-ceive all manner of 'sensations, perceptions, opinions, feelings, deeds, pictures of dreams and imaginations, representations, concepts and ideas. Illusions and hallucinations too, at this stage are equal to the rest of the world-content. For their relation to other perceptions can be revealed only through observations based on cognition.' It is of great importance to real-ize that at this point nothing can be said yet regarding the different ele-ments of our immediate experience, because any pronouncements would depend on the process of forming judgements which has not taken place yet. Having concluded what can be 'seen' at this point without prejudice, the next set of questions follows naturally. 'At what point do we begin to know? How do we determine what constitutes a percept or a concept? How do we determine what is real, what is semblance, what is cause, what effect ...?'

Assignment
Try to live into this state of consciousness, which closely corresponds to the consciousness of a baby. After all, the infant's experience is unburdened by any conscious concepts.

Two distinct parts of immediate experience
Two more quotes from *Truth and Science:*

> We must find the bridge from the world-picture as given, to that other world-picture which we build up by means of cognition. Here, however, we meet with the following difficulty: as long as we merely stare passively at the given we shall never find a point of attack where we can gain a foothold, and from where we can then proceed with cognition. Somewhere in the given we must find a place where we can set to work, where something exists which is akin to cognition. If everything were really *only* given, we could do no more than merely stare into the external world and stare indifferently into the inner world of our individuality. We would at most be able to *describe* things as something external to us; we should never be able to *understand* them. Our concepts would have a purely external relation to that to which they referred; they would not be inwardly related to it. For real cognition depends on finding a sphere somewhere in the given where our cognizing activity does not merely presuppose something given, but finds itself active in the very essence of the given. In other words: precisely through strict adherence to the given as merely given, it must become apparent that not everything *is* given.
>
> In this sense, the *given* also includes what *according to its very nature is not-given.* The latter would appear, to begin with, as *formally* a part of the given, but on closer scrutiny, would reveal its inner nature of its own accord.

What is 'not immediately experienced' within 'immediate experience'
Once again, we see how Steiner points to the direction of our search for the next step to be taken in the theory of knowledge: within all that is immediately experienced there must be a part which in essence is different, not given directly. *Concepts* and *ideas* meet the 'requirements' outlined above. When we listed what can be perceived from the 'point without prejudice,' we have seen that immediate experience actually contains concepts and ideas. On the other hand the human being must actively produce concepts and ideas within immediate experience; to do this, we have to *think,* and in that respect concepts and ideas are not given to us *directly.*

The nature of perception and of concepts/ideas
In a world without concepts and ideas our experience would consists of nothing but percepts *next to one another and after one another.* In other words, coherence would totally elude us. Just think how different our experience is when there are ideas! We all know the feeling we have when we find ourselves in a situation which is totally different from what we had expected. There is no rhyme or reason in what we perceive. Only when somebody else sets us straight or when we ourselves actively research and think do we suddenly arrive at an understanding of why things are different from what we had expected, and how they fit together. When we 'see through' something, and things 'make sense,' our thinking activity has supplied the right concepts to fit the percepts. By nature, isolated percepts are separate. Ideas connect them.

The relationship between percepts and concepts
We thus come to see that the 'activity of knowing' has two distinctly separate aspects: perception and thinking. Through our senses, we have the capacity to take in the sense perceptible world and make it our own. Through thinking, we have the capacity to make the world of concepts and ideas our own. One could also say that thinking is a sense organ for concepts and ideas (see also Section 2.2.1)

In the paragraphs above we have concluded how the world of percepts and the world of concepts and ideas have a different quality. Keywords for the world of percepts are: loose, isolated, separate. Keywords for the world of concepts and ideas are: meaning, coherence, insight. The reason for this sharp difference is that we do not produce the world of percepts, whereas we must bring the concepts together ourselves. We have to connect them within our thinking consciousness, which also implies that we have to determine how the thoughts fit together.

Having determined the qualitative difference between percepts and

ideas and given the reasons for the difference, we now turn to the question
how percepts and concepts or ideas themselves are related. Open-minded
observation shows us that a subject facing an object will begin to form
coherent thoughts regarding the perceived object. This takes place within
thinking consciousness. It has become common for percepts to be considered real, and for concepts arising in thinking to be considered subjective.
It should be stated again here that open-minded consideration of this problem shows that it is totally arbitrary to designate the concept arising within
thinking consciousness as having nothing to do with the perceived object
in the world. 'It is totally arbitrary to see the product of all that we experience purely through observation of a thing as a complete whole, and to
see the results of thinking contemplation as something extraneous which
has nothing to do with the thing itself.'

The 'pure concept'

Concepts and ideas are real and can be perceived by thinking. We can see
this from the following example. Not only can we perceive a randomly
chosen circle, but in our imagination we can 'see' all manner of circles,
and our thinking can also produce the 'pure concept' of *the* circle. 'Pure'
means free of all perceptual content here. We could formulate the pure
concept of the circle as follows: *the* circle is a two-dimensional geometrical figure, in which all points are equidistant from a point, the centre.
When we compare this pure concept of *the* circle with *a* randomly chosen
circle, we can conclude that *the* circle does not exist in the physical, sense
perceptible world, but can only exist in the thinking consciousness of the
human being. We should also note that the concept circle has a general
character. A randomly chosen circle, however, can be perceived with the
physical senses and is therefore a *specific* manifestation of the *general*
concept. The general concept contains the laws according to which the
specific manifestations of concrete circles are constructed. They all
embody the *idea* of the circle.

Experiencing the reality of thinking

Many people think the considerations above are nonsensical. For them
thinking is no more than a subjective matter or a product of the brain!
What could be the reason that the world of ideas, perceived by means of
thinking, is 'inconceivable' for so many people?

One of the most important reasons lies in the nature of thinking itself.
We meet it at the moment that we want to research it *ourselves*. This turns
out to be not so easy! Our (thinking) attention is usually focused on the
object under consideration and not on the activity which allows concepts
and ideas to appear within our thinking consciousness. When we want to

be able to perceive thinking as such, we must be conscious of actively entering into an *exceptional situation*. With this we can also make our first observation about thinking, namely that it is the *part of our mental activity which is not perceived*. At the same time, however, we may conclude that *we know thinking better than the world of percepts,* in that we do it ourselves. Because this is so, we have an immediate connection to it. Nothing comes between me and my thinking. It is totally clear to me, because I know how it is brought about. When we say this we direct our attention to the content of thinking, the concepts, which we have clear in our minds. At this point it must be stressed that in pure thinking coherence is given through the content of the concepts. Pure thinking is always an act of will, and we actively choose the concepts and how they appear in thinking consciousness.

The next step takes us to the transition from past thought to present thinking, i.e. from dead concepts which are the results of thinking done in the past to the activity of the thinking process in the here and now. This corresponds to what the scholastics termed universals *post rem* (no longer active), and universals *in re* (actively creating), and brings us to the exceptional situation spoken of in the previous paragraph: thinking about thinking. In this activity, during which the aforementioned clarity is maintained, thinking functions as a perceiving faculty, observing its own activity. In this active self-perception, thinking enters into the light of its own being, and shows itself *as a self-reliant being, translucent in and through itself.* 'It is the *I* itself, standing within thinking, which perceives *its own* activity.'[2]

At this level, the I transcends its narrow bounds; through its own activity in pure thinking consciousness, the common world of ideas and concepts appears within it. For the sake of completion, it should be mentioned here that there is a clear, qualitative difference between observing an object in the sense world and perceiving one's own active thinking. In the former, one stands 'over against' the observed object, in the latter one experiences oneself *right within* the creative activity of one's own I.

Understanding the process of knowing

To the unprejudiced observer, the concept of the object which is perceived by the senses arises within thinking consciousness. So the concept can arise in two ways. On the one hand the concept arises in an object of the physical sense perceptible world, on the other hand the concept arises in pure form (meaning free from elements of perception) within thinking consciousness. This shows that the connection between what one perceives and the acquired concept is given to begin with. At the moment we want to begin to understand the world by means of our knowing consciousness, it appears to us first as split into a world of observation and a world of concepts. Connecting percepts with the right concepts brings us to knowledge. What we mean here with the *right concept* is the one that was originally connected with the observed object (compare with what was said above about the universals). We understand the process of knowing when we realize that the *act of knowledge* brings the two worlds mentioned above together again *by our own activity.* By connecting percepts with the right concepts, knowledge arises, creating conscious experience of *reality.*

2.4 Are there boundaries to knowledge?

> Medieval scholasticism held that human thinking has the capacity to acquire concepts and ideas regarding the physical, sense perceptible world, but has not been given the ability to direct thinking in a similar way to the supersensory world. This world could only be disclosed through a firm belief in the revelations given to humanity. The boundary to the supersensory world was considered impenetrable; it could not be crossed by means of thinking.[3]

On August 14, 1872, Du Bois Reymond gave a lecture which was influential in the realm of natural scientific thinking. He talked about *two* boundaries which cannot be crossed by natural science.

> Our thinking is closed in by two absolute boundaries, marked by two unanswered questions, 'What is matter?,' and 'How does consciousness arise out of material processes?' These two boundaries seem unsurmountable for human cognition.

2.4.1 Boundaries to knowledge and Steiner's theory of knowledge

We have seen how Rudolf Steiner, in his theory of knowledge, describes cognition as bringing together percepts and concepts within thinking consciousness. There is nothing besides these two elements of cognition, hence there can be no thought of boundaries to knowledge. It should be stated clearly here that the word 'perception' is not meant to signify sense perception only, but includes psychological experiences and spiritual perceptions.

After writing philosophical and epistemological books earlier in his life,

Rudolf Steiner introduced 'his' anthroposophy. In his lectures and books he presented the results of his spiritual-scientific research in supersensory realms. He also described the path of development, a safe way to school one's latent capacities to perceive supersensory realities independently.

In *The Boundaries of Natural Science,* Steiner describes a specific form of this path of development, which applies especially to students of natural science. In this book he mentions three possible paths, which may lead to supersensory experiences (after years of practice). The *first path* concerns the cultivation of *thinking.* The initial step on this path is strengthening the thinking capacity to such degree, that it is able to think in pure concepts and ideas. After that one has to hold back the tendency to begin speculating with these pure concepts and ideas, which in turn will lead to them metamorphosing into meaningful pictures. So by redirecting thinking consciousness (the one boundary mentioned by Du Bois Reymond) one reaches the ability to perceive the world of living pictures (in anthroposophical terms: the etheric). These pictures are on the level of *imaginative* consciousness.

The *second path* concerns the cultivation of *observation.* The initial step on this path is to learn to observe exactly. After that one has to hold back the tendency to weave ideas in with these exact observations. Instead of this one has to connect different perceptions coming from different senses. The next step on this path involves bringing the totality of these exact memory pictures back to consciousness regularly, and connecting that with symbolic pictures and digesting the whole in an artistic way. This path, which is also the path we got to know in Goethe's work, will finally take us to perceptions on a higher level than the living images of the etheric. In anthroposophical terms this level is called *inspiration.*

The *third path* connects the previous two areas of insight and eventually leads to the level of *intuition.* The first path will remove the boundary of consciousness by refocusing thinking. The second path will make the boundary of physical sense perceptible matter disappear by redirecting the power of perception. With the disappearance of these boundaries the human being is lead to a perception of supersensory worlds, and with it the 'scholastic boundary to knowledge' will also disappear (see *The Philosophy of Thomas Aquinas,* by Rudolf Steiner).

2.5 A monistic, spiritual and realist view of man and world

Before summarizing where anthroposophical medicine stands philosophically, we would like to review the essence of Rudolf Steiner's theory of knowledge by placing it in the light of the aforementioned scientific views. To this end, please consider the following question: *What place*

*and value do the scientific views mentioned above assign to: observation
and concepts/ideas?*

On the basis of the above considerations, we can now come to a summary conclusion and characterize anthroposophy as a monistic, spiritual
and realist worldview. It is *monistic* in that human cognition can reduce
the dichotomy of matter–spirit, object–subject, etc. to the primary duality
of observation and concept. This *duality is conquered in the act of cognition* and the original connection is restored. It is *realist* in that ideas/con-
cepts are seen as real in the way they work and manifest in the world. It is
spiritual, because the ideas working within the world stem from the supersensory.

In conclusion we would like to once more return to something which
was mentioned at the beginning of this chapter. Where one stands philosophically has consequences for the therapeutic relationship between
physician and patient. In conventional medicine, the individual therapist's
thinking, feeling and will is seen as something that does not pertain to the
therapy *per se,* because it is considered too subjective. Placebo-controlled,
double-blind, randomized clinical trials are to guarantee a method of
approach which is not dependent on the individual, and aims to be objective, standardized and reproducible. In contrast to this, the monistic, spiritual and realist worldview enables the human being to develop and come
to something like thinking 'pure concepts.' Objective ideas become subjective within individual human consciousness, but at the same time they
retain their objective character, because they partake of *the* overarching
idea or concept. So the ideal of anthroposophical medicine differs radically from that held in regular medicine in that it depends on the individual. The individual is not merely subjective, however, but works out of
objective therapeutic ideas, which are developed in thinking and individ-
ualized and adapted to each specific situation.

This training manual for anthroposophical medicine is based on the
epistemological foundation summarized in this chapter; from this foundation, human cognitive capacities can be practised and developed. Having
established these nascent capabilities initially, work can start on both theory and practice.

CHAPTER 3

Developing Dynamic Perception

GUUS VAN DER BIE

For the exercises that follow you will need a skull or mandible of a cow (ruminant), a marmot (rodent), a fox (predator), and of a human being. If these are not available, use Figures 3.5–3.7 at the back of this chapter.

In order to experience what developing dynamic perception means, it makes sense to work from concrete objects of study, which allows us to return to perceptual content at any moment. In this instance we will use sets of teeth of different mammals and of humans. In order to become conscious of the difference between dynamic perception and regular perception, we will begin in the way we are all schooled to observe. Try to work as methodically as possible, even though that may feel a bit pedantic. Later, in Section 3.2, it will become clear why we choose to start off this way.

3.1 Types of observation

3.1.1 Analytical approach

We will start in the familiar mode of describing exactly what can be observed, the way we have all been trained to do from childhood. We know this approach from anatomy, physical diagnostics, and also from research methods where images are created such as histology and X-ray diagnostics. We can apply the same approach when we look at the set of teeth.

Assignment 1
Describe the different elements that make up the human set of teeth. Do this before reading on, to allow easy comparison with the description given below.

Description

Characteristics of the *incisors:* they are flat and wide, slightly convex in front and clearly concave at the back. Because of the incisor's width and flatness its edge is sharp. This sharp edge also explains the meaning of the word incisor, which contains the Latin word for 'to cut,' i.e. it acts like a knife. The incisor has no horizontal surface.

Molars are built up quite differently. All sides are primarily convex, both front and back, inside and outside. There is no concave surface in the vertical planes. The horizontal surface shows grooves and bumps.

The *canines* are clearly convex in front, concave at the dorsal side, and have a single point which is relatively sharp. This list of details could of course be continued. Discovering and describing as many observations as possible has its place; it is valuable to gain optimal knowledge of the separate elements.

3.1.2 The comparative approach

In the previous description we looked at each element by itself without considering the set of teeth as a *totality.* We were only interested in the details. We thus created a great diversity of details in our consciousness. We will come to a totally different picture when we start relating our separate observations to one another. To that end we can, for example, compare the various sets of teeth in the illustrations in this chapter.

Assignment 2
Give a comparative description of the sets of teeth of the various animals and the human teeth. The point is here to compare and contrast the teeth of the different species among each other.

In observing the *ruminant's* teeth we are immediately struck by the massive molars, especially the cow's. The characteristic division in three types still applies, but within the totality the molars have clearly hypertrophied in relation to the incisors and the canines. *Rodents*, by contrast, have much more prominent incisors, noticeably in the case of the marmot. Here the canines and the molars recede into the background (no pun intended).

With *predators,* it is especially the canines which are dominant compared to the other teeth. In their case, the incisors and the molars are less developed.

Human teeth show a certain degree of balance among the three sectors. None of them stand out. Their relative size and value is balanced.

The way we approach the object of study makes a significant difference to our awareness. When we are in an analytical frame of mind, we enter into the details and are aware of the particulars and their characteristics; the experience of coherence of the parts is lacking. When we compare, we constantly keep the picture of the totality in mind. Even though the picture may not contain all the details, we keep seeing the set of teeth as a whole. If we now maintain this picture of the whole, and bring in the details, we can experience how the separate elements relate to one another. Instead of separating the details out of the totality, we now see the details in their morphological context. This is in essence a synthesizing activity. The German word *Zusammenschau* ('together-view,' 'to synthesize') describes this process exactly. As a result, we arrive at the *idea* of the set of teeth as point of reference to which we can relate all the different variants. We thus experience it as a kind of primal form behind all the different manifestations in different species.

The comparative approach thus enables us to experience something, in this case a set of teeth, as a unity. We experience not so much the differences but the common basis behind all the different manifestations. This also explains why we can recognize the teeth of any animal; even though we may never have seen the animal before, we can recognize the teeth as such because we can relate them to the idea 'teeth' which we carry within us.

It is important to note that the *idea* of the set of teeth can only be experienced in our *minds*. That places it in the supersensory world, the world of the *reality of ideas*. Anthroposophical medicine sees this world of ideas as being just as real as the sense-perceptible world. This 'idea-realism' is based on the experience of self-evidence that we can achieve in ourselves within our thinking. This 'idea-realism' is thereby closely related to mathematics.

As postulated, the *idea* of the set of teeth is thinkable but not visible, yet every visible set of teeth is *one* specific example that has come to expression. Take mathematics, for example, as a comparison. We speak of the properties of the triangle, and we know that the sum of the angles is 180 degrees. But the *idea* of the triangle can only be thought. Every imaginable triangle, be it right, isosceles, acute, obtuse or equilateral, can become visible, but it is also only *one* expression of the idea of the triangle.

Assignment 3
Try to describe the experience that arises in you when you look at the sets of teeth anew. Does the comparative approach add something to your experience? If so, can you put it into words?

When one practices this approach often, one will notice a subtle change taking place in one's awareness. The perception will arise that the idea of a set of teeth is not static, but malleable. It is a pliable, generative idea. Fixed shapes only come into being when one specimen is shaped. This explains why the generative idea is called a *Fliess-Gestalt* in German. This compound contains the idea of flux in the word *Fliess,* from *fliessen,* to flow, to which the word *Gestalt* is added. (The word Gestalt has been taken into English, because there is no single word to convey the idea of both plasticity and hardening into a form). The supersensory world contains many *Fliess-Gestalts,* or *infinitely flexible shaping* forms which crystallize into an infinite variety of sense perceptible shapes. In Chapter 6 we will see that we can get even closer to the subtlety of this mobile form, and go into much more detail than can be done at this stage.

3.1.3 The dynamic approach

Having both looked at the details, and acquired an initial perception of the generative principle (*Fliess-Gestalt,* or infinitely flexible shaping form) that stands behind the different sets of teeth, we will now turn to *dynamics.* Dynamics have to do with a quality of motion. Dynamics can be accelerating, retarding, expanding, or contracting. There are countless examples which indicate how we grasp many phenomena in their dynamics. In the example above we used the term hypertrophy to describe how certain sections within the sets of teeth stand out. The word hypertrophy means 'to grow abnormally large,' implying an experience of growth dynamics. If we 'live into' the way the molars of a cow came into being, we sense how within the whole set of teeth an enhancement of the growth dynamics has taken place in the area of the molars. In the case of the rodents, it has shifted to the incisors; in the case of the predators to the canines. In a similar way, we can experience the opposite process as 'atrophying,' referring to those teeth which recede. In studies of this kind, we learn to inwardly move along, and follow precisely how one particular set of teeth comes into being. A mobile, flexible image arises in our awareness, which we can allow to transition at will from one shape into another. Of course this flexibility stays within the bounds which we have learned to recognize in the comparative approach. Through practice, an inwardly mobile image arises of the different dynamics which are possible within the bounds of the general idea of a set of teeth.

Distinguish carefully between differences in *shape* and differences in *dynamics* in studying and comparing the sets of teeth in the way described. The first is *morphological,* the second *dynamic.* The first has to do with comparing forms, the second with comparing 'movements.'

Again and again, we can discern the following threefold division:

— the *detail,* observed separately
— the *total picture,* in which the variants within the primal form (the *Fliess-Gestalt* or the flexible shaping form) must move
— the *dynamics* which are behind the eventual shape and interrelationships within the total picture

3.1.4 Further development of the dynamic approach

The more we learn to develop an eye for dynamics, the more we will notice that we no longer have a static, crystallized picture in our consciousness. Our experience of the capacity for morphological change within the blueprint of the studied object becomes more tangible. Our attention is almost automatically drawn more to the *way* the object comes into being than to the final form. As soon as we have an experience of motion, we are dealing with the generative aspects, with change and development. Experiencing development as such is based in an experience of motion. How else would we be able to form a mental picture, if it were not for the fact that we must follow along and connect the separate impressions? Whether we are dealing with the growth of a child, the full unfolding of a plant, or the genesis of an organ, we are always following a dynamic process.

This experience is fundamentally of an artistic nature. The artist must also follow along inwardly, to express dynamics and emotion for example, which in turn stirs the viewer. As soon as copying nature is no longer the sole object, a work of art always refers to a different level, one that is dynamic. We experience that level as 'higher' than the level of naturalistic copying. By *living into* the work of art we can enter, as it were, into the world from which it came. We go through the static picture and penetrate into the formative dynamics which stand behind it. One could formulate a basic law of morphology as follows: *all form arises out of motion.* Inversely, we could also say that all motion results in a form. And when we apply the right method of study we can read the movement out of the fixed form.

One of the most striking examples of this is to be found in biological processes. Even when we study living organisms under the microscope we always see moving, streaming substance to begin with. These streams slow down, substance settles and finally everything hardens into a form. Geological processes are no exception. Volcanic processes with their striking dynamics are not the only ones which show us the process of motion ending in form. All processes of solidifying sedimentation, crystallization and the formation of folds in the crust of the earth begin with motion.

When we study teeth we can also seek to reach this dynamic, 'higher' level, the level of motion creating form. In doing so, the thing is not to stray into wild fantasies, but to be guided by other observable phenomena in the animals whose teeth we are studying. This has been elaborated in an exemplary way by Wolfgang Schad in his book *Man and Mammal.*

3.1.5 The part as picture of the whole

Our examples dealt with the dynamics in the sets of teeth of a ruminant, a rodent and a predator, which we then compared with the human being. The dynamics of the teeth express something essential of each of these animals. This essence can also be found in another area.

In addition to having highly developed molars, the *ruminant* has a strikingly well-developed metabolic system which is able to digest nutrients rich in cellulose, such as grass. The molars play an essential role in the first and second phases of breaking the grass down, and the large intestine is most important in the digestive process because of its intestinal flora. Rumination, a relatively slow and clumsy motoric system, and a vegetarian diet are other typical traits to round out the picture. In the reproduction, one or two young are born each time, which are nearly always ready to move about from birth, having a well myelinized nervous system. Carrying time is long and the number of birth cycles per year is limited.

The *rodents* show a completely different picture. Their metabolic system depends on rich fatty nutrients such as nuts, seeds, or man-made products such as cheese. Their incisors are eminently suitable to gnaw through nutshells. Cellulose-rich food cannot be digested, and the intestinal tract fits this picture because the large intestine is not highly developed. Their motoric system is lightning quick and refined, noticeably so in the squirrel. Their litters are large, the young are highly dependent, myelinization is still incomplete. The reproductive cycle is short.

The *predators,* with their characteristically long canines, take up a middle position. They are often carnivores, and their metabolic system is adapted to that. They hunt for prey. The canines play an important part in catching and tearing up the animals they catch. Predators produce more young than ruminants but their litters are not as large as those of rodents; carrying time is not very long. The young need to stay in the nest for a short period of time. Their movement is gracious and supple; they do not have the stiff slowness of cattle, nor do they have the nervous twitchiness of the rodents. Their motor system in both speed and strength is ideally suited to hunting.

An animal's characteristic reactions are determined by *instinct.* It seems as if an animal body takes on the form which it needs to live out the instinct. Once again we need to look at the total picture in order to see how the most diverse details all have their place. The instinct determines what the animal actually experiences out of the totality of its surroundings, what it reacts to and how the chain of reactions takes its course. When we observe an animal, we will always note that only a limited part of the surrounding impressions seems to get through; the animal reacts exclusively to things it relates to. Only a portion of the sum total of stimuli is experienced, and one could compare this portion to a segment of a circle. *That segment is determined by the instinct and its corresponding organism.*

We can deduce from this that a correspondence can be found between the total picture of an organism, such as that of the cow, the fox, or the marmot, and the parts (including the behaviour) of the particular animal. Hence a characteristic detail allows us to imagine the whole organism. One could say that the whole expresses itself in the detail, and that the detail mirrors the whole. When we practice this discipline, certain things become *self-evident.* When we learn to pay attention to experiences of this kind, one finds that daily life supplies countless examples. A capacity to recognize characteristic signs which call forth this experience stands us in good stead in our medical practice, where reading somatic as well as psychological signs is needed every single day. Much of our diagnosis and treatment rests on our ability to recognize characteristic signs. It was not so long ago that the quality of a physician depended to a large extent on his 'diagnostic eye.' Developing such an ability, which helps us to recognize characteristic traits of a particular illness, bears fruit in practical life. We mention it here mainly to supply yet another instance of the immediate experience of self-evidence we pointed to.

Such a way of working obviously requires a radical shift in attitude. For that reason we need to examine our fundamental orientation closely and be aware of the conscious or unconscious choices we make, which we will do in Section 3.2.1.

In conclusion we may postulate that comparing many details allows us to discover essential differences between the various organisms. By adopting a comparative analysis we create a coherent picture within the context of diverse organisms. An important result of this approach is that we create in our minds coherent pictures of the specific traits of a species, both in a somatic and in a behavioural sense. All details begin to make sense within the context of the picture we build up. We can develop this approach to such a degree that we can actually make responsible pronouncements regarding the total organism on the basis of a detail. This is

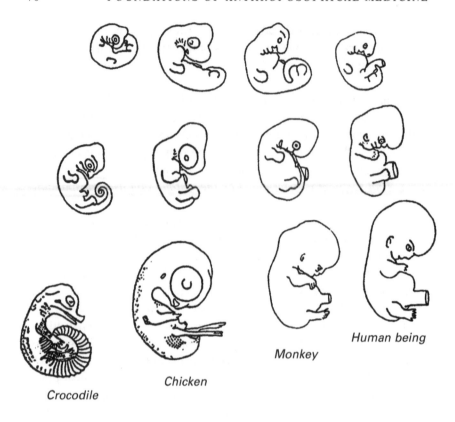

Figure 3.1. The craniocaudal curvature in various animals and the human being.

in fact the way paleontologists accurately reconstruct organisms, extrapolating from tiny remains. Finding even minimal vestiges allows them to form a reasonably reliable picture of how a certain animal was built, and how it functioned biologically and socially.

3.1.6 The human being

The human being occupies a special position. We could read from the dynamics of the set of teeth that there is no specific one-sidedness. As far as the instinctual side is concerned, we are extremely deficient. We have to learn everything, which necessitates extensive and protracted schooling. In the animal kingdom there is nothing which compares with this. This long period of growing up to learn how to cope with life is an exclusive feature of the human being. Learning basic biological and social survival strategies extends far into puberty. If premature demands are made on us to function independently, we run the risk of malfunctioning, either biologically, psychologically, or socially. In this early period the human being is therefore most vulnerable to trauma, and this can lead to permanent damage.

Assignment 4

Try for one week to remember one characteristic trait of a patient each day. Consider whether this particular trait reveals something of the whole person, with respect to either character or pathology. Writing down your observations can be a help.

3.1.7 The psychological-moral approach

We now come to the fourth level. The title might be easily misunderstood. The term psychological-moral is not meant here in a 'spiritual' sense. Psychological is meant to signify strictly what can be *experienced*. With the word moral we point to a higher level, that of human values which are common to all. Moralizing is not the intention here.

For this fourth approach, we refer to the drawings depicting embryonic development (Figure 3.2). Please note that details are not shown to scale. This has been done intentionally to highlight aspects of the motion of the development, and in order to facilitate comparing the various stages of formation. In addition, Figures 4.16 – 4.18 can be consulted.

Series A shows a lateral view of the development from day 25 to day 34 in the human embryo. The embryo goes through a development by which the spinal curvature grows. This is sometimes referred to as the craniocaudal curvature, because top and bottom seem to move towards one another. We can best enter into the dynamics of this curvature by imitating the same motion with our own bodies, by curling up as it were.

This craniocaudal curvature is a universal feature of all animal development (see Figure 3.1). Without it no animal organism comes into being. Goethe called a phenomenon of universal significance such as this one an *Urphänomen* (primal or archetypal phenomenon).

This bean-like stage of development must be one of those archetypal phenomena. This curved form always recurs in the fully grown adult, and no animal can transcend the bean stage. The primates manage for quite some time. But even though newborn primates seem to be able to transcend this curvature and become upright, the bodies of all adult primates fall back into a curved position (see Figure 3.4).

In mammals, the bean-shaped curvature shows us their predisposition to become a quadruped. We can describe quadrupeds as beings who

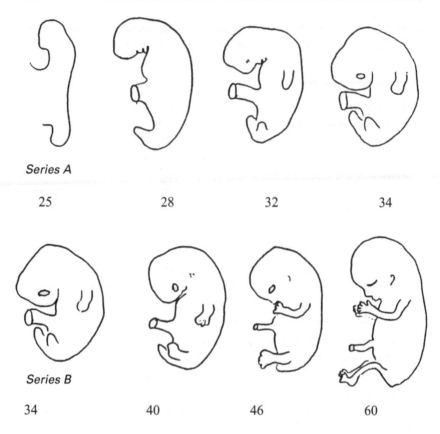

Figure 3.2. Human morphological development from day 25 to day 60.

perpetuate that bean shaped curvature. Animal development consists in ever greater specialization, within the limits of this curved shape. There are many examples of the high-level specialization that can be achieved in this respect. The final product of such a development is always an animal organism that is highly adapted to specific environments. This necessity, however, always goes together with limitation because the freedom to perform other actions has been lost. Specialization and ingenuity go hand-in-hand with a loss of all ability to metamorphose.

Series B in Figure 3.2 shows the morphological development of day 34 to day 60. This is the period in which the human embryo 'emerges' out of the curved form, straightens out and becomes upright, leaving the curved body form behind. The human being is the only creature in nature to maintain that upright position into adulthood. The occipital joint, shoulder joint, hip joint, knee joint and tarsal joint lie in one line (Figure 3.3). No animal has this, not even the penguin or the whale.

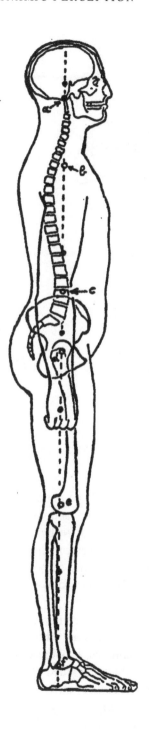

Figure 3.3. Position of the joints of the human being in the vertical.

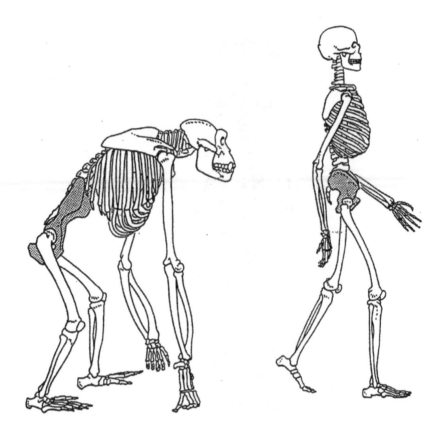

Figure 3.4. Only the human being achieves an upright position.

The continuing development of the human body results in a striking *ineptness* in performing specialized actions. The human body is *not* equipped to perform any *one* specific technical function, which is not to say that human beings cannot perform highly specialized tasks. The achievements of virtuoso musicians, acrobats, conjurors and athletes make that abundantly clear. But their skills are only acquired by arduous practice: they are never just a given.

Next to the ability to acquire these unique technical skills, the human being has another distinguishing feature: choice. We have a higher degree of self-determination than animals. It is these two aspects of the human condition which are generally disregarded by evolutionary theorists. On the one hand our actions are only partly guided by instinct, and our organisms are not geared to carry out any one set of specialized actions; on the other hand we have the ability to adapt, so that we can learn an astonishing amount.

In Section 3.2.2, we see how forms arise out of inner movements; by living into those movements and imitating the process of unfurling and becoming upright, we can experience a feeling of liberation. What kind of liberation is this? When we no longer feel the compulsion of the curve, we sense freedom and sovereignty in coming to the upright position. This feeling of sovereignty comes to expression in our language. We speak of 'getting back on our feet' after an illness or defeat has 'gotten us down.' When we 'bear up,' we're 'not brought to our knees' by the blows of fate. Maintaining our moral standards allows us to 'keep our head up.' Sayings such as these give us an immediate sense of the ego strength involved. These expressions are not about instinctual actions or servile attitudes; they're about morality and freedom. If, on the other hand, our ego strength is taxed too much, we regress to the curved gesture. We 'cringe,' when we are either appalled or in actual physical pain. Suffering can 'break' us, shame can cause us to 'hang our heads,' and for comfort we would like to 'curl up.' Language is full of images which call to mind the gesture of the craniocaudal curvature, and the expressions often go right into the physical.

The dynamic approach allows us to inwardly mimic the process of becoming an animal or human being. To experience this we need to follow series A and B respectively, living into its sequences with empathy. In this way we can experience how the animal is unfree, and how the human being has the capacity to become free and partake in a moral order. The difference between being bound and being free is a moral line.

Another striking phenomenon is that studying animal organisms directly involves our feelings. When we study the jaw of the shark with its double row of teeth turned inward, we gain a direct experience of the force of greed, and in the eagle's talon we read the drive to clutch. In such experiences we not only see instinct at work, but we also sense psychological qualities that manifest in the animal. One thing has to be kept in mind very clearly here: even though we can recognize greed and clutching, we can never judge these things in terms of good or bad. Animals really are in a separate category in this respect. Values of good and evil do not apply to the animal kingdom in the same way they apply to the human being. The curved animal remains bound to the compulsive force of a one-sided instinct, and that can be experienced in the shape of the organism. This experience is a psychological one.

It is only in the human being that we can see a morphological expression of a lack of instinctual urges and the *capacity to become free*. That is a *moral experience*. With the term moral we indicate that something purely spiritual lights up in the experience of freedom. The soul life of the human being is concerned with moral dilemmas; we have to deal with questions of good and evil. The reason for this is that the ego works into the soul, and ego experience is in essence a spiritual experience. Being self-directed and shaping our own lives is a spiritual activity, and that inevitably involves moral and social questions. There certainly is social behaviour in the animal world, but no animal has to deal with social questions, let alone moral dilemmas!

A Remark Regarding Method

As a corollary of the morphological and dynamic approach, inner experiences will arise in the researcher. Studying these experiences more closely, it turns out that they concur with what has psychological or moral meaning for us.

We can summarize the outcome of studies such as the ones outlined above in the following two aphorisms:

The morphology of the embryology of mammals shows us the embryology of specialization of necessity.

The morphology of human embryology shows us the embryology of freedom.

This last step in our approach brings us to another observation, namely that we can learn to read moral aspects in both morphology and movement. At this point this is the highest level which we can point to, and we do so in the full awareness that this whole methodology to comprehend the world around us is still in its infancy. Even though we have a long way to go in actually grasping this moral dimension, the initial experience is nevertheless a real one. It speaks to us directly, with self-evident force. If nothing else, this form of evidence gives us an inkling that the moral dimension is tangible and open to research.

3.2 Different attitudes

The previous sections describe an approach which leads to a fundamentally different view of the way things fit together, and with that a fundamentally different experience of the coherence between phenomena. It is important to realize that the researcher has different approaches to choose from. After all, we are the ones who determine which approach gives us the most satisfactory answers to our questions. The analytical approach proves inadequate when we deal with questions of life and inner experiences. We can opt for a method that gives more satisfactory answers for the strata of experience we are talking about here, where dissecting and analysing brings us no further. That was the subject of the previous considerations. This implies that we have to take a close look at our fundamental stance, and be fully conscious of it. Moreover, we must be able to justify where we stand.

3.2.1 The onlooker stance

The basic stance of the analytical, dissecting approach has been characterized as the attitude of the one-eyed colour-blind onlooker. If we ponder this, we realize that looking with one eye allows no depth perception or perspective, and that colour-blindness (in extreme cases) makes the world seem completely grey. Being an onlooker implies keeping a distance, and remaining emotionally detached. But depth perception, perspective and colour nuances are the very things that give us a richer and more differentiated picture of reality. And when we studied sets of teeth, our whole effort was directed toward connecting with the perceived object in such a way that we could live into it and move along inwardly. We observed that our experience remains shallow and two-dimensional if we restrict ourselves to separate details; the purely analytical approach bars us from true insight. The typical onlooker wants no feeling relationship and remains detached. This attitude opens up the possibility to gather a multitude of details, but allows no inner connection with the phenomena.

The paradox in this is that we have to go against the grain, because our natural reactions are based on a feeling relationship. When, for example, somebody shakes his fist at us, our gut reaction is to see this as a threat. For the onlooker-consciousness it means nothing but contracted flexors of the forearm and hand. The onlooker can make no sense of this, because this sense would be based on emotional involvement, which is 'subjective' and therefore is excluded because it can never lead to 'objective' insight. But how would we ever come to terms with everyday life if we had to make do with only an onlooker consciousness? We owe our most fruitful insights to the very feelings that allow us to relate to things! It would be extremely hazardous not to be able to read our cues from somebody's body language or attitude. In actual fact, conventional science asks us to disregard our natural capacity to live into so many things that we would not understand otherwise. Does that not ultimately demand we destroy that capacity? And all this is done for the sake of 'scientific objectivity,' namely, the analytical, dissecting approach.

3.2.2 The participator stance

Rather than destroying our natural capacity for empathetic understanding, we can choose to school our capacities in this direction, to develop and refine them in order to understand living reality. This entails conscious schooling so that *living into* phenomena becomes a basic attitude, whereby our feelings are harnessed and directed. Such a schooling broadens our whole insight. The examples given above were an attempt to demonstrate that the aim is not to supplant the systematic study of details, but to expand this approach and take it further. The accomplishments of the analytical faculties and the onlooker consciousness will actually achieve their full significance in the picture formation that the comparative approach and the participator consciousness adds. In going through the stages of forming a picture, experiencing the dynamics, and sensing the psychological moral dimension, we are given the opportunity to partake inwardly and more fully in the processes we research, in such a way that our feelings are involved. As researchers, and that really includes all of us, we make an attempt to bridge the gap between inside and outside. We try to give up the position of remaining outside the phenomena. It should be stressed that acquiring a participator consciousness requires a high degree of inner effort in order to truly enter into the processes. It is a form of immersion.

What happens when we form a feeling connection in the way described? Our own experience allows us to recognize the meaning of what we see or hear. Let us revisit for a moment the example of the clenched fist. We recognize what it means, because we've felt the same emotion that results in that outer gesture. Our understanding is based on correspondence with our own inner world of experience, which also comprises our psychological and moral findings. We recognize the outer form, because it is the outcome of an inner experience which we have had ourselves. At the same time this makes us realize that every *outer manifestation* is the result of an *inner process*. Such a realization has the force of self-evidence, and could therefore be termed axiomatic. In mathematics, the word axiom refers to something that needs no proof. The transition from an inner process of experience to an outer form is equally self-evident. We thus come to recognize the maxim: *form follows movement.*

We saw that the comparative approach allows the details to take their place within a comprehensive picture. A pictorial consciousness is more comprehensive than the analytical consciousness that stops at the details. The same goes for the participant attitude, which is also more comprehensive than the onlooker attitude and consciously includes, not

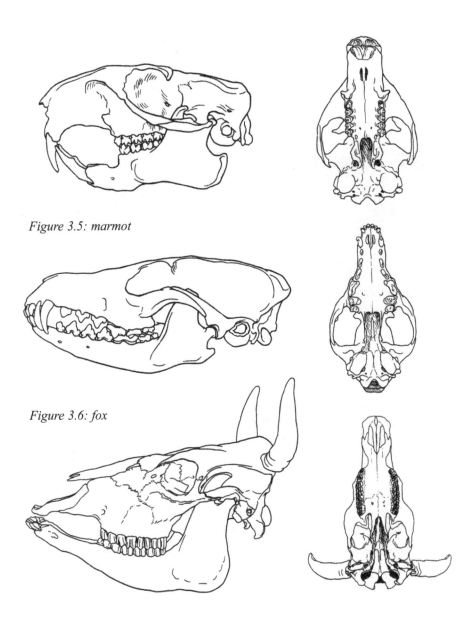

Figure 3.5: marmot

Figure 3.6: fox

Figure 3.7: cow

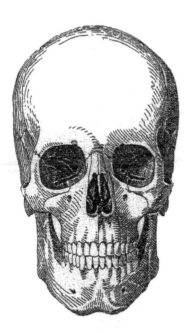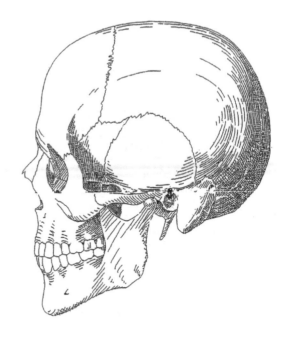

Figure 3.9: human being

excludes, the subject. Again, it is not a matter of one thing replacing something else, but of something more inclusive absorbing something less inclusive. This also shows that the words 'alternative medicine' are a misnomer, as far as this approach is concerned. We could summarize this as follows:

> The pictorial consciousness comprises the detail;
> the participator stance comprises the onlooker consciousness.

Assignment 5
Look for characteristic traits in your patients which are typical for their pathologies. These may include both verbal and nonverbal phenomena. There are distinct traits which go together with the pathology of hysteria, nervous exhaustion, and hypomania. The same goes for asthma, spastic colon, low back pain, and even allergies or stomach ulcers. In this connection, 'typical' is an interesting idiom to use when we study the relation of the whole to the parts!

CHAPTER 4

Dynamic Morphology and Embryology

JAAP VAN DER WAL

The aims of this chapter are:

— to give additional examples of dynamic morphology in order to famil-
iarize the reader further with this way of working, building upon the
phenomenological approach as described in Chapter 3 (3.1.3), where
it was termed *dynamic perception;*
— to give the reader an experience of the kinds of insights which can be
gained when one looks for *polarity* in human and natural phenomena,
taking the *participant stance;*
— to demonstrate that this scientific approach, in contrast to the regular
natural scientific approach, leads to the conclusion that nonmaterial
principles are at work in the physical world. It enables one to come to
these conclusions on the basis of observations of material phenomena,
perceived through the ordinary senses.

Since this training manual primarily directs itself to medical practitioners,
the examples chosen are mainly taken from human biology. Later chapters
(especially Chapter 6) will also apply this method to other areas of biology. The methodology and fundamental stance demonstrated in this chapter can be given a broader practical application in physiology, psychology
and pathology.

Steps and method
We will start with a brief introduction concerning the methodology of the
dynamic approach and the way the idea of polarities is used in this context (Section 4.1).

In Section 4.2 the previously described approach will be applied to human conception. Brief interludes will refer back to points made in Chapter 3 regarding scientific principles. By means of these examples the essence of the concept of polarities will be elaborated.

Section 4.3 of this chapter will deal with the human skeleton and posture, following the same dynamic approach. We will also elaborate on a central concept in the anthroposophical view of the human being, *the middle*.

Using examples of the dynamic morphology of the human embryo, fundamental principles of anthroposophy will be demonstrated once more in Section 4.4.

4.1 A minifying glass as a tool for observation

We must use the darkness
To make the light visible.
            J.W. Goethe[1]

Goethe always stressed in his scientific work how one must 'look at things in context.' This applies especially to *polarities*. After all, they can only be recognized when one looks at the whole within which the polarities appear (see quotation above).

In Section 3.1.1, where different sets of teeth were discussed, it was shown that much can be learned from observing each detail separately. There it was termed the *analytical approach*. The *comparative approach* then takes the isolated elements and places them in connection with one another, thus creating an overview. Seeing a 'higher' coherence opens up possibilities to see more of the essence of the separate parts, and discover things which remain hidden when one only focuses on isolated parts. In other words, one develops an eye for the *total picture,* which encompasses all the possible variants. Three steps were described in Chapter 3, the third of which was seeing dynamics which led to the final form-composition of the total picture. This *dynamic approach* adds a significant dimension: one begins to experience *sculptural gesture* in what one observes. By penetrating to the level of gesture, which gave rise to the outer form, one enters *via* the phenomena into the nonmaterial realm which lies *behind* the phenomena.

To elucidate the method applied here, let us now turn to the following example. Let us ask ourselves the following question, 'Why do we see the head as round?' We all experience the head that way, yet on closer scrutiny, it cannot stand up to scientific analysis. Modern natural scientific morphology cannot see the head as round anymore. In medical school, students become familiar with scores of protrusions, crests, ridges, and angular edges. No 'roundness' is to be recognized in such an approach. On the contrary, the more one focuses on the human skull, going into ever more detailed observation, the more one loses the naive perception of the head as round. The question posed above, 'Why do we see the head as round?' was meant to bring us to the following dilemma: Which of the two perceptions is more real, the naive assumption of roundness or the anatomical observations?

Many people will solve the 'dilemma' outlined above by explaining the naive perception as correct in a general sense. One can call this perception 'more or less correct,' and point to children's drawings to indicate that they always, and strikingly, represent the head as round. With such an argument, one can depict the perception of the head as round as literally *naive*. But Goethe would have opposed any suggestion to therefore apply a simplistic 'global' approach. His own observations were painstakingly exact, and his descriptions never shy away from details. On the contrary, in his scientific works he goes into minute phenomenological descriptions to document and underpin a gesture, which he saw expressed in certain organic forms, be it of individual organs or whole organisms.

In the spirit of a Goetheanistic approach, an answer to the 'dilemma' posed above, could run more or less as follows: By fixing one's gaze solely on the head or skull, one will fail to see the roundness. The context of the skull and the head belong to the human skeleton and the human body respectively. Our starting point in this approach is the entities as they occur in nature. Head and skull are analytical entities, produced by reductionist thinking and isolating them out of the whole of the skeleton or body concerned. If we start from the human skeleton or body as a whole and let our gaze wander from head to arms, back again to the head and then to the legs, back and forth, in short, if we regard the head in its polarity to the extremities, we will learn from the extremities how round the head or the skull really is.

It will be obvious that dynamic perception, as described in Chapter 3, applies here as well. The 'mobility' of perception should perhaps be taken even more literally here than in Section 3.1.3 (the dynamic approach). To be looking within a certain context, comparing and going back and forth, is meant here in contrast to the kind of gaze that fixes. However much one studies the bones of the extremities, one will never get at the character of 'straightness' as long as one keeps seeing them in isolation. Yet straightness is an essential characteristic of the extremities when one compares them with the head or skull. One will see ever more knobs, ridges, and convexities if one looks with an analytical eye at the bones of the extremities, but only a comparative approach such as the one described in Chapter 3 will reveal the character of straightness of an arm or a leg. The two approaches form a contrast. In the one case one approaches the object using a magnifying glass, which will reveal more and more detail. In the other case one takes a step back and looks at the detail in the context of the whole to which it belongs. This kind of survey allows one to view the whole, thereby practising the advice which the Dutch pathologist Louis Bolk once gave, which was to 'look at life through a *minifying* glass.' To see the head as round is not the product of looking in a general or naive way; it is the result of clear, exact, but at the same time dynamic and mobile observation.

In such an approach details are not distracting or redundant. On the contrary, they are an essential prerequisite. Once the polarity straight–round has been discerned in extremities–head, one can then go on to see, in a Goetheanistic phenomenological way, whether other phenomena fit and support the polarity observed. The gesture which has initially been discovered (inductively, if you will) can then be underpinned (deductively) by observing details. Thus an important consequence of the choice of looking dynamically, and taking the participant stance, emerges. It becomes clear that *the analytical approach which results in isolated perceptions can be included within the comparative/dynamic approach, but not the other way around. An analytical approach with its resultant perceptions principally excludes perceptions gained in a dynamic approach.*

Obviously the concept of polarities will become an important key to a dynamic morphology, understood as a morphology of gesture. After all, when one is able to discern polarities, one has already 'risen' to a different level of perception. If one stays within the narrow framework of reductionist thinking, only looking at things in isolation, polarity cannot reveal itself. For it to be recognized, one must leave the level of fixing one's gaze on a detail, and make room for mobility and comparison. It should also be emphasized that the term *morphology* was chosen here for a reason. The term anatomy is reserved here to denote the analytical approach. Thus one could say that the head is round in a morphological sense, not in an anatomical sense.

> *We have gotten used to tracing life through magnifying lenses in order to perceive matter which would otherwise remain invisible to us. How different, how much broader would our concept of life become if it were given to us to look at life through* minifying *lenses.*

> *Then we could survey all that would otherwise remain hidden for the*
> *naked eye, and rather than seeing material connections, as we do*
> *now, the interconnectedness of phenomena would become the object*
> *of our studies.*
>
> Louis Bolk[2]

4.2 From two to one — polarities in conception

We have chosen conception as the first area in which to practice observing polarities. A close study of the phenomena of the egg cell and the sperm cell will give us a chance to practice comparative and dynamic observation; a participant stance (see Section 3.2.2) will bring formative gestures to light. This example will also show us more about the nature of polarities in a Goetheanistic sense. Rather than opposites, we will see how the one is similar to the other, but 'turned inside out'; such an observation refers us to the level of a shared essence living behind the polarities under consideration. This will be elaborated in Section 4.3.

4.2.1 Polarity and contrast

Emphasizing the differences between egg cell and sperm cell is no longer customary, undesirable even, in current scientific thinking. It has become common practice to reduce living nature to the same building units (think for example of cells, DNA, molecules). Rupert Sheldrake calls this practice, somewhat derogatorily, *'nothing butterism.'*[3] This derives from descriptions like, 'traits are based on *'nothing but'* a nucleotide sequence on a DNA molecules.' Current descriptions of fertilization will speak of two reproductive cells which must merge in order to pass on their hereditary material to the resulting conceptus. The two cells derive their significance primarily from being carriers of DNA. This, then is what it's all about. The morphology of the two cells thus seems to be of little significance. This appears to be confirmed by the many modern techniques to manipulate them, accomplishing the seeming 'goal' of conception: bringing together two entities of DNA.

Now let us approach the same matter in the way Goethe and Bolk would have done, taking the phenomena for what they are and looking at the human sperm cell and egg cell in the context in which they appear. On the one hand that is the context of anatomy and physiology of the two sex cells themselves and the corresponding sexual organs. On the other hand it is the context of the *pre-conception attraction complex*. This refers to the biological complex which is formed, under normal circumstances, by both gametes together; it lasts a certain period of time before the actual penetration by a sperm cell can take place.*

Assignment 1

Using the chart on the next page, try to find as many contrasts as possible between the sperm cell and the egg cell. See also the Figure of the two gametes (sex cells) below, if needed. Look not only for contrasts on the level of individual cells with their morphology and physiology, but try to look beyond that. Think for example of the different roles the two gametes play in the process of fertilization and also of the physiology and morphology of the two corresponding sexual organs (gonads).

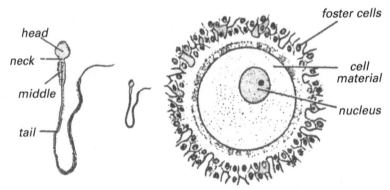

B: Sperm cell drawn on the same scale as the egg cell.

A: Spermatozoon   C: Ripe egg cell with corona radiata

Figure 4.1.

---

*   The question about the actual moment of conception is left open here. After considering the thoughts presented in the rest of this chapter, the prevailing assumption that conception takes place at the moment that the male and female pronuclei fuse might appear in quite a different light. It might need to be reconsidered altogether.

POLARITIES BETWEEN EGG CELL AND SPERM CELL

PARAMETER	EGG CELL	SPERM CELL
Size of the gamete		
Shape of the gamete		
Motility		
Metabolic relationship to the surroundings		
Condition of the nucleus, especially the DNA		
Relationship of nucleus to cytoplasm		
Number of gametes		
Vitality and biological vulnerability		
Age; lifespan		
Character (sequence) of the reduction division		
Relationship to (body) temperature		
Relationship to gonads & genitalia		

It is only through a comparative approach that one can come to the conclusion that an egg cell is big and the sperm cell is small. A quantitative description on a sliding scale of numbers and measures (head of the spermatozoon: 2–3 μm; egg cell diameter: about 200 μm) cannot express the qualitative difference between big and small. A dynamic approach to egg cell and sperm cell adds an extra dimension here. If one takes into consideration how big and how small both cells actually are and especially how they come to be big or small, an enormous polarity is revealed right away. Measured in terms of human biology, the egg cell is gigantic. With a diameter of 0.2 mm and a cytoplasm-volume of 0.004 mg in weight, it is without a doubt the most voluminous ball of cytoplasm a human being can produce. Certainly, neurons can reach formidable lengths (up to many thousands of times the average cell size, which is about 10 μm), but in terms of volume the egg cell wins out. This comes to expression in the dynamics of the way it matures. The egg cell matures in a process of both increase and maintenance of volume. The relatively large volume of cytoplasm which characterizes the original sex cell in the embryonic phase is at least maintained. During the first reduction division which the egg cell completes at the moment of ovulation, this impression of 'striving to maintain the cytoplasm volume' is confirmed by the phenomenon that the primary oocyte separates into two sister cells, which are totally disproportionate in terms of volume. One of the 'cells' — the polar body — contains the requisite DNA substrate, the other one (the secondary oocyte) keeps the cytoplasm.

Methodological remark
The observations and facts presented so far are fairly straightforward and are still only relative, because they are not the result of looking at the egg cell and its size in isolation, but of comparing egg cell and sperm cell. Through a process of looking back and forth between them, indications like 'big,' 'volume retention,' and 'expand' acquire their profile.

As a polar opposite the sperm cell shows its 'smallness.' Let us begin with the quantitative part, which is relative. The diameter of the head of the spermatozoon is about to 2 or 3 μm, and the length from head to tail is about 60 μm. Two μm is quite a small size for a cell, but 'smallness' becomes more significant, when one considers that the decrease in size of the eukaryote cell simply has a limit due to the amount of genetic material (DNA) that has to be carried and therefore be retained for it to still be a human cell. Seen in this light, the germ cell's performance is a remarkable achievement. During the last phase of the spermatozoon genesis, so much cytoplasm is discharged and secreted that at the end of the germ cell maturation very little cytoplasm, and a relatively high amount of nucleus material, remains. Moreover, the latter becomes highly concentrated. The DNA is considerably dehydrated, so that an almost pure, highly structured form of DNA remains. The germ cell shows the characteristics of a cell entering into a so-called 'programmed cell death,' *(apoptosis)*. As a consequence, the DNA becomes highly concentrated and the cell becomes pycnotic. On a submicroscopic level the DNA in the germ cell head makes an almost crystalline impression. This process of condensing or shrinking gives the germ cell as a whole the possibility to become so small.

Methodological remark

The analytical approach gives us the measurements (2 μm, 60 μm, 200 μm) and the intracellular relationships (ratio of nucleus to cytoplasm). The comparative approach shows the strong contrasts playing in here, also in the underlying processes which are part of the picture, such as the expelling of the polar body and the separating out of the cytoplasm. The dynamic approach with a corresponding participant stance allows us to experience the process of becoming large or small. Thus we live into the formative process (see Section 3.2.2), and become aware of the gesture and the movement. By taking these three steps, we become less tied to the bare material facts, which is necessary! This allows us to conclude that the egg cell is characterized by the gesture of expansion and the sperm cell by the dynamics of shrinking or concentrating. When we arrive at such a conclusion, the physical size of the tail of the sperm cell of 60 μm, (still quite big), becomes irrelevant.

Considerations concerning simple things like 'large' and 'small,' as in the methodological remark made above, bring yet another essential fact about polarities to light. Before we can elaborate, let us first return to the object we were observing. When the egg cell has left the ovary and has completed its first reduction division or meiosis, it is metabolically active. One could say that it communicates with its surroundings. This entails physiological vulnerability. An egg cell is a precarious organism which should not be manipulated by physiological force. Consider how sensitive it is to chemical, osmotic, or temperature shock. If we take the corona radiata into account as well — which we can do since we're concerned with the egg cell organism — we are dealing with a biological entity which is able to excrete substances capable of influencing the immediate surroundings, even though the amounts may be tiny. Think of EPF, Early Pregnancy Factor, for example.

By contrast, the sperm cell seems oblivious to its surroundings. That is not to say that the sperm cell does not react to its surroundings — think for example of the way the sperm cell automatically 'swims against the stream,' or how it reacts to chemotactic substances — but it does not metabolically communicate with the surroundings the way the egg cell does. Freezing spermatozoids (to temperatures as low as –60°C) does not seem to affect the life of these cells. Thawed months later, they merrily continue. This quality of remaining relatively untouched by influences from the outside fits with the cellular structure of the sperm cell. Whereas one can see the egg cell as a gigantic cytoplasm reservoir, the sperm cell is reduced to a highly structured nucleus package (DNA package) with a relative lack of vitality.

Which morphologic concepts would apply in this situation? To sum up the dynamics of the polarity described above, one could characterize the sperm cell as *closed,* and the egg cell as *open* to its surroundings. Now if one really lives into the dynamics of this situation, one can bring them in line with the previously mentioned dynamics of large and small. After all, expanding and striving outwards goes together with being open, whereas concentrating and centring goes together with being closed.

Methodological remark

At this point we invite the reader to try to find even wider and more encompassing terms to characterize the gesture we have discovered. To point the way, we offer the concepts *centrifugal* (towards the periphery), and *centripetal* (towards the centre). One could also attempt to approach the phenomena by asking the following question, Which of the two gametes shows the dynamics of 'being fertile,' which of 'fertilizing'? This may seem trivial from the perspective of basic biological knowledge of today. But the point here is to try to imagine the underlying gesture. Later on in this chapter we will return to this inevitable corollary of an approach such as this one. Describing dynamics and gesture increasingly pushes the boundaries of language, as one progresses beyond the level of form to that of process. One starts off by describing characteristics of the two cells; from that basic level one proceeds to get at the formative process by thinking and describing more in terms of the typical forces that shape the egg cell or sperm cell, and after that one penetrates to an even higher level. At that point one begins to need abstract words such as 'centre' and 'periphery,' 'open' and 'closed,' whilst getting ever nearer to the essence of the dynamics.

4.2.2 Polarities and turning inside out

The above phenomena could still be described in terms of contrasts. Yet it may have become obvious that more is at play here than contrasts in terms of polarity, of repulsion, and of inequality. In the case of the processes and dynamics of the egg cell and sperm cell discussed so far, there is an additional factor. It was shown, for instance, that the egg cell with its dynamics of 'cytoplasm retention' carries out a highly asymmetric division in reproduction (meiosis), whereas the sperm cell must expel cytoplasm. If one looks at this in terms of the dynamic characteristic of egg cells or sperm cells, one can postulate that the egg cell casts off the sperm cell principle ('sperm-cellness') at the moment of its first reduction division and that the sperm cell, in turn, excludes the egg-cell principle ('egg-cellness').

> *Methodological remark: corroborative data from pathology*
> Knowledge of pathology often helps to gain a better insight. If the sperm cell does not succeed in ridding itself of superfluous cytoplasm, it does not function properly. It would be too heavy and hampered in its mobility by the bag of cytoplasm attached at the height of the neck. When one looks for polarities, pathology shows the following pattern: *What is good and fitting for one pole and promotes its function, is disturbing for the other pole and makes it dysfunctional.*

One could describe the egg cell as a cell which has an inside; there is a content. The sperm cell has sacrificed its inner side, it has given its content away. In that (dynamic) sense the sperm cell has no 'inside.' The egg cell absorbs light (to which end it has its mass) but the sperm cell refracts light, a phenomenon directly observable under the microscope. In that sense it fits that the separated polar body is strongly light-refracting. Moreover, the polar body is no longer characterized by the optimal fertility which is so characteristic of its sister cell (the secondary oocyte). In human beings, it is highly questionable if a polar body would still be capable of human development. If such a thing occurred it would only be rare and sporadic, in which case it would be a very rare form of fraternal twinship.

Even more captivating is the phenomenon of *mobility,* which we mean here in a literal, physical sense. Indeed, one cannot fail to notice that the sperm cell is highly mobile. Pathology shows that sperm cells which cannot swim will not function. The characteristic ability of sperm cells to go against the current and determine their direction that way is foreign to egg cells. An egg cell cannot move independently. It is passively carried along in the stream of ovarian fluid. Again we see a contrast, but is this also a polarity? Up to now we observed *outer* movement, but what is going on inside? Almost absolute quiet reigns inside the sperm cell, which is due to the structure (in the form of the DNA formula), but we hardly see any intracellular metabolic dynamics. The situation inside the egg cell is quite the opposite. Plenty of cytoplasmic dynamism of cell organelles and metabolic activity reigns there. It could be postulated that the sperm cell shows mobility on the outside, whereas this is internalized in the egg cell. In their interaction with the surroundings, the two cells are polar opposites. In their manner we can see a parallel with the 'open' vs. 'closed' gestures signalled above. Whereas the sperm cell relates to its surroundings by pushing *against* them, the egg cell communicates with and is open to its surroundings; it moves *along with* them.

The latter brings us to the phenomenon of *turning inside out.* Deeper consideration reveals that the observed contrast is at heart a commonality. This can be easily demonstrated in biological terms for the spermatozoon and the ovum. Both cells are derived from primordial sex cells which have the same shape at the cellular level in a six-week old human embryo, even though they each contain a different genome (either XY or XX). After this commonality at the beginning, the spermatozoon and the ovum become one-sided and go their separate ways. *Seen in terms of morphological dynamics, one could postulate that the sperm cell specializes in 'nucleus,' and the egg cell in 'cytoplasm.'* This is in complete harmony with the biological principle that a spermatozoon, just like the polar body, is incapable of producing a cell (an organism). An ovum does have that capacity (in principle), as can be seen, for example, in parthenogenesis.

Methodological remarks

These observations mark a clear break between this approach and the current reductionistic, dissecting method. For most of today's biologists it would be undesirable to proceed in this direction, they would even consider the territory we have entered 'out of bounds.' To call a germ cell a 'nucleus-head,' or to designate an egg cell as a 'ball of cytoplasm,' is only justifiable within the framework of the phenomenological approach practised here. It could be objected that the sperm cell also contains cytoplasm (even if it is not much), or that the egg cell also has a nucleus, and that they both have the trappings of a proper cell. Fair enough. But if one remains at the level of details, one will never see what this approach opens up. If one stays within one basic paradigm, these observations are indeed not 'true.' The dynamics of the germ cell as 'nucleus' and the egg cell as 'cytoplasm' simply do not reveal themselves within that framework.

Calling this a break is justified, because the analytical approach would exclude insights which can be gained through the dynamic approach. *The reverse, however, is not the case.* These remarks run along the same lines as the conclusions we reached when we talked about 'seeing the roundness of the head' at the beginning of this chapter. This strongly underpins the postulate that *facts are not value-free,* but that a perceptual content is always intertwined with interpretation.

The following considerations supply further support to show that we're dealing with polar gestures between 'nucleus' and 'cytoplasm.' Of course the egg cell has a nucleus, but it is embedded in a completely different process from that of the sperm cell. The DNA in the egg cell is metabolically active; it is 'rolled out' as far as is necessary and involved in well-known processes of transcription, translation, etc. One can postulate that the egg cell shows the processes of a cell in *interphase.* By contrast, the biological dynamics of the sperm cell have the signature of a cell in the *mitotic phase.* The DNA is ordered and structured, the nucleus is correspondingly pycnotic and metabolically resting. In the current analytical, 'magnifier' approach the sperm cell and egg cell have both nucleus and cytoplasm; in the comparative, 'minifier' approach the sperm cell is 'nucleus' and an egg cell is 'cytoplasm.' Viewed this way, an interphase bears the signature of cytoplasm and could thus be characterized as peripheral, centrifugal, and open. In other words, it is like an egg cell. The mitosis bears the signature of the nucleus and could therefore be characterized as central, centripetal, and closed; in short, it is like a sperm cell. In that sense it could be postulated that if constant cell division were to take place in a living human being (every second, day in day out, a whole life long), we could call this a huge breathing process. There would be a large rhythmical alternation of cells closing themselves off from the surroundings and turning towards the replication of the 'inner' ('sperm cell gesture') and cells opening towards the periphery ('egg cell gesture') and so on.

> *Methodological remark*
> Recognizing such a gesture in the process of cell division obviously requires a rather high degree of 'dynamic perception.' But imagine where this can lead. It enables us to gain a first glimpse of cells in a larger breathing process. First, they open up to influences from the surroundings (periphery). Then, they turn to concentrate on reproduction, so that they can stamp those influences from the surroundings onto the inside of the cell (the process of cell specialization and differentiation). The dynamics of the two gametes which are involved in conception resound like a first chord in a symphony. The first manifestation of the living organism!

4.2.3 Preliminary conclusion — polarity and unity

One can look at ovum and spermatozoon as one-sided, polar developments from one many-sided, common origin. By forming a concrete image of the original sex cell it is even possible to picture the original unity out of which the two gametes polarized. Building the image up in thought, one can transform the one into the other, that is to say, the polarity exists in fact within a unity.

'Egg-cellness' can manifest because 'sperm-cellness' is cast off, and the other way around! If we take a step further, we could say that they owe their existence to one another. They belong together. Understood in this sense, it is no wonder that sperm cell and egg cell meet one another. They complete one another! How they manage to do that (by means of the pre-conception attraction complex), will be dealt with later. In the dynamics of cell division with its alternating mitosis and interphase we can see a rhythmical 'repetition' of the gestures of the ovum and the spermatozoon, which indicates that we are beginning to gain insight into a higher level which is at work in the formative gesture of the particular egg cell and sperm cell.

4.2.4 More polarities in conception

Why can we think of the sperm cell as 'straight? Thinking back to the corresponding question we asked with respect to the naive assumption of the roundness of the head, this question is relevant. For that waving 'creature' is of course straight in that it has the form of a *radius*. The spermatozoon is a radius with a beginning and an end; the ovum is a *ball*. The anatomical facts make this obvious: there is hardly a more perfectly spherical cell. Spherical cells are an exception. Maybe this is so because cells are never found on their own, but always form tissue together with many others. The ovum is a solitary cell. Egg cell tissue does not exist. The sphere is a self-sufficient form, it has no beginning and no end.

Assignment 2
Imitating the found gesture by acting it out and thus experiencing it physically can often be a great help. One can 'play' spermatozoon by standing upright and stretching up as far as possible, and feeling how that is. After that one can withdraw into oneself and roll up into a ball, thus getting a sense for that condition. Apart from sensing the sphere and the radius, there's also an experience of dark and light. The sphere can be felt as a self-contained form. The sphere has no direction, no beginning and no end.

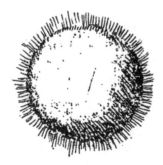

Figure 4.2. Preconception attraction complex
Drawing from Appenzeller, Genesis im Lichte der Embryologie

Assignment 3

Form drawing can also support one's own experience when one recognizes the gestures. Draw a circle with a pencil, do it in a large format and repeat the circular motion for quite some time. Accelerate the movement and then slow it down. Notice how you feel, pay attention to your consciousness.

In drawing this kind of 'perfect' circle, which you're quite likely to succeed in, you will find that you make the centre of the circle visible even though you do not draw it. After all, everything revolves around that point. Is the circle not a collection of points equidistant (radius) from a chosen centre? And that centre is an 'invisible' point. Now take a new piece of paper, concentrate on the central point and try approaching it from every direction, swooping down to the paper, landing, going through that chosen centre, and then lifting off from the paper in the same movement. Try this several times and once again notice how you feel, paying attention to mood, consciousness and inner experience. Is it not very different? How easy or hard is it this time to exactly draw a point? This time, too, the radii make visible a sphere, which also 'is not there.' Can you sense how these are two ways to deal with a centre? Try to experience how these are literally two 'approaches,' substantiating the press of the turning inside out of sphere and radius.

The analytical eye might have difficultly seeing the radius character of the sperm cell, but for comparative and dynamic perception it is clear as daylight. Moreover, it is an impressive thing to witness the process of turning inside out. In a geometrical sense, there are myriad radii within the sphere of the egg cell, only they have not manifested in a physical form. The sperm cell makes the radius visible. In that sense the two cells are polar opposites again, and at the same time the one is the other one turned inside out. The egg cell shows what the sperm cell hides, and the other way around. What can we read in the whole preconception attraction complex? In Figure 4.2 we see the unity formed by hundreds of sperm cells and the single egg cell, which lasts for hours before penetration of the sperm cell can take place. Do the sperm cells not make visible what the egg cell carries invisibly within? Sperm cells literally radiate that invisible dimension back to the egg cell. Do the sperm cells not form one large sphere, consisting of rays?

We will now go on to discover even more polarity. For conception in the normal definition of the word (the fusion of two pronuclei), one sperm cell and one egg cell would suffice. If one looks at what actually happens, however, one sees how during the period of the preconception attraction complex hundreds, even thousands of spermatozoa need to be present. With fewer than that it does not work. The numbers supplied by fertilization physiology confirm this. When a man is not able to produce 20 to 40 million spermatozoa per ejaculation, he is physiologically infertile. Tens of millions of sperm cells are produced every single day! That means hundreds of them per second! Out of every 10 to 20 primary oocytes which commence the final stage of maturation prior to ovulation, the majority will perish. One ovum will be released, at most two.

Now let us consider the concepts *one* and *many,* or *a lot.* Do they form a polarity? Here the same principle applies as in the case of 'small' and 'large.' In ordinary thinking, these words are used to denote quantities or measurements; in the series 1, 2, 3, 4, ... and up, we progress from the number 1 to *many,* i.e. a large number. But there is a different way to look at this. *One* is also a dimension, a quality. In the Middle Ages, people regarded *one* as the largest number. Something (or somebody) of which (whom) there is only one, that is a lot. *One* human being is not much in terms of physical matter, but very much when considered as a unique entity. One could say that a unique entity 'fills the cosmos.' In contrast, one can think of the cosmos as being filled with countless material Milky Ways, galaxies, stars and planets, usually experienced as *many.* Seen this way, *one* and *many* are polar opposites. The one form of *many* is material, in the sense of a lot of physical presence. That could be viewed as *many* in the spermatozoic way. Over against that there is the other *many,* or rather *much:* the immaterial vastness of something unique. That could be viewed as *many* in the ovum way. As qualities, *one* and *many* are poles, whereby the one is the other turned inside out.

Methodological remark
Perceptive readers will have noticed that there is more that distinguishes the polarity of egg cell and sperm cell — or rather 'egg-cellness' and 'sperm-cellness' — more than mere contrast. We have already remarked on the principle of turning inside out; this is not a simple matter of + and –, but rather of +/– and –/+. One also has to keep distinguishing at which level one makes the comparison, and within which parameters. Thus, when focusing

on the *metabolic*, we spoke of an 'open' egg cell and a 'closed' sperm cell dynamics of the cell. But if one uses the concepts 'open' and 'closed' to express *formative* dynamics, then things are reversed. At the level of form (sphere–radius), the egg cell is the one that is 'closed,' and the sperm cell is the one that is 'open.' This methodological remark aims to point out once more that one is dealing here with a higher 'Gestalt-level' where polarity manifests.

To round this off, we now turn our gaze to the dynamics of 'sperm-cell-ness' and 'egg-cellness,' but this time at the level of the gonads. Directions and qualities of the gestures are again reversed here. The dynamics of the ovaries versus those of the testes portray a kind of 'counter image.' Whereas the sperm cell as a cell has the gesture of con-centration and the egg cell of expansion, the testes and the ovaries show us the reverse in dynamics. The testis is an organ which bursts with bubbling vitality, displaying an enormous mitoti activity. The sperm cells are also relatively 'young.' They will exist for 65–70 days at most, after which they are reabsorbed. Much calmer dynamics prevail in the ovaries. We cannot speak of productivity here. Already during the foetal life of the woman, egg cells lose their mitotic capacity and from that moment (the sixth foetal month) the number only decreases. The ovaries preserve and protect; the gesture is more centripetal, one of a slow 'decease' until the number of egg cells is reduced to zero when menopause is completed. The bubbling, explosive, centrifugal, radia-tion sensitive dynamics of the testes contrast with the quiet, imploding, centripetal dynamics of the ovaries. Macroscopically, the testis is a hard, shielded organ; microscopically we see a vast surface opening up to the outside. With 200 metres of seminiferous and efferent ducts plus 12 metres of epididymis, the testis is all surface and openness. The ovaries are tender, but massive; the egg cells are embedded in them, and hard shielding off is a pathology here, as the Stein-Leventhal syn-drome demonstrates.

Methodological remark
It will have become obvious by now that it becomes more and more tricky to find concepts and terms for the gestures one begins to track. More and more concepts are needed in order to express the dynamics manifesting here, and the concepts are not synonymous, each one capturing a different facet of the gestures.

Take for example the sequence mentioned above: centrifugal/
centripetal — open/closed — periphery/centre — radius/sphere —
light/dark — explosive/implosive. The researcher can get the
somewhat unpleasant feeling of using a plethora of concepts while
hardly, if at all, being able to name the central concept or the all-
encompassing gesture. At that point it feels as if one loses the firm
ground of clear facts and concepts. Yet at the same time one can
begin to gain a definite sense for the concept (see the consideration
below). The orthodox materialist might feel at this point that things
are getting too nebulous, but for the phenomenological approach
this experience indicates one is penetrating to the heart of the
matter. The essence cannot be caught in words, but is nevertheless
palpable.

Metaphorically speaking, the researcher is 'treading water' in
the world of concepts. A form of certainty can yet be found when
one keeps moving. The fact that we need to 'tread water' now can
be regarded as inherent to the level we are beginning to reach.
We're no longer concerned here with shape, nor with process, but
with Gestalt, gesture. With this one reaches the world of formative
forces, which are at work behind every shape which has come to
visible manifestation. Spiritual science calls this the *etheric world*.
This level can only be perceived in pictorial form, using
imaginative consciousness. This exercise of 'treading water' is a
prelude to this.

Considerations regarding Sensing and Seeing
Blaise Pascal made a distinction between the esprit de geometrie *and
the* esprit de finesse *(the spirit of geometry and the spirit of finesse).**
The esprit de geometrie *is needed for visual discernment. In the
natural sciences the esprit de geometrie is the basis of every method.
Its main feature is communicability. ... It can be made clear to
anybody that a papillionacious flower has an undivided corolla, 10
stamens, one pistil etc. ... But that flowers are 'passions of the earth,'
as Goethe calls them, can only be communicated to someone who
already 'sees' it.*

J.H. van den Berg[4]

---

*   The *esprit de finesse* refers to that part of reality which one 'sees' in a different way, and which can be just as tangible as that which can be communicated. Pascal puts it like this, *'On les sent plutôt qu'on les voit,'* 'It is more
sensed than seen.'

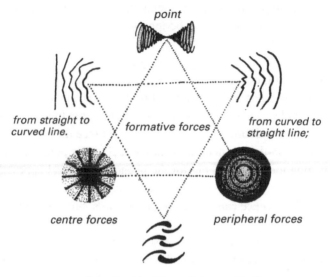

point

from straight to
curved line.

formative forces

from curved to
straight line;

centre forces

peripheral forces

mixture — rhythm — interpenetration

Figure 4.3

Assignment 4

From Sphere to Radius — An Exercise in Transformative Thinking
We have been working with the polarity of radius and sphere
(straight and round). Were not those the dynamics of head versus
extremities? The extremities can be seen as radii made manifest.
Yet it is those very arms and legs which are able to describe a
cone shape by spherical movement. Thereby the form is moved,
placed in space; it becomes external movement. Is the head not
spherical movement come to rest? If so, where are the radii? Are
they the invisible dimension of the head, in the same way that the
sphere or cone is the invisible dimension belonging to the extremi-
ties? And what is the movement which belongs to the head? Is that
external, spatial movement, such as arms and legs can perform, or
is it more inward, nonmaterial?

Figure 4.3 is part of a 'meditative drawing' by Karl Heinz Flau.
The assignment is to come to an experience of the geometrical
principles of point, curved and straight line, centre and periphery
as 'mathematical gesture language.' The task here is to try to
transform one thing into another in thought, turning them inside
out. One literally 'comes out at the other end.' Please note the
process indicated with the word 'mixture' in the drawing. This
concept will be elaborated in the next chapter.

Assignment 5 *Drawing Exercise to Experience Transformation Turning 'Sperm-cellness' into 'Egg-cellness' (and vice versa). Take a piece of paper, and first put down three points which will form the ends of three sides of an equilateral triangle. Do not draw the sides straight, but curved slightly inwards. The idea is now to experience a force pushing in. Continue drawing the sides, whereby the force pushes them further in each time. The lines will curve in further and further, making the enclosed triangle smaller and smaller, more and more like a sperm cell. Once one has the feel of a rhythmical movement, moving through the line segment, coming to rest in the point, moving through the next segment, coming to rest in the next point, and so on from angle to angle, one almost gets into a circular movement and loses the feeling of the* angular *shape of the triangle.*

If one analyses the resulting drawing, one can see the still point, the transition where the form is turned inside out. *After that, one comes out 'on the other side,' and another triangle slowly emerges, this time with the base up, and 'bulging out' on all sides. Is this not how a concentrating, sperm cell movement is turned into an expanding, egg cell movement?*

In Figure 4.4, the series drawn by Karl Heinz Flau, note that he uses a totally different terminology, speaking of sucking *and* welling, *and from the* outside *and from the* inside.

Encore
At the end of the drawing exercise, one could continue the lines, taking them from the angles and extending them out in thought. It will appear that it is thus possible to imagine the continuation of the lines into an infinite periphery.

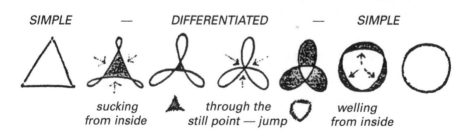

SIMPLE — DIFFERENTIATED — SIMPLE

sucking
from inside

through the
still point — jump

welling
from inside

Figure 4.4

Assignment 6
Try finding characteristics of 'egg cellness' and 'sperm cellness' in individuals. This is best done by looking dynamically at pairs of individuals and comparing them. This is a good practice especially when one is considering children.

First concentrate on the way the chosen individuals are built, and consider posture and/or constitution. Keep a list of points of comparison between the two, and note down what you think the characteristic gestures are.

The next step could be to compare the found gestures with soul dynamics. What is inner, what is outer? For example, are there people who externally seem to be always on guard, hiding their inner feelings? And are there also people who are socially very accessible, but couple this with deeper psychological dynamics of reclusiveness?

It would be harder still to go on to examine the relationship between 'soul dynamics' and outer appearance. One could ask the question, for example, whether a person who outwardly has an open attitude also has inner psychological and social openness. Do outward appearance and inner reality go together?

4.3 One plus one makes three — the middle

One conclusion we could draw from the foregoing paragraphs is that *polarities exist within a unity.* Having seen that polarities are transformations of one another we can surmise that a higher principle connects or unites them. In this section we will begin to research the nature of this principle and see if it can be known. To that end we will direct our attention first to the human skeleton.

4.3.1 Polarities in the human skeleton

In Chapter 3 we studied teeth, looking at their different elements both on their own and comparatively. Our focus now will be on the totality of the human skeleton (and human bearing), within which we will look for polarities. The main one is between *head-skull* and *arms/legs-extremities,* so we are operating in the dimension of *centre-periphery.*

Assignment 7

Once again, as in the case with the polarities between egg cell and sperm cell, it is a good thing to start with our own observations. On the checklist on the following page first note down polarities, using the approach we chose. Start from the principle of transformation, consistently thinking through to 'the other side'.

As we know, the skull bones are a set of flat plates of bone tissue which can be regarded as the surface of a sphere, manifesting in bone. Together, these plates form a round container which holds the brain and is known as the neurocranium. One could comment on this by pointing at the viscerocranium. Such a comment, it could be postulated here, would come out of an analytical approach, something which we will come back to later in this paragraph. The flatness of the skull bones and the spherical character of the skull as a whole will only come into perspective when we direct our attention to the bones of the extremities. For there we are dealing with long tubular bones. They do not form a sphere, but rather a long stretched out chain of skeletal elements.

The skull bones form close connections. The sutures are known for their tightness. Although, histologically speaking, we are dealing with connections built out of ligament (syndesmoses), they are extremely tight and hard to break due to their complicated jigsaw structure. In infants the connections can still be severed; in adults a skull will be more likely to rupture or break in case of trauma; the seam is unlikely to become disconnected. We could postulate that tightness and form retention are the normal function here, whereas mobility would be pathological. With the bones of the extremities, the situation is reversed. Here we are primarily dealing with *synovial connections,* which rather have the character that they are not really connections, for there is a space in between. This is functional because the joints need to be free to move. Tightness, characteristic of the physiology of the skull, would be pathological here. Concrescence within the connections would cause malfunctioning of the extremity.

In connection with this, a striking feature of the skull should be mentioned: it is an exoskeleton. Through the skin the bony skull can almost be directly examined in vivo. An individual's typical physiognomy is reflected in the bone structure of the skull. The bony elements of the extremities, on the other hand, are hidden from view. They are an endoskeleton, mostly covered by soft tissue, especially muscle. The

POLARITIES BETWEEN HEAD AND EXTREMITIES

	HEAD/SKULL	EXTREMITIES
PARAMETER		
Bone Shape		
Nature of bone connections		
Mobility of the parts		
Degree to which bones are recognizable in vivo		
Relationship to temperature		
Open or closed		
Internal vs. external mobility		
Vitality		
Blood flow		
Relationship to consciousness		
Relationship to outside world (periphery)		

presence of muscles in the extremities and the seeming absence of muscle in the head goes with this. The facial muscles are not meant to move the separate bones of the skull in relation to one another. The chewing muscles seem to be an exception, something which we will return to later on. A striking feature of the skull is that it is an exoskeleton; the soft parts (brain) are located on the inside. In the case of the extremities it is the other way round: the soft parts surround a hard centre, they are on the *outside*. Whereas the bony elements of the extremities are embedded in muscle tissue directly involved with movement, in the case of the head, movement is harmful for the soft contents. This is illustrated by the fact that the brain malfunctions (temporarily) in case of a concussion.

The head has an 'inside.' The skull encloses that, which goes with its spherical shape; the skull is *closed,* in contrast to the extremities, which 'radiate' out, have a beginning and an end, and are *open* in character. Here we once again meet the polarities of sphere and radius. The pathology of (now rare) rickets gives us the picture of the reversal: the round head becomes the *caput quadratum,* the straight extremities become bent.

The character of extremities is to diverge, split and fan out. If one follows the series of bones down the arm, one sees this pattern clearly: 1 humerus, 2 forearm bones (ulna and radius), 3 proximal carpals, 4 distal carpals, 5 metacarpals and corresponding phalanges. In order to characterize the dynamics expressed in skull and extremities, one could use the terms **concentration** vs. **divergence.** The extremity diverges out to the periphery, and 'opens out' to it. Each in their own way, the extremities are turned to the outside world, ready to adapt to it or change it with their actions. The extremity finds its centre 'out there.' By contrast, the head closes off, concentrates, and finds its centre 'here.' The extremities exist and develop gravity. The head encloses a space which is free of gravity, within which the brain is suspended in the cerebral spinal fluid.

Methodological remark

It is hard to find the right terms to sum up the gesture which is at play here. Does the skull form a picture of detachment? Do the extremities make a gesture of shooting out towards the periphery? How is the relationship of the human being with the environment and the world expressed in these two areas? Do we not in our head reflect about the world, whereas with our limbs we act in the world? Perhaps the words *separate* and *connect* would be fitting terms to express the two gestures.

In this connection, we should further pursue the theme of mobility, and try to find out about being active inwardly and outwardly. We found this equally helpful in order to understand the gesture inherent in the sperm cell and the egg cell. The extremities clearly move, they move in space and they are subject to gravity. In the extremities, the human being moves in a physical, material, sense perceptible way. In the physical body, the human being moves *with* his arms or legs. As indicated above, the head has a different relationship to movement. Outward, material, sense perceptible movement is limited to a minimum here, it even hampers proper functioning of the brain and the senses. In order to observe accurately with eyes and ears, one holds the head still, otherwise perception is disturbed. This goes for other functions performed by the head as well. There is, however, a quiet mobility of a nonmaterial kind. If one observes the brain and the skull, one notices that they are strongly formed and shaped. In making that observation, we think not only of the fact that the skull is highly 'chiselled,' but also of the neurons, which lie in a strictly neuroanatomical order. Even the movement of stimuli thought to take place along the neural passageways is only a semblance. In 'reality,' spatial structures, which neurons are, depolarize. Whereas we move *with* matter in our extremities, in the head we ***relate to*** matter with a different movement. That type of mobility, characteristic of thoughts and imagination, is of a very high order. In fact, the mobility inside our heads is much more subtle and ephemeral than any motor movements of our actions can ever be. We recognize this in common expressions — one can 'change one's mind,' ideas can 'come' or even 'hit' in a flash. Imagination has no bounds, and thoughts can move anywhere they want.

The extremities are radii which have become visible, and the head is likewise a sphere which has manifested in the visible world. The extremity, however, is invisibly connected to the sphere. This underlines once again that the extremities are polar opposites of the head, because the mathematical centre lies in the periphery, whereas the spherical head actually has its centre within. The extremities have their centre 'out yonder,' but the centre of the head is 'here.'

Assignment 8
At this point it would be good to go over Figure 4.2 and
Assignment 3 and either review Assignment 6 once again, or take
it up anew.

It may have become clear by now that the range of polarities which unfold between the head on the one side and the extremities on the other, is inexhaustible. This is no wonder, because they have to do with the nature of the way we relate to the world, which is indeed quite different for different areas of the body. The nature of cognition is in many ways the polar opposite of the nature of action (or volition). To be conscious and awake are two prerequisites of cognition, without which we are dealing with a pathological situation. In the sphere of action, the domain of volition, there is of course a certain degree of consciousness also. However, if one wants to be fully conscious when one carries out an action, and be fully awake in every facet of the motion, one would actually hinder its fluidity. It is even so that someone who fully masters a motion, say, of playing an instrument, will say, 'As soon as I stop and think about it, it goes wrong.' At a certain point, it is 'in the fingers,' and no longer in the head. Experiences of this nature point to a certain degree of unconsciousness as being beneficial for uninterrupted motion and adequate action. We might well be dealing with a totally different relationship between body and spirit in these two spheres. There will be more to say about this in Section 4.3.6.

To round this off, let us make some observations concerning blood flow and temperature. The blood supply in the extremities is less precarious than that in the head. This is illustrated by the fact that it is possible to operate on an extremity for quite some time in a 'blood vacuum.' Cutting off large vessels in an extremity does not immediately lead to necrosis. The vascularization of the head is very different. Blood supply to the different regions is regulated with great precision. Interruption, even if only for a few minutes, will soon lead to damage (necrosis). In that respect, the head is much more vulnerable than a limb. Apparently the buffers of vitality are greater there than in the head. Later in this chapter, we will return to this question of the connection of vitality with consciousness. With respect to body temperature, extremities differ from the head. The extremities really are further out, which goes together with a lower temperature (34°–35°C). The head, together with a large part of the trunk, has the core temperature (37°–38°C). If this is reversed, it is clearly unhealthy; 'keeping your head cool' is a well-known expression, and everybody is familiar with the fact that fever can lead to unclear thinking. A hot, feverish head is not the place for wakeful consciousness! But the extremities do not function well in the cold. In physiotherapy, many applications are based on the wholesome effect of warmth on muscles and joints.

With these initial observations, we focused on the polarity of head and limbs. The aim of the chapter, however, was to find the way in which they form a unity. It will have become obvious that looking at head and extremities confronts one with the difficulties of the reducing, 'minifying' lens, by which we mean that one has to be very precise about the level at which one applies the comparison.

4.3.2 Connecting polarities — the lemniscate

We would like to go on now to the realm of the *middle,* and its importance with regards to polarities and threefoldness. First, however, some considerations about the *lemniscate* as a connecting figure.

Assignment 9 *Transformation in a Lemniscate*
We would like to begin by recalling Assignment 3, which dealt with the sphere and the radius.
Using a large piece of paper draw a large lemniscate, like a form drawing, i.e. keep moving as you draw. As in Assignment 3, take note of how this activity feels, and notice your consciousness.
Once you have the shape, begin to bring in a variation by expanding one loop, and making the other loop correspondingly smaller. What do you notice?
Try drawing a lemniscate with several parallel bands of colour.

Strictly speaking, the lemniscate is not a shape but a movement. If one only concentrates on the shape of the lemniscate (see continuous line in Figure 4.5), one might fail to see the polarity which is so characteristic. Only by following the line, moving along with it through the drawing, can we distinguish the different character of the inside loop and the outside loop. When we follow the direction (along the dashed line), it becomes obvious how that takes us from the inside to the outside. Doing that, one also will realize how the midpoint is a *turning point,* where the transition takes place from 'outer' to 'inner.'

The 'secret' of the lemniscate is that it is a movement which combines and transcends the polarities of sphere (here a circle) and radius. At the periphery (point *P*) the movement is circular; the centre (*A*) is not actually drawn, but is invisibly and necessarily there for the circular movement to be able to be carried out around it. After all, a circle is a combination of all the points which are equidistant to a given central point (remember Assignment 3). In drawing a lemniscate, the circle with centre a is not completed. One could put it this way: before the circle could be completed, another point begins to attract and pulls one away from a one-sided circular movement, and this point *B* 'wins out' and takes over. This time, however, the movement is similar to the one of the radii moving through the centre of drawing Assignment 3. A straight line moving towards middle point *B* now gives direction to the pencil and this time one does go through the visible central point *B*. This straight movement could potentially be carried on to the periphery in infinity, but the invisible centre *A'* now attracts the movement

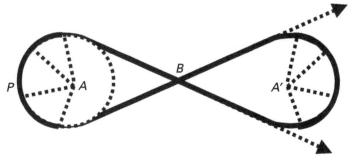

Figure 4.5

and bends it into the circular movement around it, and so on. In this lemniscate movement, the central point alternates all the time, shifting from *A* to *B* to *A'*, back again to *B,* etc.

The lemniscate is, so to speak, a 'breathing' figure, one that transcends the polar one-sidedness of radius and circle (sphere) in a movement which connects both polarities. The lemniscate is neither circle nor radius, while being both at the same time. The lemniscate is the continuum which combines the two, yet also stands 'above' them.

The concepts 'transcend' and 'connect' can help one understand the unity within which the polarity does in fact exist. The one polarity helps us recognize the other. In the quote at the beginning of the chapter, Goethe said, 'We must use the darkness in order to make the light visible;' to this we could add. 'and also the other way around.' We showed this in a dynamic and comparative approach to ovum and spermatozoon, and to head and extremities. If we were to imagine a dimension which would simultaneously be light and dark, it could be no other than one which *carries* both light and dark 'inside,' without *being* either light or dark. Were this dimension to be *either* light *or* dark, it would present itself as one of these. Goethe called it *sinnlich-übersinnlich* (sensory-supersensory);[6] he pointed to a dimension which is not exactly visible, yet can be known. Polarities could thus be looked upon as two manifest extremes of a middle dimension which can be surmised from the extremes. The two poles are visible, the middle transcends the visible.

In the case of the sperm cell and the egg cell one can even form a concrete image of this in thought. Are sperm cell and egg cell not one-sided, polar developments of something like a primordial sex cell? Out of that sex cell they have developed into polar opposites: the egg cell as 'cytoplasm,' the sperm cell as 'nucleus.' To help us imagine this in the example of head and extremities, study the drawing below.

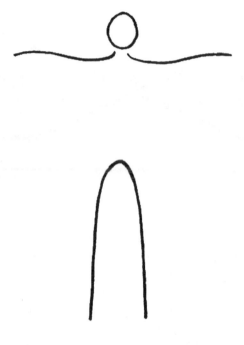

Figure 4.6. The human form
Let us recall the two poles into which a lemniscate can diverge. On the one hand there is the closed-off circle, focused on the centre (A), on the other side there is the open radius, focused on the periphery. The drawing illustrates this principle at work in the human figure.

4.4 The middle as a place of meeting and interaction

The exercise of thinking through the lemniscate brings home how one pole is the other one turned inside out. The other thing it teaches us is that the two poles are in fact connected. That is a general law of polarities. The poles are to be seen as one-sided (specialized) manifestations of something which lies between them, a middle dimension, to be thought of dynamically as being of a higher level, straddling and uniting both poles, not coming to manifestation itself. One could postulate that the two poles reached 'form,' whereas the middle dimension remains in the 'process.' So the middle carries within it the potential for both polarities *(and-and* character), while at the same time standing above the poles and being neither *(neither-nor* character).

Bearing in mind that all shapes come into being through movement (discussed in Section 3.1.3), we can postulate that the two poles are one-sided manifestations of one single dimension which comprises and unites the movement (process) of both.

This realm of the middle is characterized by *rhythm*, which will be shown below. Rhythm can be understood when one pictures breathing. The two extreme poles of breathing are inhaling and exhaling. In themselves, these are 'deadly.' Breathing, which is closely associated with *life*, connects these extremes in a process of rhythmical alternation between the two. Breathing is not a fixed thing, but a process; being *within* that process and maintaining it is essential.

Goethe described this connecting dimension of the middle as being on the *sensory-supersensory* level. The feeling of 'treading water' that was mentioned before, is naturally connected with this dimension, due to the fact that it is not visible, unlike the two poles. However, it can be *known*, and we will now look for manifestations of it in the skeleton.

4.4.1 Ribs

The individual rib should initially be classified as an 'extremity.' Even though it is bent, it does have a beginning and an end. In anatomical nomenclature one speaks of caput, collum and corpus as one does with regular long tubular bones. When one looks at the rib cage as a whole within the totality of the skeleton, the picture changes. The thorax then appears to us as a 'head.' The soft parts are inside, and, inspectable and palpable as it is, the rib cage is unmistakably an exoskeleton. The connections are not as rigid as those of the sutures, but neither are they as flexible as the joints in the extremities. The rhythmical movement of breathing in and out is limited; it is a mixture of quiet form on the one side and movement on the other. The cranial ribs are almost exclusively enclosing, as is the head. Going down, they gradually become less connected to the sternum until finally, in caudal ribs 11 and 12, they end in two pairs of loose 'extremities.' The lower ribs are also more mobile. The thorax thus occupies a kind of middle ground between head and extremities. Cranially, we see the closing, spherical gesture of the head (skull), caudally we see the radiating openness of the extremities. We're dealing with more than a mixture, however. Neither are we looking here for a middle in the sense of a dimension on a higher level. The mixture as such is a sense perceptible reality in the shape of the thorax. But we can also look at the rib cage as a *function* of the activity of the two polar qualities, whereby the whole is more than the parts. With this we mean to say that individual ribs are certainly like extremities, but transcend that quality in their total function of the thorax, wherein they become a head. The skull is an anatomical given; it remains intact long after death even though its 'enclosing function' within the living organism is no longer needed. With ribs, it is different. Soon after death, when the body has decayed, they 'return' to what they also are, namely a collection of loose 'spokes.' The 'thorax head' is something one can see not so much *in* the parts, but *from* the parts. The thorax head is on a higher organizational level.

4.4.2 Vertebrae

What is the place of the individual vertebra within the polarity of skull and extremities? Spina bifida shows that 'openness' is pathological. The vertebral arch closes itself off into the vertebral foramen, like a mini-skull. The spinal cord, which lies within the spinal canal formed by these foramina together, is enclosed as the brain is in the neurocranium.

Taking a step up and looking at the vertebrae within the totality of the human skeleton, we see the *spinal column*. Over thirty vertebrae together form a firm yet flexible column which physiotherapists sometimes call 'the fifth extremity.' Just as with the thorax, one sees how the individual components transcend their individual nature and together build their counterpart. The vertebrae have built something that has the character of a radius in this column. The 30 odd 'heads' make an 'extremity.' The fact that the spinal column is unmistakably an endoskeleton fits in with this observation. In vivo, all that is noticeable of the whole complex spinal column are the spinous processes. The enormous muscular columns of the erector spinae cover the rest. The resulting column, however, does not have the rigidity typical of the long tubular bones in the extremities. The radius character here is not one of shape, but of *process;* the spinal column 'achieves' the form of the radius in its totality. The possibilities for movement are quite different from the extremities; no angular movement is possible, the spinal column as a whole can bend into curves, whereby the rhythmical element stands out again, which we also recognized as a characteristic of the thorax. We thus recognize the spine as an extremity not in the parts, but from the parts. The spine is extremity at a higher organizational level.

4.4.3 The unity of rib and vertebra

Looking at rib and vertebra together, the similarity to a lemniscate is striking. The vertebra can be seen as a head, the ribs as extremities. Heads have minimal mobility (too much movement is actually pathological); for the extremities movement is possible, in fact, they *must* move. This unity as

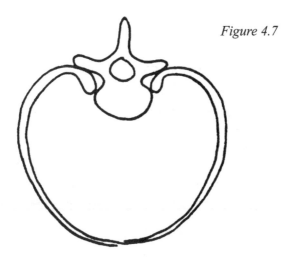

Figure 4.7

such does not reveal the essential character of the organization of which it forms a part, namely the trunk. When we picture the trunk, it turns out we can speak of the head and extremity dimension again, but *reversed* this time. Head is now extremity (spinal column), and the extremities are head (thorax). The trunk is head and extremity at the same time, but not only in the sense of 'in between.' In the dynamics of the shape of the trunk we see the anatomical manifestation of the process which is both head and extremities simultaneously, while also being neither. But this process of 'coming to manifestation' does not go as far as it does in the case of the two poles. The thorax, for example, never becomes an anatomical 'enclosure.'

4.4.4 The concept of *Steigerung*

In a case like this Goethe used the word *Steigerung,* intensification, progression, enhancement, rise, or increase.[7] In the meeting of the qualities 'head' and 'extremity' a higher organizational level becomes 'visible.' One is faced here with a dimension which *is* neither of the polarities, yet *has* them. Goethe derived this concept from his theory of colours. After countless experiments and a long period of research, he came to the conclusion that colours manifest where light and dark meet. The colour grey is the mixture, the passive confluence of light and dark. Colours, however, are the active middle, the active meeting of those two qualities. If one would have asked him the question of what preceded dark and light, Goethe might have answered something like this, 'Light and dark are *expressions* of a dimension of a nonmaterial order which is neither light

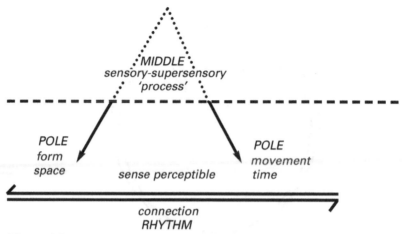

Figure 4.8

nor dark and at the same time both light and dark. Colours are that non-material dimension made visible.'

Thorax and spinal column are the *picture* of the dimension which can be 'seen' in every lemniscate. This dimension itself does not become visible, but is at work 'behind' the visible phenomena and can only be known as such. That is what is meant here by the *middle,* a supersensory quality that can nevertheless be experienced, and thus be understood and known. In Figure 4.8 the relationship between the two poles and the middle with its rhythmical quality is expressed in a triangle.

4.5 Rhythm as the quality of the middle — rhythm and life

Next to the polarity of closed and open (sphere and radius) we came to see in head and extremities* the polarity of rest (form) and movement. These two qualities are united in rhythm. Rhythm is a constant swing of the pendulum between the boundaries imposed by form and the radiating out of movement.

We have seen that poles are one-sided. This one-sidedness is transcended in the rhythmic quality of the middle. The realm of the middle expresses the quality of not falling into one-sidedness; it mediates, because it both connects and creates space between the two polarities. We have seen

---

*   One could ask the question here why there is only one head but several extremities. An answer might lie in what was said above concerning the dimensions one and many in our discussion of the sperm cell and the egg cell.

this above in the shape of the skeleton, and the picture gains considerably in richness when we think of the rhythmical processes of inhaling and exhaling, of systole and diastole, of contraction and relaxation, etc. In this example breathing is the process of life. Continuing in the one-sided activity of inhaling leads to death. This also goes for exhaling. Life gets stuck in the extreme polarities. This example also shows that the middle is much more than 'mean,' or 'average.' In the middle there is a process which comprises both poles and is of a higher order, which is certainly not present in a kind of halfway point between inhalation and exhalation.

Life is a process, a 'breathing' between poles. Life is rhythm. Much is contained in this statement. Rhythm is always **threefold.** There are three parts to it, two of which, the polarities, are manifest and visible. The middle, by its very nature, remains invisible. Therefore visibility implies polarity.

4.6 Making the invisible middle visible

In all these considerations the following question plays in, 'To what degree can the dynamic, participatory stance contribute to achieving supersensory perception?' Having arrived at the middle sphere, it may have become clear that this quality has taken us one step further in grasping gesture. In the poles one seeks to discern the results, the end products, of the formative forces. Those are the visible phenomena. Dynamic perception sees *through* the physical manifestations and penetrates to the level of gesture. Once one pushes through to the quality of the realm of the middle, one has reached a dimension which is unmistakably both sensory and supersensory, and enters the level of the original process behind visible phenomena. In the case of the skeleton, one has the calcified bones in which the formative gesture can be recognized. The gesture of the Gestalt which expresses itself in the threefold division into *head — trunk — extremities* can only be recognized when one starts from a higher systemic level. If one restricts oneself to an analysis of the parts, one has no access to the experience of this Gestalt or process. Once again, Goethe summarizes this concisely:

> In the palm of his hand he holds all the sections,
> Lacks nothing, except the spirit's connections.
> [*Dann hat er die Teile in seiner Hand,*
> *Fehlt, leider nur das geistige Band.*][8]

Towards the end, we introduced the notion of threefoldness. Dynamic perception was a necessary prerequisite for recognizing polarities, and once one sees the polarities, the perception of threefoldness follows logically.

In the following paragraph we will go on to demonstrate this approach in another example of human anatomy.

Interlude

Conception seen as a meeting in the middle

Before conception proper takes place (i.e. before the pronucleus of the egg cell fuses with the pronucleus of the sperm cell), one single egg cell and several hundreds (even thousands) of sperm cells form a biological unity, which exists for several hours. This preconceptual attraction complex (PCAC) is a necessary prerequisite for actual conception, which starts with the penetration of the sperm cell. PCAC lasts several hours, and it is a crucial period of choice. Much hangs in the balance; both egg cell and sperm cells have to meet very specific conditions before a specific sperm cell will penetrate. This is a period in which a very fragile equilibrium exists. When optimal conditions are reached the whole 'mechanics' of penetration, melding etc. happen in a flash. Before that, it is a time of 'putting out feelers.' There is no obligation and everything is open. Both sides are in a precarious balancing of probing conditions.

With regard to the biological relationship one can see a transformation taking place. One must imagine that both gametes are derived from an original sex cell. The one gamete has become a one-sided 'nucleus-head,' the other has turned into a 'cytoplasm-ball' (see Section 4.2.2). During this time, ordinary biological conditions are totally reversed; normal cell conditions have turned inside out. In normal cells, the nucleus is both structured *and* structuring *inside a dynamic, active and changeable periphery of cytoplasm. But during PCAC, cytoplasm is the quiet centre with the nuclei moving around in the periphery.*

One can picture this as follows: Imagine turning the cell inside out the way one does with a glove, and think this through to the end. Eventually this leads to the situation of the preconceptual attraction complex. (Compare also Assignment 5). It is as if the two gametes create 'the cell' at a higher level during this subtle and fragile play of reconnaiscence. PCAC is a joint achievement: the two polar components progress together to 'the cell,' bringing it about anew. In contrast to the cell as we normally know it, this one is of a higher order. One can imagine that something else enters in during this stage of openness and meeting. It is as if matter is lifted outside normal biological circumstances. In this state (less biological, less like ordinary matter), it makes itself accessible for another, nonmaterial dimension, which can connect with substance (incarnation).

4.7 Threefold perception

4.7.1 Introduction

Perhaps the title 'Threefold Perception' does not quite correctly characterize our methodology. In this chapter we have practised the dynamic approach up to now. This is inseparably connected with discerning polarities. As indicated in Section 3.1.3, dynamic perception includes three aspects: 1) describing *details;* 2) including the *total picture* within which the various details must move; 3) perceiving the *dynamics* resulting in the eventual proportions of the forms within the total picture. Recognizing polarity is not possible without comparing. That, combined with the dynamic approach, gave us insight into the *gesture* behind the polarities. Going further, one inevitably comes to the dimension of the middle which bridges and unites polarities, something which is both sensory and supersensory. The two poles appear in the sense perceptible realm, but by its very nature the middle lies in the realm of the invisible. Whereas polarity therefore always implies the visibility, the middle always implies a rhythmical process.

When we speak of threefold perception, we mean an approach to nature and the human being which recognizes that creation manifests the polarity of *spiritual principles* and *matter.* In the anthroposophical view of the human being and the world, this spiritual reality is the starting point. Although this spiritual reality does not lend itself to conventional 'proof,' it is, however, verifiable in observed phenomena of threefoldness in the human being and nature. The dynamic approach demonstrated here, combined with thinking and observing in polarities, is the minimum requirement for perceiving this threefoldness. In the next paragraph we will give another example of how to direct our observation and thought, followed by a summary of the consequences of this approach.

4.7.2 Upper and lower pole

To begin with, let us posit the polarity *cranial–caudal* in the human being. In that framework, let us compare the dynamics of the head/skull on the one side with the dynamics of the belly/pelvis on the other side. Many of the polarities we discovered when we looked at the 'axis' of head in contrast to the extremities, will be recognized here too. Next to that, other polarities become manifest. Once again we suggest starting with independent observations. In the chart you will find a number of criteria offered as a guide to discovering the polarities. It will be obvious that the head forms a polarity with the 'counter-head' pole of belly and pelvis along this axis, and also that the principle of turning inside out is recognizable again.

The chart uses the term 'anti-head,' because this axis of *upper pole* and *lower pole* should be seen in connection with the aforementioned axis head–extremities. In that case we were dealing with centre (head) and periphery, here we are dealing with upper (head) and lower. This also makes it understandable how the terms *upper pole* and *lower pole* are often used in anthroposophical terminology to indicate the *nerve-sense pole* and the *metabolic-limb pole*. Within such a frame of reference one does away with the dissecting approach. Most current textbooks of anatomy and physiology treat limbs and intestines in completely different chapters. With this approach one sees connections between domains which are currently seen as belonging to completely different disciplines. Threefoldness in the human being is not so much an anatomical framework, at best it could be seen as a morphological framework: we are dealing with the spatial relationship of *process*. It would be better to speak of 'spheres.' These spheres (or poles) do exist in space, but not in a Cartesian sense. Recognizing threefoldness automatically leads to seeing connections with the field of psychosomatics and different disciplines and makes a connection between different and now separate disciplines visible. Later on we will show how the polarities of threefoldness can be seen in more than one axis or direction. Take for example the unity of the rib and vertebra. Dorsally, it has the character of the upper pole and ventrally the character of the lower pole. Moreover, once we have learned to see it in one place, we will recognize the principles of threefoldness if manifesting within each part of the body, and within every organ and on every level which can be perceive macroscopically or microscopically. Think of the nervous system which has its upper pole in the neurocranium (above) and the spinal cord (behind) and its lower pole in the peripheral nerves on the axis centre–periphery, whereas the vegetatively autonomous intestinal plexus forms the lower pole on the axis centre–intestines.

This gives a little indication that one can see threefold polarities in several directions and dimensions and the more one sees, the more the certainty of topographical space falls away. We may feel we are treading water, but we will find a new foothold in the *topography of processes*. This topography stands 'above' physical anatomy, while weaving 'through' it at the same time. Here we enter the sphere of the sensory–supersensory again.

CRITERION	HEAD POLE	COUNTER-HEAD POLE
Form (spherical or radial)		
Concentric–centrifugal		
Motion–rest		
Temperature		
Exo/endoskeleton		
Articulation (one–many)		
Hardness/consistency		
Closed/open		
Smell		
Sound		
Colours		
Degree of moisture (relation to water)		
Degree of consciousness		
Degree of vitality		

4.7.3 Three levels of consciousness

Two of the criteria mentioned in the chart will be elaborated here, because they can help us to understand the polar relationship between the spiritual and the physical, working in the two spheres. The polarity *vital–non-vital* is one which obviously goes through the whole of human morphology. On the axis upper–lower, the non-vitality of the nervous system stands opposite the belly/pelvis area with its predominating vitality. One manifestation of this is the fact that nerve tissue is far less able to regenerate itself. The scope of this polarity widens when one takes into account the criterion of sensitivity to radiation. Apart from nerve tissue, striking examples of tissues which are totally or almost totally insensitive to the mutagenic effect of radioactive radiation are fat tissue, muscle tissue, and collagenous connective tissue. By contrast, bone marrow, testis tissue, and almost all epithelia (skin and intestinal tissue among others), are very sensitive to radiation. Presence or absence of mitotic activity is evidently related to this difference. In the one type of tissue, cell division, growth and regeneration (signs of vitality) have become lost, which is a hallmark of the upper pole. The organs concerned are fully formed. *Form* and *structure* predominate, which is a characteristic tendency of the upper pole. In the opposite type of tissue, time is still a factor in the biological process: the anatomical form is a shape in time. The physical representative of these organs and their tissues is a passing one. The lower pole tendency of *process* still predominates. We use the word 'still' here because we know of the history of the embryo that all organs and tissues have partaken in processes of growth, transformation and regeneration. In the upper pole the process comes to rest and hardens into form. In extreme terms, the brain is all but dead. In the lower pole the process remains active and vitality predominates. Think of it this way: the organs and tissues of the lower pole remain 'embryonic' in a certain sense. This also helps us to understand why the human body as a whole is sensitive to radiation in the embryonic phase. In this phase the whole of the human being must be like the lower pole.

The polarity vital–non-vital is related to the polarity *conscious–unconscious.* Where there is vitality, only sleeping consciousness is possible. Sleep is so much the state of consciousness connected with vitality, that it is actually pathological when the functioning of the lower pole organs and tissues comes to consciousness (think, for example, of a stomach-ache). On the other hand, vitality must apparently recede to enable consciousness to light up. An absence of vitality is a necessary prerequisite for consciousness. *Vitality and consciousness are opposites.* Where things are broken down and where there is form, consciousness can arise. In this polarity of waking–sleeping, one can imagine a middle realm of dreaming consciousness, having on one side the wakefulness of sense perception, on the other side the sleeping character of sinking into unconsciousness.

All this throws a new light on the threefold organism of the human being. In the anthroposophical paradigm the human being mediates between spirit and matter, and the relation between the two apparently varies inside the body. 'Form follows movement' was the adage of

Chapter 2. The dynamics living in the upper pole and the lower pole confirm this. The upper pole — characterized by form, structure, and lack of vitality with corresponding wakeful consciousness — is *secondary*. The lower pole comes first; process is *primary*. Consequently, death is no longer primary, but comes forth out of life; not only does this totally reverse current dogmas, but it throws new light on the two different ways in which the relationship between body and spirit can manifest. In the sphere of the lower pole the relationship between shaper and shaped, i.e. the relationship between spirit and matter, is close, like hands shaping clay. In this sphere where the formative processes disengage from matter, like hands leaving the sculpture when the final product is achieved, process stops, form 'appears,' and the spirit is freed. Viewed this way, consciousness is like a waking up *from*. Where spirit disengages itself from the body and 'leaves' it, consciousness lights up; where the closeness of the lower pole relationship remains, spirit submerges into the unconscious.

This view has tremendous consequences; it totally changes the way we look at the human being. It enables us to see that the spirit is not exclusively linked to the nerve-sense system (upper pole). It is not limited to that; the human being is also present and active as a spiritual being in the lower pole. The nerve sense sphere, with its upper pole relationship between spirit and matter, can now be understood as a 'carrier,' which enables us to have waking consciousness. In this view, spirit is present throughout the body, but there is a different relationship in different areas. In the lower pole, spirit works *with* matter (process; shaping; metabolism), there is no consciousness, and the sleeping quality of the embryo is retained. In the upper pole, spirit can free itself from the body, one of the consequences of which is waking consciousness. Here spirit works *from* matter. When one follows this train of thought, threefoldness acquires its true *psychosomatic* meaning: it is about three levels of relationship between spirit and body. Roughly formulated, that comes down to a tripartite division of human consciousness into

waking — dreaming — sleeping,

which, in the respective spheres of

upper pole — middle realm — lower pole,

allow the soul functions of

thinking — feeling — will

to work in three distinct levels of consciousness.

More of this later in this training manual. Here we just wanted to show that a participatory stance, practised together with the dynamic approach, can be the key to seeing sense perceptible, physical data quite differently. These data need not lead inescapably to a materialistic worldview;

through this approach, those very data allow us to recognize the spiritual dimension of the human being. Whether one penetrates to the reality of the spirit does not depend on the facts by themselves, but is determined by one's orientation. It all depends on where one stands.

Assignment 10

Read the article in the Appendix titled 'Heart and Turning Point in Time,' by G.H. van der Bie.

Reading this article can be seen as a form of self-evaluation. In essence, the article deals with the threefold human being. Once one has digested the previous chapters, one should be able to grasp the content of this article, which deals with the nature of the heart as an organ of the middle.

Consider the verse by Rudolf Steiner below. When one has studied and considered what has been written up to now, one might have a good foundation for understanding this verse, which is a pithy condensation of the threefold view of the human being. Try to live into the 'directions' which sound in the verbs. Note that this verse, which aims to summarize what makes us human, starts with the middle.

ECCE HOMO
In the heart feeling weaves,
In the head thinking radiates,
In the limbs will surges.

Weaving of radiant Light,
Strength of the Weaving,
Light of the surging Strength,
This is man.

In dem Herzen webet Fühlen
In dem Haupte leuchtet Denken
In den Gliedern kraftet Wollen

Webendes Leuchten
Kraftendes Weben
Leuchtendes Kraften
Das ist der Mensch.

4.8 Four phases of human development

This section deals with prenatal development, with human embryology. We set ourselves two aims:
— The first is to give an example of the phenomenological, dynamic approach to the human being. We will deal with the central question, 'What is the human being involved in during the embryonic phase?'
— The second is to demonstrate the dynamics of the four *members* of the human being in embryonic development.

This section presupposes familiarity with the dynamic, comparative approach as explained in Chapter 3 and Sections 4.0 to 4.3.2.

Our focus is as follows: we will specifically look at the *somatogenesis* of the embryo as a whole, i.e. the process whereby the outer form of the body comes into existence and develops during the embryonic phase. We will thus limit ourselves to a specific aspect of this development; the formation of the different organs and organ systems *(organogenesis)* will remain outside our focus.

4.8.1 The four kingdoms

By way of introduction, we would like to give a brief sketch of what is at work in the four kingdoms of nature. This is a subject in itself, worthy of a much more thorough treatment than can be given here. This chapter will also describe the dynamics of the four members of the human being. These dynamics resemble the dynamics in the four main phases of *individual* human development — *ontogenesis,* which in turn are mirrored in the four large phases of the development of humanity *as a whole — phylogenesis.* We will start with a brief summary of the four phases of human development as they are distinguished in anthroposophy.

As an entry into these four phases, we should first recognize the dynamics of the four kingdoms of nature. Anthroposophy recognizes these as 'precipitations' of an evolutionary *process* which has taken place in the course of time. As stated before, every shape is the end product of a process and in every form one can 'read' how it came into being, by empathetically living into the formative processes. The gestures of the four kingdoms therefore bear the stamp of the underlying evolutionary process. This is also where the link to embryonic development lies, because the dynamics have a related signature. In the course of the chapter it will become clear how the study of the dynamics of the great phases of evolution deepens our understanding of embryonic development and vice versa.

Anthroposophy recognizes an increasing separation into the different members, taking place in the course of evolution. This goes for the whole Earth, nature, and humanity. The *mineral kingdom* is characterized by the presence of pure (dead) *matter.* The higher kingdoms (of plants, animals and humans) have *life* in addition to matter. To distinguish animals from plants, we recognize the presence of *soul.* Next to matter, life, and soul, the human being is permeated by *spirit.*

	physical body	etheric body	astral body	I
spirit				human being
soul			animal	
life		plants		
matter	mineral			

This chart presents only a rough indication, which will be elaborate.

The visible kingdoms are the result of the activity of formative forces.

The mineral kingdom

As stated above, the *mineral kingdom* is characterized by the presence of a physical or material body. Here, the spiritual levels which have induced the formation of the minerals, have as it were 'released' their 'product.' The spiritual entity which has formed the mineral does exist, but does not dwell inside the mineral. Of course the physical characteristics of the mineral do show us which spiritual being shaped this matter. In essence, minerals are pure form, occupying space. We are dealing with a formed end product. One could best describe it as an 'upper pole process' which has been carried all the way to the end (see Section 4.7.2). In that sense matter can be compared to an organism which has died. The members which were shaping it have 'left it alone'; shaped matter (mineral kingdom) is all that remains. In what is left, only the laws of matter, of physics and mechanics, rule. In anthroposophical terms, the mineral 'only' has a physical body. Note that the concept 'physical body' is not totally synonymous with the concept 'material body.' By physical body we mean that body which is only subject to the laws of lifeless nature. In the present phase of Earth development, those are the laws of matter.

The plant kingdom

We look upon the plant as a living being. In anthroposophical terms this means that there is an etheric body. In this kingdom, matter is not only subject to the material laws of physics and mechanics; it partakes in a higher level, namely that of a living organism. In contrast to minerals, time plays a part in the living plant organism. The plant also interacts with its surroundings, which is an interaction in the sense of metabolism. The ether body is sometimes described as a *time body* or *body of formative forces*. Having a physical body, the plant is of course also subject to, say, the law of gravity, but in essence it strives against these laws. The apple falls from the tree because of its material character; it grows and ripens on the tree because of the life forces.

The animal kingdom

The plant organism is characterized by life; the animal organism has an additional dimension or level, in that living matter is *ensouled.* In contrast to the plant, the animal has an inner life which can interact with the environment. The plant certainly does have a form of 'behaviour,' but that is expressed in its morphological outer shape. The animal has the possibility to behave by moving that outer shape. With animals, we can begin to speak of perception and consciousness. In anthroposophical terms, the astral body is what distinguishes animal from plant. One can know this new dimension from the whole complex of instincts, behaviour, and actions which animals present. One also speaks of *sentient* body, or *soul* body. The metabolism of the animal organism becomes dominated by *catabolism,* which is an expression o the fact that soul processes, perception, and consciousness cost energy an lead to the breaking down of 'life.' The ether body, by contrast is *anabolic* because it is permeated by vital forces which build up.

The human being

Anthroposophy speaks of the incarnation of the individual, who, like the animal, has this inner world of instincts, sensations and experiences, but can also face them and become aware of them. Self-awareness and independence are hallmarks of the *I.*

This summary introduction to the anthroposophical view of the four kingdoms of nature can never do justice to the complexity of the subject but it is one way to enter into the dynamics of the four members. There are several ways to read the signature of the four kingdoms. One of them is the approach which starts with the *four elements* of earth, water, air, and warmth (see Chapter 7). We can connect the mineral kingdom with earth,

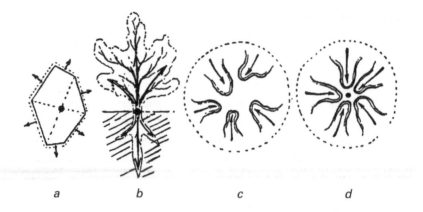

Figure 4.9. In these illustrations, the basic directions which the four natural kingdoms have in relation to space are represented. These are respectively: Centre and periphery; Outer and inner; Direction out from the self; Direction towards the self. a. Crystal; b. Plant; c. Animal; d. Human being. Notice the reversal of direction and the polarity between plant and animal. Derived from O.J. Hartmann.[9]

the plant kingdom with water, the animal kingdom with air, and the human being with warmth. Students are referred to this as a topic of independent study.

Our starting point in this section will be the approach of O.J. Hartmann (see bibliography). He describes the relationship of the 'organism' (insofar as one can speak of an organism in the case of minerals) to its surroundings and expresses that in the relationship between *centre* (point) and *periphery*. Figure 4.9 is from Hartmann and to begin with, we propose that the reader try to meditatively feel into the dynamics of the four kingdoms represented here.

The schematic representations of Figure 4.9 characterize the *directions* of the four natural kingdoms with regard to the relationship of periphery to centre. We intend to elaborate on these four directions and elucidate them further in the course of this chapter. We are dealing here with directional processes and dynamic principles which are characteristic of the four natural kingdoms and distinguish them from one another. The recognition of these dynamics will enable us to get to know the gestures of the four natural kingdoms.

For the considerations below, it is important not to see the four members as 'stacked on top of one another,' either in the course of evolution or in the sequence mineral, plant, animal, human being. It is important to stress that the dynamics — 'direction' in Hartmann's terminology — of one level is opposite to the dynamics of the next one up. So the dynamics of the plant do not come out of the mineral; they are not a continuation or 'more of the same.' A new principle manifests in the plant which stands in direct opposition to the mineral. One could think here of entropy (the striving of dead matter to reach the lowest energy level), and the contrasting striving of the plant to reach a higher level of energy. The ether body is not a product of the level below, which is the physical body, but stands in opposition to it in a sense. Hartman expresses this in his chart of the dynamics of the various directions. With the mineral, the point is the physical centre. Growth and expansion come about by repeating that point. Space is filled with more and more particles (points) which are as many physical repetitions of the same. L.F.C. Mees refers to this kind of 'growing' as accruing, or adding on, whereas the plant, by contrast, grows out from a starting point, which is the seed. It does not come about through physical repetitions of the initial point, but through the metamorphosis of the initial point, repeated *in the course of time.* There's no such thing as a plant particle which repeats itself and has one form. This also helps us to understand that the animal is not a continuation of the plant. Once again, we can speak of opposition.

As noted above, the animal distinguishes itself by the presence of an inner life, which we could simply call 'inside.' This should not be taken only in the anatomical sense (the inner world of the organs) but also in a psychological sense; the animal has an 'inside,' which gives it independence from the world around it. Instead of growing out as the plant does, one could speak of growing *in.* This happens literally in the embryo (gastrulation), which distinguishes it from the seed. Plant and animal, *etheric* and *astral,* form a polarity; they are 'opposite in direction' Hartmann would say.

In the human being, this 'inside' further acquires a centre, serving as a point of orientation for the inside. In contrast to the starting point of the crystal, that point is not physical, but spiritual. That does not mean it cannot be perceived; everybody is familiar with the *core experience* of the I in the human being. So once again one can speak of an opposition. The animal's inner life is 'undirected,' the human being has a centre towards which the inner life orients itself. The same principle applies as before: the human being is not a continuation of an animal principle. Something different takes the stage. Self-awareness presupposes an object (the self) which one becomes aware of; it is not the product of awareness.

So much for the first general characteristics of the four natural kingdoms and their dynamics, or 'directions.' Before we go on to look at the dynamics of the human embryo in order to deepen the highly summary observations given above, we insert an exercise for the reader to consider, and a methodological remark.

Assignment 11
The chart below contains key words relating to the four kingdoms of nature. They are partly from this text, and are partly inspired by the work of O.J. Hartmann and L.F.C. Mees. Going down, they try to characterize gesture and dynamics of the physical body, the etheric body, the astral body and the I respectively. Try to live into the indications and also connect them both horizontally and vertically.

MINERAL	PLANT	ANIMAL	HUMAN BEING
dead (body)	life	soul	spirit
grow on (= accrue, add on)	grow out	grow in	grow out of
...	extent (exterior)	content (interior)	...
maintain self	form self	feel self	know self

Methodological note
The problem of finding words for observations such as these has been remarked on before, in Section 4.2.4. There are many ways to indicate dynamics or gesture, say, of 'the plant,' or 'the etheric.' Each describes a different aspect of the dynamics. It is practically impossible to find universal concepts for the gesture of the mineral world as a whole, or to indicate what lives in plants. The feeling one gets, which we called 'treading water' in Section 4.2.4, is literally one of losing the ground under one's feet, but it belongs with the territory. It is inherent to the conceptual level which one enters, namely the level of gesture.

4.8.2 Our mineral nature

Figure 4.10 depicts human embryonic development in the first week. The fourth drawing in the top row represents the *morula* stage which under normal circumstances is reached around the third day after conception. The last drawing (right below) depicts the situation just before or during *nidation* or *implantation*. This is the *blastula* stage. All this takes place during the first week of human development.

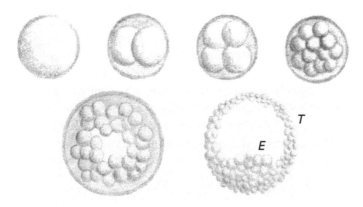

Figure 4.10. Stages during the first week of embryonic development, going from zygote (top left) to blastula (bottom right). E = embryoblast. T = tro-phoblast.

It is very important to realize that the last two drawings are not in scale with the first four; they are considerably enlarged. In reality there is no increase in mass or volume during the whole of the first week. It is characteristic for this first phase that all cell divisions occur within the mass of cytoplasm given with the *zygote* (fertilized egg cell). This finds expression in the word *cleavage* which is sometimes used for segmentation. There is as yet no growth, otherwise so characteristic for a living organism. The *zona pellucida* which surrounds the egg cell only dissolves in the last phase of the first week. Only from that moment will the embryo begin to grow. As stated, during the first week all cell division takes place within the fertilized egg cell. After about three days the stage of the 16-cell *morula* is reached, and after five to six days the embryo has been divided into about 100–120 smaller cells *(blastula)*.

The total process has the character of a sub*division. In other words: The* whole *zygote splits into ever smaller* parts.

Remembering what has been said about conception in Secton 4.2, we could postulate that the egg cell after conception behaves like a sperm cell. For example, immediately after fertilization, the zona pellucida undergoes a change. The 'open,' communicating character of the egg cell turns into 'closed off' and inaccessible. The metabolic character of the egg cell disappears and it becomes a separate space, just like the sperm cell. It is no longer open to its surroundings. As a 'result,' we see cell divisions and segmentation. We begin to see even more 'sperm cellness,' because every new cell means another nucleus, more DNA and also more cell membranes. At the same time there is a loss of inner malleability, which used to distinguish the egg cell from the sperm cell, and an increase in *structure.* We could 'prove' this as follows. Whereas the egg cell was vulnerable and hard to manipulate, a morula can easily be frozen with state-of-the-art technology; at least it is not as hard as freezing an egg cell. Was this not a typical trait of the sperm cell? The relationship of the nucleus to the cytoplasm slowly goes in the direction of what typified the sperm cell. One could formulate it as follows: what was still *outside* the egg cell before conception — and had its physical representative in the sperm cells — now appears as process *inside* the fertilized egg cell. It is a bit like an island; it gives the impression of a 'spaceship' which floats in the Fallopian tube and the uterus without having any particular metabolic exchange with the environment. In a sense the fertilized egg cell slowly dies; it begins to show characteristics of death and goes towards the form-pole. Some cells in the centre even die (lysis), and a space with fluid is created (blastula stage).

We can imagine how such a process, if carried to the end, would be final. Predictably, development would come to a halt if there were more subdivisions, and the conceptus would change into a mass of DNA (like a sperm cell). Without the impulse of a new principle, development would stop here, which it actually does in many cases (modern estimates mention 30 to 50 percent of fertilized egg cells). Nidation does not occur, or is not sufficiently successful, and with the next menstruation the remainders of the embryo are 'removed.' Further on in this chapter we will discuss the new impulse which becomes visible in the embryo when nidation is successful. It is important to note here that this represents a critical stage. If the development of the first week were to continue in the same way, there would be stagnation.

What speaks to us in the dynamics of this first phase of embryonic development? We are clearly dealing with a living entity. The fertilized egg cell is not just one cell, but an organism consisting of one cell. The morula and blastula are the next manifestations of the living organism which is the human embryo. It is a living organism, but shows more and more signs of death. Can we see tendencies of the mineral here?

Something which supports this is the fact that this phase always lasts a week, both in mammals and the human being.* We reiterate: the phase up to the implantation *(blastula)* stage always lasts 'a week' *regardless of the total time of the pregnancy!* This total time can be twenty-one days for a mouse, twenty-one months for an elephant, or nine months for a human being. There even are animals, such as deer, in which development starts right after fertilization, reaches the blastula stage, but then halts in a kind of hibernation. This stagnation lasts from mating season until implantation is continued in the spring! All this goes to illustrate that *time is not there yet* in this first one week. Did we not just recognize time as a hallmark of life? It seems as if this stage, in which the embryo is floating like a 'spaceship,' is deprived of life, like a mineral. Of course this is not correct if it is taken literally (the blastula is after all a living organism), but the observation is correct, when it is understood in terms of gesture, or as a signature. Remembering how Hartmann describes the characteristics of the minerals, it is easy to see how the beginning of the process can be described as a splitting into a number of the same elements. Is that not a trait of the mineral, this being subdivided into identical particles, this repetition? We also see the verb 'maintaining' of the chart borne out: the whole is kept from falling apart.

If we return for a moment to the chart with Hartmann's drawings of Figure 4.9, we can say that the morula shows the gesture of the 'crystal'; it has a mineral character in that it is like a point in space, a particle which repeats itself. The aforementioned 'accrual' is a repetition in space of the same thing. We see the same dynamics in the zygote when it splits into equal segments, albeit in a reverse sense, so to speak.

If we read this gesture correctly, it is plausible that the moment of nidation represents a break. After all, something new has to happen if it is to continue. This break could thus be compared to the chasm existing between dead and alive in the mineral and plant, as explained in Section 4.8.1. There we postulated that life does not come from death, and that the plant is not a continuation of the mineral. Here we see something similar, a turning point which marks the transition to a new principle in the development of the embryo. The next sequel in the story of the embryo does not follow straight from the first week. Before going on to elucidate the next stage in human development, we insert a few remarks about the concept of differentiation.

---

*   We should realize that a week is a variable concept in biology. In human beings it is known that nidation can occur after five days in some cases, in other cases only after eight to nine days.

Differentiation

The last drawing of Figure 4.10 shows that more has taken place than a mere splitting into equal parts. It is highly likely that the 16-cell stage still contains equal cells, but just before implantation a differentiation between 'inside' and 'outside' has formed within the population of about 100–120 cells; there is a centre and a periphery. The whole of the conceptus has separated into an *embryoblast* in the centre, containing about 10 cells, and a *trophoblast* in the periphery, containing about 100 cells, which forms a mantle around it. Between the two, cell fluid has accumulated, partly osmotically drawn in from the surroundings, partly the residue of cells which have died.

This is an excellent example of the process which characterizes the (embryonic) development of all organisms: *differentiation*. We are used to thinking that organisms are built up out of separate parts, so we think in terms of the whole being the sum of it parts, and with those parts, their characteristics. This way of thinking is deeply anchored in all of us; embryonic development serves as a constant reminder that this thinking model is not true to life. Ever and again, one sees how the *whole* splits into *parts*. There is an endless series of differentiations, following one another in the course of time, creating the organs and the different parts of the body. It is never the other way round!

An anatomist starts from the separate parts and thinks in terms of building blocks, out of which the human being is assembled. But even in anatomy we once started 'at the other end,' and separated the whole into parts. Think of the Greek roots *ana-temnein,* to cut into separated parts; compare also the word *ana-lysis.* In our *thoughts,* we then put those parts together. It should be stressed once again that this is a *mental picture,* not actual fact. In the reality of life, the *undivided entity* comes first; *division* follows. The embryologist Blechschmidt hits the nail on the head when he says that the 'law of the preservation of the individuality' applies to the embryo. One might question the word individuality, but the tenor is clear. 'It is the *appearance* which changes, not the *essence,'* he says. In the desert of modern-day thought-life, it is the embryo which cries out that *wholeness* comes first in living nature.

4.8.3. Our plant nature

After the phase of the first week the unity of the zygote has developed into a duality: the *embryoblast* and the *trophoblast* as an inside and an outside. It would be better to speak of a centre and a periphery for the embryoblast and trophoblast. We will now go on to discuss the next phase, using Figures 4.11 and 4.12.

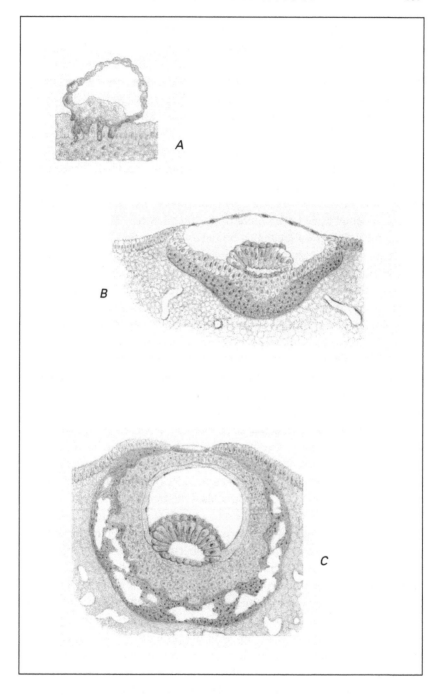

Figure 4.11. Stages of human embryonic development. A. Directly after
nidation; B. Day 7/8; C. Day 9/10. All drawings are in the same scale.

In the days that follow, the development of the embryo undergoes a radical change in character and dynamism (the 'direction,' in Hartmann's terminology). The periphery especially begins to show a completely different development. A huge activity in growth and metabolism manifests there. The trophoblast expands enormously. The activity of cell division is so vehement that cells on the outside even lose their structure and merge into a kind of cell-syncytium (the syncytiotrophoblast). It all even makes an almost malignant impression, because the trophoblast transgresses its boundaries, entering the maternal tissue. With many enzymes the endometrial tissue of the mother is 'digested' and the embryo nestles further and further into the mucous membrane of the uterus. The character of transgression is emphasized even more by the fact that the maternal organism puts up no defences by creating a boundary: after a few days the embryo even 'eats into' the maternal blood vessels. The embryo, however, reaches out even further into the periphery, beyond the anatomical boundaries of the syncytiotrophoblast! The trophoblast excretes quantities of hormones which may be tiny (best-known is the HCG, the hormone of pregnancy), but which do have enormous consequences in the far periphery. The whole maternal organism is influenced by them and brought into such a state that it can accept the new organism, which is in fact foreign to it. It seems as if the basic gesture of pregnancy is one of relinquishing the boundaries of identity and immunity, which the maternal organism does in order to give the embryo room to nestle and expand within it.

This trophoblast is much more than the anatomical externals. Its dynamic gesture is one of striving outwards, being without boundaries, of growing beyond itself. It flows out and merges with its surroundings, while at the same time showing characteristics of taking root and attaching. One could rightly call the trophoblast the outer body of the embryo. The outside is where it interacts with its surroundings, where it has metabolism and growth, and where it expands. In the outer body the embryo grows and lives, reaching from centre to periphery. The change from the first week is evident. We have gone from a state of being a closed off 'spaceship' to a growing, expanding and interacting organism. Do we not come upon the same concepts here which were used in Section 4.2.1 to characterize the ovum? Do we not see once again how a 'cosmic pole' is at work? Once again we meet up with the problem of finding adequate words; there are many ways to describe the gesture which one can experience here. The gesture comes out more clearly when one takes the centre of the embryo into consideration. The *embryoblast* does show changes, but the dynamics are totally different. What occurs is a differentiation into (pre-)*ectoderm* and (pre-)*endoderm,* a polarity which we will not go into here. The growth, however, and the relationship to the periphery is entirely different from that of the trophoblast. What we see here is slow growth with a slight differentiation, but not the loss of form and the expansion of the trophoblast. The dynamics are not directed outwards; rather, they turn away from that and the amniotic cavity comes into being, and thereby the bilaminar germinal disk loosens itself from the trophoblast.

An enormous internal tension now arises in the embryo. On the one hand there is the periphery (the trophoblast) striving outwards, on the other hand there is the centre (the embryoblast), directed inwards. This tendency continues into the second week, even though the parts change and new differentiations change the details. Inside and outside of the embryoblast and the trophoblast have now become manifest as *endocyst* (inner egg) and *ectocyst* (outer egg). Endocyst denotes the complex comprising the amniotic cavity, the yolk sac, and the bilaminar germinal disk; ectocyst denotes the trophoblast, which in the meantime has differentiated further. Even though the parts have changed, the dynamics are unmistakably the same. The embryo is striving outwards during the second week; it *grows out continually.* The core of the embryo — the bilaminar germinal disk of ectoderm and endoderm — is the *centre around which everything revolves.* The periphery predominates in the embryo; it does not *con*tain, but '*ex*tains.' It reaches outwards so strongly, stretching to form roots in the outer world, that the centre stays considerably behind in growth. A whole new space comes into being, lying between the expanding ectocyst and the endocyst which stays behind. A cavity comes into existence which mediates and creates space, called the chorionic cavity. The mesoderm which lines this cavity (see Figure 4.12) forms a *body stalk,* which maintains the connection between 'outer' and 'inner.'

Extrapolating this gesture further, a being would come into existence only consisting of 'outside.' Such beings actually do exist, but before dealing with them we first return to the gesture of this second week. The dynamics manifesting here are the polar opposite of those of the first week! At that point the predominating tendency was all that characterizes space, lack of growth, division, splitting into parts and turning in. The embryo of the second week is striving outwards, is reaching beyond. It loses the compactness of the morula. It also begins to grow in the way we are used to seeing in living creatures: there is increase of volume and also metabolism. This embryo does have a centre, but it is no more than a starting point for peripheral striving. Everything seems to revolve around the centre (the germinal disk, or embryonic disk), like a wheel around an axis.

In the meantime the factor of *time* has become fully present in the development. With metamorphosis, differentiation and growth going on, the embryo has begun to partake in time; it now shows the dynamics of life. Referring back to Hartmann's chart in Fig. 4.9, the dynamics may be

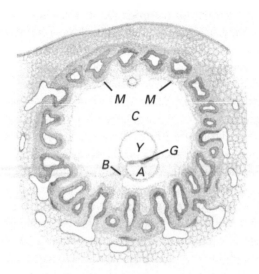

Figure 4.12. Two week old human embryo. Note this figure is to a smaller scale than Figure 4.11. A amniotic cavity; Y yolk sac; G germinal disk; C chorionic cavity; B body stalk; M mesoderm.

clear: this embryo shows the characteristics of the plant gesture, which is more outward moving. This could be called the 'outward human.' A conclusion such as this one is only revealed when one takes the phenomenological approach. We can characterize how plants extend themselves fully to the world around them; they offer themselves and open up, having little possibility therefore to emancipate themselves from their surroundings. Their morphology shows this. The roots extend and open up completely to the earth, while leaves and flowers do the same towards the atmosphere, towards air, light and warmth. Plants are so open that they are also basically defenceless, and completely given over to influences from the outside. We can put a plant in a greenhouse, where it will respond to any artificial influences. The gesture of opening up can not only be seen in its morphology, in branching out and unfolding towards the periphery, but also in its physiology. The plant completely surrenders to its surroundings and has practically no way to close itself off from influences coming towards it. The plant is also usually bound to the seasons, it is being lived by the rhythm of the year. So one could say that the plant is more 'out there' than 'here,' in itself. Plants are creatures of openness.

When one has lived into Figure 4.9b, and lives into the gesture of the embryo during the second week with equal empathy, one becomes aware of this tendency to be 'out there'; this being is obviously not fully present yet here on earth. Added to this, one can observe that the bilaminar germinal disk of the second week is not only the centre around which everything revolves, but is flat and two-dimensional in appearance. At this stage the embryo is no more than two surfaces meeting, which are the two epithelia. So one cannot yet speak of 'content,' especially when we know that there is as yet no mesoderm, i.e. the dimension of tissue and filling is still missing. Being two-dimensional, the flat bilaminate germ only has outside, periphery, surroundings. Its 'direction' goes from centre to periphery. Key words to characterize the human being in the second week are thus: extending, planar, and plant-like.

One could well imagine that if this tendency were to continue unabated, development would stagnate and come to a halt. We met something similar when we looked at nidation. If the mineral tendency that seemed to manifest in the first week had continued, further development would not have been possible. Nidation marks a turnaround in the direction of the development and the gesture of growth. To a certain extent, nidation is thus a moment of crisis, and many embryos do not 'make it.' Is there a similar moment for the embryo in the second week? Living into the dynamics of the strong expansion outside the central body, one can sense the danger which threatens this embryo. The tension which exists between the endocyst and the ectocyst threatens to become a rift. It is also understandable biologically because the 'outside' dwells in optimal feeding conditions for growth and expansion — in the mother's mucous membrane, whereas the inside remains more and more behind and lacks the source of nourishment. At the end of the second week or the beginning of the third, a chorionic cavity has come into being with tissue of a kind that mediates, connects, but also creates space. It connects the two dimensions through a body stalk, which is mesoderm. What would we get if this tendency were to continue? The so-called *hydatidiform mole* clearly shows that. Technically, we can still speak of pregnancy because through hormones the extended 'outer body' has been created and the amniotic sac is visible on an echogram (the later manifestation of the outer body). There is no heart, however, no real embryo, no 'inside' body. The thread is broken; the embryo only has an outside, and there is no human being 'here.' Just as the plant has no 'self' or soul, but only a physical and etheric body, the hydatidiform mole has not made it 'here,' but it remains out 'there.'

The essential gesture of the second week becomes more and more pronounced. The word 'plant-man' might give a partial indication of the character of the conceptus at this stage. One could also say that the embryo manifests the signature and tendencies of the *etheric*. This word denotes the life principle, which is at work wherever we see growth and metabolism, form being dissolved, opening out to the periphery and inviting or even forcing matter to change towards a higher level. The first week of the embryo bore the marks of the physical, the mineral, showing tendencies of hardening, densification and a centripetal direction; in the second week we see the opposite: opening, centrifugal motion towards the periphery.

This whole impression is reinforced by something else we can observe in the second week. We can see a special trait which will be lost afterwards, which is that it can still be divided; up to and even in the second week identical twins can still come into existence. After that the embryo cannot be divided anymore; there is only a short span of time during which a Siamese twin can come into being as an in-between phase. Cannot be divided anymore: Is that not literally *in-dividual?* The embryo is not yet individual in the plant phase. Could one speak of two human individuals within one body in the case of identical twins? In our sketch of the four natural kingdoms we indicated how we can only begin to speak of the soul in the animal kingdom. That makes it plausible that something else still has to be added for embryonic development to continue.

Rudolf Steiner indicates that the human being 'is not there yet' in this early embryonic phase, but moves around the physical kernel and targets the centre from the periphery. He describes this from the vantage point of supersensory perception. The embryo of the second week certainly makes that impression of 'not being here yet.' This could even mean that Rudolf Steiner indicates something like the existence of a 'pre-embryo,' decades before regular embryologists came up with the same idea (incidentally, using much more questionable criteria). The big difference is that regular biologists conclude that the human being 'is not there yet' — a conclusion with vast ethical consequences! — whereas Steiner speaks of the individual being definitely present, but reaching out from another dimension to its physical kernel; the human being is present, but not yet 'here.'

When *does* the human being 'arrive' more? In order to tackle that question, we need to focus on the next phase.

Before taking the next step, we first need to make an observation using Figure 4.9. The animal stands in polar opposition to the plant. The animal does have inner life, something which the plant does not have. What is the fundamental difference between a *seed,* the starting point of plant development, and the *embryo,* the starting point of animal development? The seed *grows out* — from the seed comes a leaf and the beginning of roots, and they both unfold out into the periphery — whereas the embryo *grows in* (gastrulation) and unfolds the world of the organs within. The plant lacks that inside dimension. The root system 'becomes' intestinal surface; the crown of leaves 'becomes' the bronchial tree; rooting in the earth (the world around) 'becomes' independent movement in relation to the surroundings.

Emancipation goes further: an inner environment begins, relatively independent from outside influences. The animal's temperature differs from that
of the surroundings; the pace of life no longer follows the rhythm of the
year. During animal evolution, this tendency is developed and perfected further and further. More about that later. These observations may suffice for
now to point out that the animal chooses to go in a new and different direction. The animal is not a further developed plant, it is the opposite of a plant.
Thus begins the process of emancipation and *individuation*.

4.8.4 Our animal nature

Once again, embryonic development approaches a critical moment.
Perpetuation of the developmental dynamics which characterized the
embryo during the second week, would lead to a 'hydatidiform mole', an
'exterior human being.' If that were the case, the tie between outer and
inner would rupture; the central point on the inside — the germinal disk —
would disengage from the outside and atrophy. From the polarity between
plant and animal which we studied in the paragraphs above, one could
almost predict the turn that is about to occur in the embryonic dynamics. A
look ahead shows significant developments at the end of the third week.
The embryonic disk is still flat, but there is a crucial difference. Between
the ectoderm and the endoderm — the aforementioned two epithelia, a
combination which Blechschmidt calls *Grenzgewebe,* border tissue — an
intermediate layer appears, the *intra-embryonic mesoderm.* Blechschmidt
characterizes this as inner tissue, *Innengewebe.* The mesoderm is no border
area, no epithelium, but is a tissue with a third dimension. It creates space
and connects at the same time. So one could say that the trilaminate germinal disk, in contrast to the bilaminate germ, now has the new element of
'content.' Its predecessor only had surface and surroundings, the trilaminate embryo has inner content in addition to that. This mesoderm has
entered *into* the germinal disk, by growing *in* from the *primitive groove.*
That process started in the middle of the third week of embryonic development, as shown in Figure 4.13. We are obviously dealing with a radical
turn in direction. Where do these new dynamics originate?

When the chorionic cavity has formed at the end of the second week (see
Figure 4.12), the so-called extra-embryonic mesoderm covers the inside of
the ectocyst and the outside of the endocyst. The former is called *parietal
mesoderm,* the latter *visceral mesoderm.* The body stalk links the 'inner
body' (endocyst) with the 'outer body' (ectocyst). At the beginning of the
third week the first blood islands and blood vessels (capillaries) originate
inside this extra-embryonic mesoderm. The formation of blood vessels and
blood is the very first functional differentiation of the mesoderm. Within this

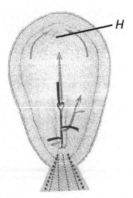

Figure 4.13. Germinal disk in the third week, seen dorsally. The arrows indicate the direction in which the inter-embryonic mesoderm grows. The body stalk (caudal end) has been drawn in. H origin of the heart.

very primitive system of blood vessels a hesitant circulation begins. This flow finds its 'cause' in the metabolic processes on the periphery of the embryo, the trophoblast (ectocyst). In the adult body the movement of fluids on a capillary level is also initiated by the life processes inside the tissues themselves; this is parallelled in the movement of the blood which takes pace in the third week of embryonic development, when it begins to flow from the periphery to the centre. After all, the activity of metabolic processes takes place in the periphery. The blood streams through the capillaries from the parietal mesoderm in the direction of the body stalk. By means of a variety of growing movements which we will leave out of consideration here, this body stalk has moved in the meantime to the caudal end* of the germinal disk (see Figures 4.12 and 4.13). This primordial blood streams towards the cranial end of the embryo, flowing alongside the 'flanks' of the germ disk, then dorsally along the amniotic cavity and ventrally along the yolk sac. There it cannot go any further and reaches the most central part of the embryonic body (see Figures 4.12 and 4.13).

Another reversal of direction arises in the embryo. Up to now growth was predominantly directed outward; at this point we see a first indication of 'circulation' going in a different direction. The blood flows from the metabolic periphery of the trophoblast to a central point, where it comes to a halt. The flow of blood turns around when it has arrived at this central point which lies cranially in the germinal disk. It flows back along other capillaries to the periphery of the trophoblast, where it goes back into the metabolic processes as tissue fluid. This point of reversal, where the flow comes to a

---

*   It is only at this point that the polarity cranial–caudal appears in the embryo. On the caudal side are the body stalk with the blood flowing to and fro, on the cranial side lies the future cardiogenic area.

standstill, turns, and acquires a rhythmical character, is the first indication of the origin of the heart. Here the first real centre arises in the embryo, which is different from the almost virtual, point-like centre of the second week around which everything revolved. By contrast, this is a real anatomical centre, which places itself *over against* the periphery of the outer body. It is the heart. The heart arises out of the circulation of the blood! As is so often the case, this approach places things in a different context, allowing one to gain a perspective which differs from current approaches. Movement is primary, the heart is *secondary*. First there is flow, and where this holds still, the form arises. There are good reasons to look upon the heart as the 'upper pole' of the blood circulation,* and the capillaries as the 'lower pole.' This is in accordance with the relationships existing within the whole of the embryo at this stage. The trophoblast on the outside is the lower pole, the heart with the germinal disk on the inside is the upper pole.

In every respect, the origin of the heart marks a turnaround of the dynamics within the embryo. As 'predicted' above, the developmental dynamics become more like those of the animal; now the direction goes from the outside to the inside, from periphery to centre; an inner world is formed over against the outer world. Biologically one can put it this way: the continuation of the inner body, which otherwise would have become detached from the periphery, is now guaranteed. Nutrition flows from the periphery back to the inner body. In the wake of the genesis of the heart area, we therefore see a large number of developmental processes which from now on have their starting point in the germinal disk. The most essential thing is that, starting from the caudal end of the embryo, inward growth starts. Through the primitive groove, ectoderm grows dorsally into the embryo and metamorphoses into mesoderm. The embryo ends its existence as a flat, two-layered disk 'without content,' becoming a three-dimensional entity because it now has real inner content in the shape of *intra*-embryonic mesoderm. All the impulses to form organs arise in this mesoderm. When one looks at the dynamics of the morphology of the heart within the embryo, this whole process is a model for the way all organs form. The impulse first arises in the periphery, then moves into the centre where it finally comes to rest, manifesting in the final shape of an organ. The developmental dynamics go from the periphery to the centre.

Halfway through the third week we can mark a new turning point in the

* Note that we speak of 'blood circulation' for lack of a better word. There is no closed circulatory system yet at this point. Blood is being 'produced' in the periphery, flows to the centre, whence it returns and is absorbed again as tissue fluid in the periphery. There is no closed capillary system. Only in the fourth week can one speak of a first placental circulation.

development. More and more clinical data have reinforced this in recent years. Up-to-date research shows that pregnancy is more frequently interrupted at this point than had hitherto been assumed. The 'missed abortion' is a clinical manifestation of the fact that the embryo has to take a hurdle at this point in its development. If there is no origin of the heart, followed by the formation of all the organs, the embryo will not survive this crisis. This is not without significance, as we will substantiate below. The processes after the third week do not follow in a straight line from the second week. This becomes even more poignant when one takes into consideration what Rudolf Steiner said about this phase from the standpoint of supersensory perception. At the beginning of the twentieth century, when orthodox science knew nothing yet about these stages of human development, he pointed repeatedly to a turnaround in human embryonic development 'around the seventeenth day.' He put it this way:

> Whereas the incarnating soul-spirit entity was more present *around* the physical kernel up to this point, the 'astral individuality' of the human being now incarnates into the physical kernel itself.

In other words, the human soul comes a step closer 'to the earth,' with the heart as the organ of incarnation! All this becomes even more coherent when we realize that the dynamics which arise 'around the seventeenth day' in the embryo are of an animal *(astral)* nature. Only now can we speak of a real inner entity which can stand over against the outside world and become independent. Does this not run exactly parallel to the dynamics which marked the division between plant and animal, as we discussed above? (Refer back to the chart in Fig. 4.9.)

4.8.5 Reading the gesture in evolution and embryonic development

We will now review the three phases, gestures, or directions we have covered so far. We started from the characteristics of the three natural kingdoms, that are akin to the dynamics of the physical, the etheric and the astral. In the description of the embryonic development of the human being we have so far described three phases, and more is to come concerning the third phase. The point is to find out in how far 'translating' the phenomena which characterize each of these three embryonic phases is helpful. Can we gauge whether we gain a fuller understanding of what is at work, when we cross-reference the essential dynamics to the characteristic signatures that can be 'read' in the natural kingdoms?

The physical body

The following nouns characterize physicality: compactness, three-dimensionality, death, mineral. To what extent do we recognize these traits in the human being at the morula stage? Imagine taking a round ball of clay in both hands. Feel how it rests in itself. Sense the coherence, the mass, and the gravitation. Compare your findings with the way Hartmann's chart gives expression to these qualities. To conclude, we could sum up as follows: The physical rests 'in itself.'

The etheric body

Imagine a kind of material which you can pull out towards the periphery and spread out, disperse. The being of the plant opens out to the periphery, and what is of a mineral nature in the plant is absorbed by forces of a higher level. Life counteracts the mineral, physical laws. Life works against gravity, and we now also see interaction with the surroundings (metabolism). We notice a parallel process in the embryo. The way it opens out and strives outward, nearly losing itself in the periphery, is matched by the 'selfless' way the plant relates to the environment.

The astral body

Life is broken down, a catabolic tendency appears. Inwardness is created which can hold its own against the outside and emancipate. A different state of consciousness arises in the animal. An inner environment has now been established, leading a life which is independent of the surroundings. It can move of its own accord and establish a relation to the environment.

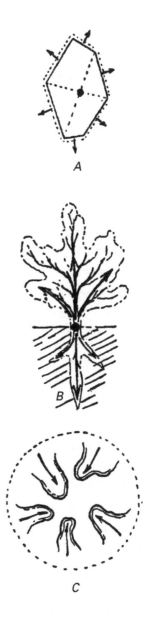

Figure 4.14.

Another thing that the dynamics of the three embryonic phases teaches us is that there is no even transition from one phase to the next. On the contrary, the dynamics of each subsequent phase do not come from the one which has gone before, but stand in opposition to it. The line of development is interrupted, there are marked transitions. Can those be recognized in the dynamics of the three natural kingdoms? Current biology does indicate transitional forms between death and life (think of viruses) and between plant and animal. However, the comparative approach clearly shows that one cannot think the plant as continuous from the animal, or of mineral as continuous from the plant. The etheric is not some sort of diluted materiality; a totally different principle is at work. The astral is not a further refinement of the etheric; it is a new quality. Seeing polarities alerts one to this. Assignment 12 is given as a suitable preliminary conclusion.

Assignment 12

Make a list of as many polarities between plant and animal as you can name. Do the same for dead matter and living creatures.
When you have done this, check whether the polarities you found also apply to the corresponding three phases in embryonic development, which we found to be akin to mineral, plant and animal.
Make another comparison, this time between a dead person, a sleeping person, and a waking person.

4.8.6. More on animal nature — emancipation and individuation

The trilaminate embryonic disk has only a preliminary independence. More is to come in terms of emancipation and individuation. It is still flat and very open. For example, the flanks make a smooth transition into the layers of tissue of the extra-embryonic cavities. The three layers flow into it as it were (see Figure 4.15a). The embryo obviously has a long way to go before it has truly become emancipated enough from the outer body of the mother to separate itself from it and live as an independent entity. At the tail end, the embryo is linked openly to the periphery through the body stalk. Steiner called this phase of human development *Paradiesmensch* (paradisal human being), indicating that this is only a first step towards emancipation from the surrounding world, with which the embryo is still connected quite naturally and openly. Is that not what the ancient story about paradise describes in pictures? Human beings had emancipated from their cosmic and divine origin, but 'were still linked to God.'

During the third, but especially the fourth week of human embryonic development, the process of delamination occurs, also known as 'folding.' Interestingly, the Germans call this same process *Abfaltung* (folding off). This folding process, characterized by *curving* movements marks significant progress in terms of emancipation. The flat trilaminate embryonic disk is folded into a somewhat *cylindrical* embryo, whereby the folds *roll around*. In ventrolateral direction, the ectoderm — and with it the initially dorsally positioned amniotic cavity — undergoes an enormous expansion in relation to the ventrally located yolk sack with its connected endoderm (see Figure 4.15). Apart from this so-called transverse folding, there is the longitudinal folding in craniocaudal direction (see Figure 4.16).

With the emergence of the embryo out of the two-dimensional plane (delamination means 'coming out of the plane'), we can now speak of a real, spatial outside and inside in an anatomical sense. The term ectoderm now comes into its own: what was behind (dorsal) in the flat disk is now outside. Consequently, what in the endoderm was ventral is now inside. It also becomes clear that the terms 'inner' and 'outer,' until now referring more to direction (Hartmann), or quality, now acquire anatomical meaning. One can easily live into the gesture. Drawing it is one way to do so. Better still, it can be imitated with the body, as outlined in Assignments 13 and 14.

Assignment 13
Stand upright and spread both arms out. Bend over, and at the same time bend your arms and bring your hands together. Check if and how your awareness of the surroundings and your own 'inner space' changes. Can this be put in terms of 'from extrovert to introvert'? From 'open' to 'closed'? Go back to your original position. Repeat this exercise a few times, doing it slowly.

Assignment 14
The embryo at this stage is kidney shaped. See, for example, Figures 4.16 and 4.18. Try to find as many kidney forms as you can in nature, the environment, but also in the world of the organs. To what extent is the relationship between outer and inner the same as it is in the embryo? Or is the gesture of closing off (outer, ectoderm) and streaming in (inner, endoderm) recognizable as a polarity, just as it is in the embryo?

The motion which the embryo performs here is a further continuation of the gesture which characterizes the turnaround of the seventeenth day. The *animal/astral* gesture is further completed here. The embryo emancipates still further from the periphery. It is important to realize that these are *growth* movements, not muscle movements. The formative process of the whole body is involved. It is *somatogenesis*. A growing gesture such as this is a necessary precondition in order to form a human body. One can even enter into the movement and continue it up to the point where one notices that one 'gathers up' the inner body as it were; this 'creasing,' one can feel, has the inherent danger of cutting off. If this process were to be brought to full completion on all sides (cranio-caudal, left-right), it would surround the whole embryo with amniotic cavity and ectoderm, blocking off the nourishment from the periphery and the placenta, which is the outer body.

It does not go that far *yet!* Because there is one place where the inner body is not completely closed off, remaining open until birth. That place is the navel. It is around the navel that two elements gather, from the tail end and the cranial end. These two elements are the body stalk and the heart. Consulting an embryology book to follow the process in the craniocaudal direction will lead to the logical conclusion that there has to be a concomitant process whereby the heart 'descends.' This is the so-called *descensus cordis:* as the heart and the cranial top end of the embryo exchange places, the heart moves in the direction of the navel. On the other side, the body stalk 'rises' from caudal to ventral, and only now can it really be called *umbilical cord.* And it is through this that communication between the inner body and the outer body is safeguarded. At least for the time being.

We are dealing here with the gesture of growth, as we have stressed before. One can try to follow the tendency of this growth and think ahead to the moment of *birth*. At birth the umbilical cord is definitely (anatomically and physically) cut. One could not think of a more definitive physiological emancipation! The German language calls delivery *Entbindung.* Literally, this means 'unbinding,' so what was bound is now unbound. One could safely say that the dynamics of this process already start in the fourth or fifth week. Morphologically, these dynamics are repeated at birth. The curving processes by which the embryo creates an inner world, with all the organs, could be seen as the further consequences of the *astral* impulse to which the embryo is subjected. This is highly characteristic of our animal nature.

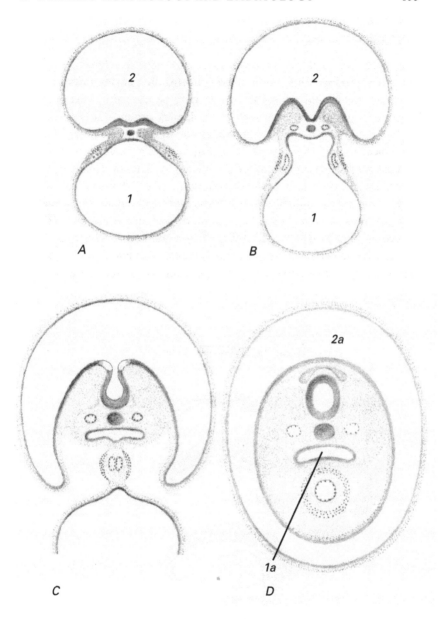

Figure 4.15. Diagram of transverse folding in the embryo during delamination. The dorsal side is up, showing the amniotic cavity (2), the ventral side is down showing the yolk sack (1). Figure A depicts the trilaminate embryonic disk before the folding process. Figure D depicts the completed folding process, where the folds have rolled around to create a roughly cylindrical embryo. Now the ectoderm is outside, surrounded by the amniotic cavity (2a), and the endoderm is inside, having formed the wall of the primal intestinal tube (1a).

4.8.7 What's next?

One more step needs to be taken to complement the dynamics of the embryonic process. This fourth phase concerns the transition from animal to human. Or should we speak of a turning point again? This question brings us right into the present-day polemics around the question of whether the human being is an animal or not. Recalling the Figure 4.9, we can expect to find the gesture of opposition again between animal and human. In order to understand this, we need to distinguish between *self-awareness* and awareness of the *surroundings*. In our deliberations above, we have seen how animal (astral) emancipation simultaneously enables consciousness to arise. With the creation of an inner world over against the surrounding world, the possibility of *awareness* arises: the outer world can now be perceived. This is easy to imagine. The condition for having this awareness and perception is separation. A similar thing can be

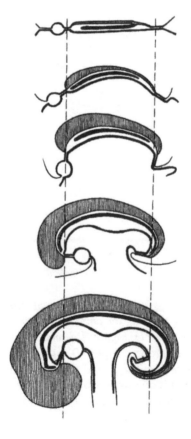

Figure 4.16

observed in the dynamics and the morphology of the embryo which we have discussed. Hartmann shows in Figure 4.9 how the human being takes a fundamentally new turn. The new direction could be described as finding a *standpoint* towards one's own inner world, i.e. all one's experiences and feelings. The word standpoint could be taken almost literally here. Hence the point at the centre of the human diagram in Hartmann's chart. We can experience a centre in ourselves which is conscious of the fact that we are beings with a consciousness.

Teilhard de Chardin put it this way: *'An animal knows, but a human being knows that he knows.'* One could follow up on this saying with numerous additions, such as, 'An animal thinks, but a human being knows that he thinks; an animal feels, but ... etc. '. Anthroposophy points to the *I* in the human being with this. This is the element that is capable of commenting on itself, or, in other words, that can stand over against itself. That what is meant with the 'point' in the figure, the stand-point.

Is this the new direction we were talking about? If one lives into the astral gesture of curvature of Assignment 13 once again, one can experience that that is finite. It finds its completion in a state of being closed off. The movement of delamination ends in a close circle with an inner space. What movement stands in opposition to that and liberates us from this state? The Dutch physician L.F.C. Mees characterized the animal with the words grow *in* and the human being with grow *out of.* What movement gets *out of* 'the astral'?

The corresponding morphodynamics are *stretching,* or *getting up.* The upright position is a uniquely human achievement. Although this topic is too large to be covered fully in this chapter, this statement is supported by everything that is written about evolution. When we talk about uprightness here, we do not mean being a biped. Human beings share this feature with penguins and kangaroos, for example. What is meant here is that the head balances on the trunk which in turn balances *above* the lower extremities. The centre of gravity of the trunk above the hip joint is not a little bit in front, as is the case with apes, or straddling, as is the case with kangaroos. In order to acquire this position, the necessary bodily conditions have to be met. Therefore one can anticipate a process of stretching in the course of *somatogenesis* during embryonic development. When we discussed the birth process, we saw how this was anticipated in the curving of the fourth or fifth week of embryonic development. We recognized a similar tendency in growth, and characterized this as becoming 'unbound,' a process of freeing. Similarly, the tendency towards uprightness, which distinguishes the human being from the animal, has been anticipated in an embryonic gesture. The curving and pursing gesture, with the corresponding organ formation and the further emancipation of

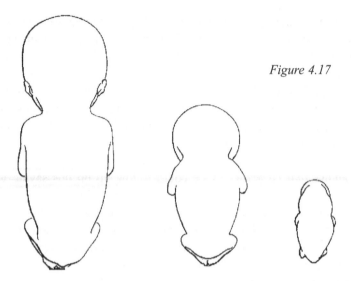

Figure 4.17

the amniotic cavity and the umbilical cord, continues into the third month. Simultaneously, the stretching gesture, the upright tendency which is so typical of the human being, already begins to manifest in the fifth week.

During the process of stretching, the head and the pelvis emancipate out of the round/oval entity which the embryo still is in the fourth week. Gradually, the neck and trunk emerge (Figure 4.17). The side view (Figure 4.18) shows this even more clearly. Both head and pelvis come 'out.' The head grows cranially away from the trunk, whereby the neck is formed, the pelvis 'turns' caudally 'away' from the trunk and comes to lie *under* it, whereby the waist is formed. This constitutes the visible stretching. The impulse to this is given from the inside by the elongation of the brain, whereby the characteristic flexures between the different parts of the brain come into existence. This is typical for the human being. With it, the development of the brain frees itself spatially, and is no longer a continuation of the trunk axis. The whole process could be described as *un*-folding; the rolled up embryo opens out. The process proceeds from the cranium starting from the brain, then the whole head, followed by the neck. Then comes the formation of the waist and the 'emancipation' of the pelvis from the trunk.

Is it not remarkable how this *craniocaudal gradient* (predominant in many embryonic processes) is repeated in postnatal motor development? The head goes up first with the maturation of the primary senses, then the baby sits up, the pelvis is turned under the trunk, and standing up comes last. Once again, it is as if the embryonic morphological development *(somatogenesis)* was 'practice' for physiological functional development after birth. Once the head and the pelvis have turned out of the curvature,

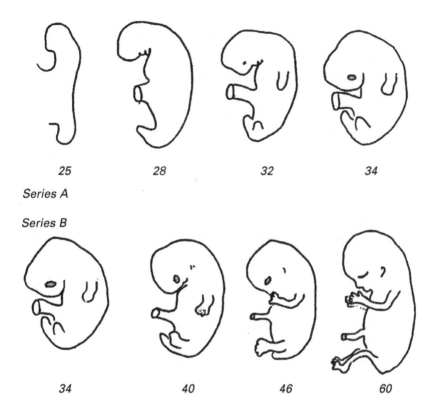

25   28   32   34

Series A

Series B

34   40   46   60

the necessary prerequisites have been created for the upright position of the human being.

What is going on is more than stretching, however. A polarity begins to develop between the head on one side and the extremities on the other. The emancipating tendency of the animal (astral) process is apparently preserved in the head. This is actually a condition for proper functioning of this 'pole' in the human being (see Section 4.7). Over against this the extremities begin to develop. Up to now this predisposition was as good as absent in the embryo. At the same time that the stretching process is happening in the head (upper pole), the extremities (radii) are streaming out into the periphery. It is as if the human figure polarizes between closure ('here'), namely the head, and openness ('there'), namely the extremities. One does not have to try all that hard to recognize the two poles of the polarity in the gestures of the head and the extremities (see Section 4.7). Stretching and walking upright are likewise a picture of a balance between these polar tendencies: turned towards or away from the earth. This represents yet another manifestation of the polarity of the radius vs. sphere, which we dealt with when we discussed conception.

Assignment 15
Take your head in your hands and sense how much 'inside' there is. Shift your consciousness to your arms and legs and experience how different they are in that respect. Try to focus on the relationship 'inside/outside,' and 'here/there.'

The polarity between cranio–caudal (head–pelvis) also extends to both sets of extremities (arms and legs). In the fourth to the fifth week the hands are positioned with the hand palms turned in on the heart (which at that time is relatively large). The feet are turned slightly outwards (with the soles turned inward) against the umbilical cord. In other words, the extremities are part of the predominantly round and curved gesture of the whole body at that time; just try it. (Come on folks, this is nothing worse than a little bit of eurythmy…!) Subsequently, however, the hands and arms grow outwards, and the legs and feet inwards. The hand palms turn to the ventral side, the foot soles to the dorsal side. This contrast of the *endorotation* of the arms and the *exorotation* of the legs leads to the polarity which is so characteristic for the human being (because it belongs with uprightness); it manifests in the anatomical posture. This anatomical posture, one could say, is embryonically incorrect.

Assignment 16
Start in an upright position with your arms bent and the palms turned slightly inward at the height of the heart. Now carry out an exorotation, stretching the arms. Continue this movement until the arms are stretched up alongside the head with the palms turned dorsally.

Now bring the arms back, rotating inward, continuing until they are stretched alongside the trunk, with fingers down and the palms of the hands turned to the dorsal side. Imagine your legs doing this movement.

In conclusion, we might say that the 'embryological posture' is one in which the human being is fully stretched and unfolded.

The upper extremities turn away from the earth, the lower extremities turn towards the earth. The latter are connected with the earth and gravity. Poppelbaum explains it as follows, 'No animal achieves the total harmony with gravity in the lower extremities which the human being achieves.' It is because the pelvis and the legs are able to completely carry us that our hands are freed up. They are freed from locomotion, which brings the arms and hands totally within the domain of *manipulation*. Goethe postulated that the polarity between arms and legs in the human being is an *essential* distinction; arms and legs differ both in function and physiology, which is the case with no animal.

What does this tell us about the dynamics of the I and the question of human being versus animal? The gesture of stretching and unfolding has to do with becoming freed from the 'inside.' We are looking for a new trend, for something which is not a continuation of the animal/astral (expressing itself in the highly typical curvature with its corresponding dynamics). Is there something which opposes that and frees itself from that? We find this in the stretching motion with its corresponding dynamics. One could say that a new dynamic centre arises in the strong polarity between head and extremities, which is neither the one pole (head/astral/animal/closed), nor the other (extremities/etheric/plantlike/ open). In having to maintain the upright posture, the human being is a creature of *balance*.

One can find this tendency in all higher animals; various forms of stretching and unfolding occur in their embryonic development. But there is one difference: they are never brought to completion. Following the line from lower to higher mammals, through apes to the human being, the tendency to continue stretching and *maintaining* that gesture manifests more and more strongly. The essential polarity of the two extremities (Goethe) *does not appear* in quadrupeds! The anthropoid apes (Pongidae) come very close, but they soon lose the human traits which they have when they are very young. In other words, the morphogenesis of the human being is typified by stretching and becoming upright, accompanied by the unfolding and polarizing of arms and legs, head and pelvis (all the upper and lower parts); all of this is necessary in order to stand straight and *maintain that upright position into adulthood*. Standing upright is more than just an anatomical gesture, it is also a *spiritual* gesture. It is a gesture of holding back, maintaining an equilibrium in relation to gravity. In the animal, the centre of gravity always lies in front of the spinal axis and it surrenders to its force. At the point where the animal gives in, the human being remains upright. Perhaps being upright is a primary, being a quadruped a secondary quality, but that would go beyond the scope of this book! This implies a view of the relationship between human being and animal which is radically different from the prevailing biological viewpoint. This has been worked out in more detail by authors such as Poppelbaum and Mees. 'Opposition distinguishes the human being,' a revolutionary slogan says. It points to a quality which is a hallmark of the I. The point is not to postulate that 'the human being is no animal,' the point is to recognize that 'the human being is *different from* the animal.' What we have described above gives us a picture of the difference. The different 'direction' (Hartmann); becoming upright; maintaining that position; finding a standpoint: these are key phrases to fill in this picture. Embryonic stretching shows us the corresponding gesture.

4.8.8 Closing Remarks

Having gone through all the complexities of this chapter, we will now return to Hartmann's scheme in Fig. 4.9. The aim of this chapter was to highlight four gestures which are characteristic of the way the outer human form comes into being. Corresponding gestures were sought in the four natural kingdoms. The link between these two domains is found in the series of principles which in anthroposophy go by the name of *physical, etheric, astral,* and *I;* these are found to be progressively present and at work in the four kingdoms. These four spiritual qualities are likewise to be found working in human development. In order to make these visible, we have tried to live into the directions as indicated by Hartmann, and 'translate' them into 'somatogenetic' gestures. It is probably inevitable that this approach only leads to increased questions for the reader. The intent of this chapter, however, was not to give answers but to stimulate further study. This approach opens up vistas which lie far beyond the discipline of embryology.

CHAPTER 5

Polarities — Projective Geometry

FERDIE AMONS

In the previous chapter, the figure of the lemniscate was used several times in order to help the reader picture and experience how polarities can be turned inside out. Drawing exercises were also given to clarify the process of thinking one's way through from one polarity into the other. Chapter 4 discussed the polarity between what anthroposophy calls the spiritual world and the material world. Anthroposophy sees these areas as complementing one another, yet forming a unity. In this chapter an attempt will be made to give the reader an experience of the reality of this polarity — and mutual interdependence — by means of geometrical descriptions and representations. This may seem a rather theoretical pursuit, far-fetched and removed from daily reality. Yet these mathematical imaginations are a help to gain access to this realm which is hard to penetrate. Therefore this should be regarded as practice material.

This chapter's approach aims to make clear that the anthroposophical concept of a 'spiritual world' is neither grounded in free associations of the imagination, nor in unclear raptures about 'energy clouds' and the like. We have the capacity to get to know a spatial world of a different kind from the material world with its characteristic measurable quantities. This capacity rests on mathematical thinking, which all of us can use to a certain degree. We can get an initial glimpse of the supersensory world when we try to do this with the kind of clarity which is only granted by mathematical thinking. Mathematics is the only exact science which is totally perspicuous, by virtue of the fact that it is completely unconnected to the senses (it is abstract) and basically cannot err.* Through the inner power of the activity of thinking we can thus transcend the inherent limits of the sense world.

---

* Of course we can make errors, but by the same token we can trace them and acknowledge them.

In anthroposophy the level of life, which lies directly next to sense perceptible reality, is called the 'etheric world.' Although it is invisible, it can be grasped as an idea. The examples dealt with in this chapter aim to get to the beginning level of an initial experience of this etheric world, as it relates to physical-material reality.

5.1 Point–circle: turning inside-out

In Chapter 1 of the book *Extending Practical Medicine,* Rudolf Steiner and Ita Wegman described how the *forces of attraction* are characteristic of the physical world. The centre of the earth is the primary place from which this power of attraction works, namely the force of gravity. When we look more closely at several physical phenomena, however, we see that many centres of forces can be at work within the inorganic world. These do not always have to be forces of attraction, but can also be forces of repulsion. The essential point is that in principle one can always point out the *place* where these forces are at work, in other words: they are located in *physical, earthly space.* Even when we're dealing with forces which emanate from heavenly bodies (forces whose source is far away), they are still located within this same space. Even forces which by nature are not really mechanical — such as light, chemical effects, phenomena of warmth, etc. — have a point of origin which can always be located somewhere in space. All these forces of the physical world work on things from the outside.

In the plant world (the organic world) other forces are at work too. Of these Steiner says, however, that they do not emanate from a central point, but radiate from out from the whole of the periphery of the cosmos into this centre. Thus the direction of these forces is diametrically opposed to the forces mentioned earlier. Steiner calls these *etheric forces,* which belong to the ether world, a supersensory world, and the origin of these forces cannot be pinpointed; we can only do that with forces belonging to the physical world. It is these etheric forces which, for example, make it possible that plants grow up, against gravity (contrary to the laws of the physical world). Living nature does not live in conflict with the laws of dead nature, but works in spite of these laws. Generally speaking, we can say that we can distinguish two kinds of mechanisms which are at work, namely those characterized by forces of pressure (in physical space), and others which are characterized by forces of suction (in etheric space). How are these two related? Do they coexist, or are they perhaps far removed from each other?

Let us now look at the significance of such questions for our picture of space; we could very easily pass these questions by, overlooking their implications and not truly experiencing them inwardly. Everything on earth has its place, or is moving from one place to another. In the process of checking how such a mental picture comes into being under the influence of thinking, one will notice that in forming mental pictures there is *no escape from physical space.* I am placed in space together with every object or thing I consider, however far removed, and that includes the living plant. Our mental picturing is therefore apparently bound to physical space.

Now we do have the possibility — which exists within our thinking only — to call on the concept of 'infinity' to take us a step further. We thus indicate, with a word for the time being, that there is a boundary to physical space. Even though this concept may go beyond our powers of imagination, it is a concept nevertheless. Our capacity to form mental pictures is earthbound after all, and cannot take in anything which is not *also* earthly in character.

So what do we do with this statement that there are forces which stream in from out of a cosmic periphery? Where do *they* have their source? After all, we only know diverging forces. We cannot determine the origin of *converging* forces; at most we can point to the place where they take effect. This is disorienting.

We started out with the question, Where does the physical (material) world border onto the spiritual (etheric) world? Are they in fact worlds which lie next to one another? However familiar we may be with the look of the plant which stands in the pot on the windowsill, it lives only partly in the space we are familiar with, namely insofar as it is a physical body. What distinguishes it from the objects in dead nature lies in a supersensory (spiritual) world, of which you cannot just say that it is 'somewhere else.' Entering that world demands the development of a different kind of thinking (Steiner calls it 'pure thinking,' *reines Denken),* which does not suffer from the limitations of our earth-bound thinking, tied to the brain. It is possible to do thought exercises which, starting from normal thinking, bring us closer to experiencing the boundary between the physical and the etheric world. Mathematical thinking is eminently suitable to escape physical space. After all, our thoughts themselves, which we use to practice mathematics, cannot be said to exist 'in space' anymore.

In Assignment 1 we see what happens with the circle when the centre moves away from us: it becomes ever bigger and bigger. At last it will be so big, that the distinction between it and a straight line no longer exists. The centre is then at infinity.

We can now continue this process in thought, and why could we not? If the centre continues to move further away, what happens to the circle?

Assignment 1: *An exercise in thinking (see Figure 5.1)*
Imagine a circle, which has a radius and a centre. In thought,
position yourself on the circumference and let the centre move
away from you. It moves further and further away. What happens
to the curvature of the circle?

Of course the centre does have a specific location, but direct
your attention especially to the direction in which it moves away
from you. The curvature of the circle becomes less and less and we
can see the eventual outcome: a straight line! This will only hap-
pen when the centre arrives in infinity. From every point on the
circumference a radius goes to the centre, so from the place where
you are standing you can at least indicate the direction in which
that centre must be located. In this case it is perpendicular to the
straight line which the circle has now become.

Now consider the following: 1 m (or 10 m, or 10 km, etc.) fur-
ther on someone else stands on the same circle. She does the same,
she also looks from her point of view at the same centre. Are we
now looking at the same *point in the direction of infinity? Both per-*
sons are oriented in the same direction, their gaze runs parallel!

Repeat the same exercise a few times in your imagination. The
point is to experience it! How would it be if somebody were to
stand on the circle, but who is facing the centre perpendicular to
your own view? Would both orientations still be perpendicular to
one another by the time the centre arrives at infinity?
And, as a last example: how would it be if two people would face
one another?

Here we need the help of logic. We have seen the movement which the
curved line of the circle made. This movement in turn has to continue.
What used to be concave will now become convex, and the other way
around. This means that the direction into which the centre has vanished
will now be opposite. It will approach us from behind and a new circle
will come into being, which, as the centre moves further, becomes smaller
again.

It is important to note here that the first and the second circle are the
same. Their identity is clear: there is a continuous transition from the
one to the other. But the similarity stops here, *because what used to be*
inner world in the first circle, becomes outer world in the second one.

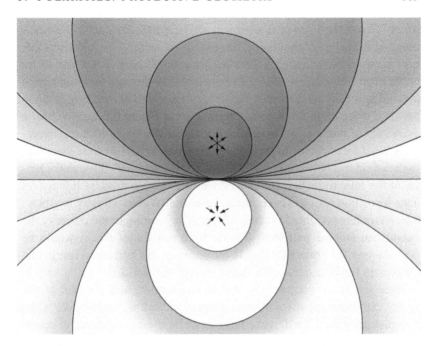

Figure 5.1. Circles turning inside out. Dark: inner world. Light: outer world. Top arrows: diverging (central) forces. Bottom arrows: converging (universal) forces.

The limitless (light) field outside the first circle in turn becomes the limited inner world in the second one.

So far this thinking exercise has mainly led to a reaffirmation and a re-experiencing of what was said about polarities and turning inside out in Sections 4.2 and 4.3. (Compare Assignments 4 and 5 in Section 4.2.5). The point here, however, is to take the mental picture further, in order to come to an experience of the 'border territory' between the physical and the etheric worlds.

As stated before, all forces which emanate from one point in physical space take a diverging course. Taking into account what Rudolf Steiner said about the forces in the plant kingdom, or more generally speaking, the etheric realm, those must be *convergent* in their direction; they were described above as *radiating in* from all around the cosmos). The question then becomes where *those* forces originate. Their origin could not logically be located in a place which we can imagine concretely; we would not be able to point it out. It would be located in the second circle indicated in the example given for practice. This would be the strict mathematical consequence of the behaviour of the diverging lines of force (the radii in the first, upper circle), which became evermore parallel as the centre approached infinity. When the lines of force run exactly parallel, the centre (here representing the origin of the forces) lies exactly in infinity. We know that this must be true, even though we cannot imagine it! Now when the centre moves even *further* than infinity (we are breaking through the boundary of physical space, in other words), the lines of force will *of necessity* begin to converge if we think this through to the end. In Figure 5.1 we saw how a second circle forms as a consequence, and that the origin of the converging lines of force comes to lie in the centre of this second circle therefore. So the circle can only come into existence when we break through the barrier of the infinite surface (line). And we cannot even imagine infinity, let alone a position which is even further removed! Within our drawing, however, it remains possible to survey all this. The location of the centre of the second can still be indicated, but we must not forget that it would be located *under* the horizontal line. In the drawing, this horizontal line in fact symbolizes the boundary of the sense perceptible world.

Since the space enclosed by the second circle* runs *counter to* our earthly experience of space in every respect, we call it *counterspace*. (The examples given in 5.2 will make this clearer by means of projective geometry.) Nowadays modern physics, especially theoretical physics, is in the vanguard of groundbreaking research. It has come so far that it is beginning to form a picture of this counterspace, even though it may be hypothetical at this point. It posits the existence of negative matter, for example.

As indicated above, in physical space, forces work from the outside and influence one another that way; the sources of strength which are situated in counterspace, however, *work from the inside.* Therefore they have an internal point of application, and bring substances in line with the laws of the etheric world. This can be observed best in growth processes which are totally subject to physical laws, in contrast to those in living nature. When we follow the growth of a crystal we see that this happens by means of *apposition* of material, so it accrues on the outside. A living organism grows because of *internal* growth processes.

We find the origin of etheric forces which ray in: they originate as it were in the centre of the second circle. The horizontal line (see Figure 5.1) separates two spaces from one another, the one lying inside the circle, the other outside. The circles themselves delineate a boundary between two spaces, which cannot be crossed; crossing it is only possible in infinity, that is to say in a realm which we cannot picture concretely. We can only determine this boundary mathematically, we have no physical access. This has consequences for the way we have to view the relationship of the

---

*   Of course we can imagine the circle in three dimensions, where it would be
     a sphere.

etheric body to the physical body in living creatures. The spaces which these bodies occupy do not have *topographical* boundaries! These boundaries can only be grasped as ideas.

When we inject a substance (for example medicine) subcutaneously into the living body of a human being, we are inclined to view this as introducing that substance *into* the body. However, this is only correct in one sense. The space outside the skin — physical space, that is — borders directly on the space which is enclosed by the skin, so they form a continuity. By contrast, when we mean etheric space, we are dealing with a discontinuity between the two spaces. The substance only enters inasmuch as we regard the body as belonging to physical space. With a physical injection needle we principally have no *direct* access to the *living* part of the body. Injected substance has to be taken into life, that is to say into *those* processes which lie within the domain and guidance of the ether body. Physiology and biochemistry describe how a substance fares when it is introduced into the body. Advanced technology allows us to have detailed knowledge of how that substance is transformed or broken down, where it goes in the body, etc. Please note, however, that the substance under consideration has then been reabsorbed into the physical-material body of the human being.

In current biology and medicine it is said that sodium chloride is subject to the same laws, no matter if it is inside or outside the body. When one researches the processes inside the body only using the knowledge of the laws of physical space, it will also be impossible to escape from this space. However, once a substance has been absorbed by a living organism, that means that it is also in etheric space, in counterspace. When a substance has been brought into the body through the skin, i.e. 'here' in the physical worlds, another boundary is simultaneously crossed, namely the one into infinity. In order to assess how a substance influences the body — and that also goes for nutritional substances — one constantly has to be aware of the aspect under consideration. One has to bear in mind whether one has a physical focus, and therefore dealing with central forces, or an etheric (living) focus, dealing with the peripheral forces. In fact, medicine and biology are constantly researching effects originating in counterspace. But these effects are not recognized as such. Therefore they are explained on the basis of knowledge of the material world. This usually succeeds, even though hypotheses are sometimes needed which cannot be verified. Therefore a materialistic worldview never really comes into conflict with manifestations of life. The fact that plants grow upwards can also be reconciled with the laws of thermodynamics. The growth gestures which plants exhibit indicate that they belong to another realm, but such a statement no longer fits in such an interpretative model simply because a concept like 'gesture' does not belong in the realm of matter.

5.2 Projective geometry

In the previous paragraph we referred to the world of lifeless and of living nature. In actively completing certain trains of thought which take infinity into account, one can get a first inkling that these two worlds only meet in infinity. Our starting point in carrying out these thought exercises was the familiar space around us, which led us to the initial idea of *counterspace,* also called *negative space.* These mental pictures are derived from projective geometry. This is a mathematical method which is relatively young in comparison with other branches of mathematics, one which only began to blossom in the nineteenth century. It lends itself very well to the tracing of formative processes. As a result, one can follow these processes more easily and has the possibility to live into them. Projective geometry is a particularly apt method for elucidating and describing metamorphoses. This geometry deals with phenomena in 'projective space,' i.e. the space in which the special nature of the location of points, lines or planes in infinity is not taken into account as such. So they receive the same treatment as finite points, lines or planes.

Projective geometry can lead to the insight that everything which appears to us as living forms in sense-perceptible space has a necessary parallel in a different world. These *living* forms can be experienced as 'not of this world,' which necessitates seeking the origins of such forms in a different world. That is to say, a world which lies *beyond* our earthbound capacities of mental picturing. If this is indeed the case, namely that appearances which I can look *at* have their correspondences in another realm, it would be worth the trouble to research the relationships between these two 'spaces,' I would then be perceiving this 'something' in another realm from the inside, in contrast to looking at it from the outside, the relationship being that the one realm behaves like the other one turned inside out. For we concluded that the two realms mentioned were qualitatively the opposite of one another. If we imagine the circles in Assignment 1 as spheres in three-dimensional space, we can experience how the first surrounding sphere will ultimately metamorphose into another one, whereby what used to be 'inside' now becomes 'outside.' This viewpoint will give us an important perspective which allows us to penetrate to the essence of living organisms.

Assignment 2: An exercise in thinking and imagining
Taking Assignment 1 as our starting point, we can take a different
initial position by placing ourselves in the middle of the sphere.
Now we allow the surrounding sphere to become ever bigger until
it approaches infinity. As a result, the curved inside of the sphere
which we are looking at will become a plane. This will happen not
only in front of us, but also to our left and right. It will also hap-
pen behind, above and below us. The result, however, remains a
plane!

Repeat this exercise many times and try to experience it as
intensively as possible.

With this exercise we have made a groundbreaking discovery: wherever we find ourselves, we can feel surrounded at all times by a plane. We can call this 'the all-embracing cosmic plane.'

Present-day explanations of the genesis of an organism are based on mechanistic laws. In that domain, however, only point-based forces play a role, as we have just seen. These are all surrounded by the cosmic plane at infinity that we have just discovered, so it is 'where the finite ends.' We can surmise that the sources of everything which has living formative capacity lie behind that. There would be the origin of the *peripheral universal forces,* which we saw were converging, in contrast to the diverging forces of the physical world. Once we know how to escape from the constraints imposed by orthodox models of explanation the way is free to approach the morphology and dynamics (physiological processes) of living beings in a different way.

One example is the current embryological tenet that limbs grow out of the body. The final form of the hands would thus come into being because growth processes simply cease. But why would a hand not come into being because the *shape* of the hand was there first, so growth processes would cease when that shape would determine it? In this case the aforementioned peripheral forces would be exerting their pull. The difference with the current assumption would then be that this shape of the hand is not the *product* of physical and chemical conditions of cells etc. (which also play in, of course), but a *manifestation* of a non-material, dynamic formative process. To explain shapes and processes, there are always *causes* to be indicated in our familiar physical space. However, when unprejudiced observation allows us to see that an arm or hand grows into a final form, could we not postulate that cause and effect may be conceived as reversed in time? So in fact there are two equally valid ways of explaining phenomena, which can be seen as contrasting or parallel explanations:

1. There are intrinsic, programmed, (genetic and epigenetic) growth processes *(cause)*. There is as yet no definitive form, but there is a progression through developmental stages resulting in the shape of the hand *(effect)*.
2. The shape of the hand is there first *(cause)* and it sets processes in motion *(effect)* which are brought to an end by the formative principle.

Here we see two diametrically opposed explanations for the same manifestation. They seem to be mutually exclusive, but there is as yet no reason to be tempted to mark either as the only correct one. There is a substantial difference between the two, however. That they can coexist nonetheless, is due to the fact that they have been formulated from two different points of view. The first explanation stems from the world of the point-based forces (mechanistic forces), the second from the world of the peripheral forces that stream in. The latter can be taken as a dynamic-creative gesture, a meaningful language which never comes to a standstill. Both principles are in harmony with one another and take each other into account within living organisms. What we meet here, in fact, is a problem which has been known since the Middle Ages: what comes first, the ideal form or the actual matter? It is possible to escape from this dilemma when we take the following into consideration. The physical-material world (the dark area of Figure 5.1) is gripped or penetrated by formative forces originating in the area of the 'all-embracing plane.'

We can learn to see through this with the help of projective geometry. We will now go on to give a few vignettes which do not pretend to be an exact logical argument, but appeal to a common sense of self-evidence which we all share. In this process it will be inevitable to make leaps in thought, and we cannot go into mathematical proof here. For readers who want to penetrate this material further, see the bibliography.

This geometrical method allows us, for example, to construct two kinds of circles. One circle can come into being by drawing an infinite number of *points* equidistant from a centre. This circle is determined from *within,* and extends no further than the length of the chosen radius. But likewise a circle can be formed by an infinitude of *tangents,* coming from infinity and returning there, just touching the circle from the outside. This circle is

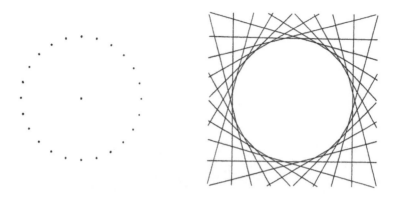

Figure 5.2. A circle built of points and a circle built of tangent lines.

determined from *without*. In both cases we see circles as a result, but each one has a totally different origin* (see Figure 5.2).

Projective geometry allows us to penetrate countless phenomena in living nature in a way which differs from conventional methods. This is not only true for the observation of definitive forms (morphology), but also for the genesis and change of forms (morphogenesis). In this way it is possible to reach a more essential feeling for and experience of the true nature of an organism. An organism lives both in space and in time, or, put in different terms: in actuality. Modern streams in biology, as proposed for example by Sheldrake, Lovelock, and in *structuralism,* present all-embracing views which conceive of the earth as one organism. Discoveries such as these point to far-reaching connections.

A typical trait of projective geometry is that this is a discipline dealing with the *qualitative* aspect of things. It does not express distances in centimetres, nor does it count angles in degrees. All constructions can be carried out with a straightedge and compasses without measurements, in contrast to the more quantitative character of 'ordinary' Euclidean geometry (see the circle built up of points). Projective geometry deals with points, lines and planes which can be seen as *projections* of other points, lines or planes; hence the name. Dual and polar relationships and definitions form an important basis; an example of this in two-dimensional space is the polarity between a line and a point.

---

* If we imagine this in three-dimensions we would be dealing with a sphere instead of a circle. In that case the tangents will no longer be *lines,* but *planes* coming out of and returning to infinity.

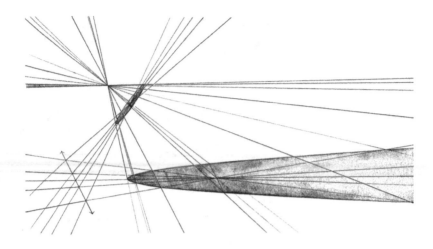

Figure 5.3. Perspective transformation

Two lines determine a point (the crossing point) and *two points determine a (straight) line.*

Or, in three-dimensional space, between line and plane: *two intersecting lines determine a plane* and *two intersecting planes determine a line.*

Point and plane are polar opposites, they are mutually exchangeable, whereby the line functions as an intermediary. These are examples of the so-called *duality-principle* (polarity-principle would be a better term for this, but the concept of polarity in projective geometry is used in a more specialized sense). This duality-principle clearly shows that two definitions can both be valid, the only difference being one of perspective. Different standpoints give rise to different definitions.

Figure 5.3 demonstrates the projective character of this type of geometry.

Here we see how a point (formed by a light source for example) throws a shadow of a circle on to a plane positioned at a certain angle to the plane of the circle. The situation in the illustration has been chosen in such a way that the line connecting the point with the upper edge of the circle runs exactly parallel to the projection plane. Under such circumstances a shadow results which has the shape of a parabola. Other positions of the circle in relation to the projection plane will result in ellipses, different circles, hyperbolas, or parabolas. That is to say, they are all conic sections. We can conclude from this that these figures all belong to *one* family, that they are related and also that they can stem from a single principle.

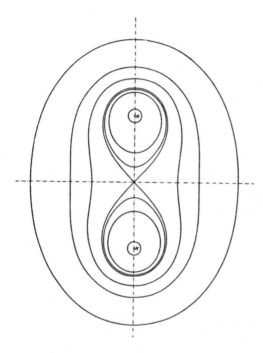

*Figure 5.4. Threefold
metamorphosis in a
family of curves*

Investigate what positions give rise to the conic sections mentioned above.

By choosing different initial positions, while keeping the constructions the same, many different curve shapes can be obtained. The relationship between the separate curves is the result of their common origin, as shown for example in Figure 5.4.

In Figure 5.4 the so-called curves of Cassini are represented.* They are only six examples out of an infinite possibility of curves, all answering to certain geometric formulas. By choosing different initial positions forms can come into being which are nearly elliptical, and others which show a narrowing on the side. The well-known lemniscate will be recognized as well, it being another member of this family. Furthermore, there are egg-shaped pairs of curves, which form a single curve together in spite of their discontinuity (they are connected through counterspace). One can let this family of curves expand in thought; it will then the approach the 'all-embracing plane.' If one lets it shrink, it will disappear into *one* point (the all-relating point). Such a family of curves together forms one species, which can express itself

---

* Constructing these curves is quite complicated and demands exact drawing. Interested readers are referred to Louis Locher-Ernst, *Urphänomene der Geometrie* (Basic Phenomena of Geometry), from which this illustration was taken. This book also contains the procedure to construct the curves.

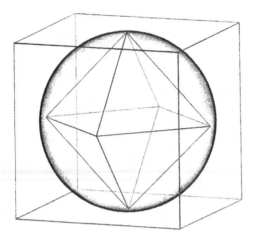

Figure 5.5.

in various manifestations, analogous to the classification 'dicotyledon,' or 'mammal,' for example. The figures shown here are all still two-dimensional, they are projected onto a plane as it were, but in their perfect forms they are in fact three-dimensional shapes. The pliability of these spatial mathematical figures can be compared to metamorphoses in living nature. Although they have very different manifestations there, they still have things in common; in the one case they correspond to the requirements of geometrical rules, in the other case the requirements of the morphogenetic principle which Goethe calls *Typus* (type). For every body in physical space a corresponding body can be found in counterspace. In projective geometry this can be shown with constructions, even though they could become very complicated. In that case we are dealing with *pairs* of spatial bodies, which not only have a *polar* relationship, but are also located in different spaces. With this we introduce the real concept of *polarity* in projective geometry. This phenomenon of polarity is facilitated by an intermediary, in relation to which the projection is carried out. An example of this is the spherical form,* whereby one spatial body is located *in* the sphere, the other one *outside* the sphere (think of Assignment 2 above). Figure 5.5 shows a simple example.

Figure 5.5 shows a cube with inscribed sphere in such a way that this sphere touches the inside of the planes of the cube. Inside the sphere an

---

*   The intermediary role between the two pairs of spatial bodies does not have to be the spherical form; this is only chosen because it provides an easy demonstration of the phenomenon. Therefore we confine ourselves here to this simpler case.

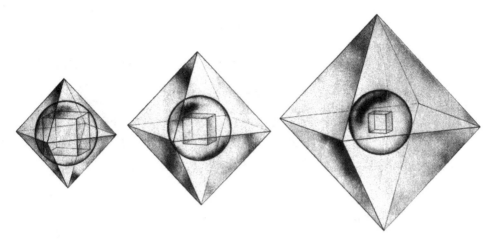

Figure 5.6. Expansion and contraction of a cube and an octahedron

octahedron can be inscribed. The mutual relationship between the two bodies is such, that the octahedron forms a point where the sphere touches a plane of the cube. Thus the polarity is between *plane* and *point,* in accordance with the described duality-principle in projective geometry. The relationship between the two bodies is subject to one law. That implies, that the opposite must hold as well: when one draws the octahedron outside the sphere, there will be a corresponding cube inside the sphere. This goes not only for the bodies which touch the sphere as a plane or a point, but also for larger or smaller bodies* which do not touch the sphere, for which it *is* an intermediary, however. From Figure 5.6 we can deduce that this relationship also shows a quantitative reciprocity: when the cube decreases, the octahedron increases correspondingly and vice versa. If we take the polarity between point and plane as our starting point, the polar relationship between cube and octahedron retains its validity if we let one of them decrease in size. The other one has to increase correspondingly, as indicated above. Thus basically all kinds of shapes can be translated into their polar counterpart (counter-image). This means that very small organisms, such as the flea, a seed, or the zygote, are likely to correspond to very large counterparts in the dimension of peripheral forces. Through projective geometry, we thus

---

*   In the case of two-dimensional figures instead of three-dimensional ones, we are dealing with the polarities of *line* and *point* rather than *plane* and *point.* (Compare the circle built up of points and the circle built up of tangent lines in Figure 5.2.)

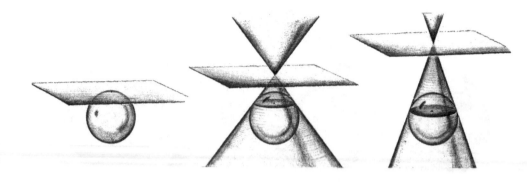

Figure 5.7. Point and polar plane. Reciprocal movement.

find the same principles which we met before in Sections 3.2 and 3.3, where we found them in a totally different way — namely by looking at the human organism using the comparative, dynamic approach.

The general laws of the polar relationship existing between point and plane can be demonstrated with Figure 5.7, even though the scope of this chapter does not allow us to enter into the subject deeply.

Every *point* of the polar plane outside the sphere corresponds to a *plane* inside the sphere (and the other way around). This plane inside the sphere is determined by a conic section which has the point on the polar plane as its top and touches the sphere. Another point on the polar plane gives us yet another plane inside the sphere. Where the two planes intersect on the inside, they form a line. The third point on the polar plane makes yet a third plane inside the sphere, which has *one point* in common with the line thus formed at the intersection.*

It is a rare occasion when this polar plane touches the sphere itself, but when it happens point and plane coincide. The polar point then lies on the polar plane. Where would the point be when the polar plane is in infinity?

In Assignment 3 it will be obvious that the plane and point are always located on either side of the sphere. Here, too, the surface of the sphere represents a boundary which cannot be crossed, just as we saw

---

*   Note once again, that the duality principle with regard to the exchange of point and plane applies here also. Three *points* on the polar *plane* correspond to three *planes* in the sphere. Three *points* determine the (polar) *plane* and three *planes* determine the (polar) *point* inside the sphere.

Assignment 3

Imagine a point inside the sphere and imagine its polar plane outside the sphere. What happens to the polar plane when the point moves towards the centre of the sphere, when it is at the centre of the sphere, and what happens when it moves towards the outside of the sphere, and when it touches the sphere itself?

in Section 5.1 in the case of the circle turning inside out. The sphere — even though it is itself placed in space — determines two separate worlds. Thus we have to look upon the intermediary sphere as the boundary between space and counterspace (positive and negative space respectively). Everything contained in one of those spaces will inevitably have its correspondent in the other in such a way that the polarity of point and plane is met. It probably goes without saying, that when there is a finite spatial figure (not an infinitely small point) within the sphere, that this can be conceived as being composed of a large number of (an infinitely large number, actually) *points,* each of which has a defined place and corresponds to as many *planes,* which form a mirror image as tangent planes on the outside. Such a shape can look quite different in certain cases, while retaining a quite definite relationship to the figure inside the sphere. Since one can think every spatial body as being built up either out of points or planes, this means that every body in sense-perceptible (positive) space has a corresponding (but visually different) body in counterspace (negative space), and vice versa. So there is not only an inversely proportional relationship, which we mentioned before, but also a qualitative form relationship, or metamorphosis relationship. In the case of mathematically (or geometrically) defined bodies, it is still relatively easy to construct the one on the basis of the other. In principle, *every* body is related to a counterpart, and that also goes for the human body! It is quite an amazing thought that every individual human being has a corresponding nonsensory body in a different space, which is not a hypothetical possibility, but a reality which can only be grasped as an idea. That body has just as many specific traits as the ones we can perceive in the physical human being with our senses.

5.3 Projective geometry and morphology

The two concepts of point and plane bear the principles within them for a new morphology. When we look around us in nature, we always encounter both in more or less recognizable form. It is a matter of recognizing the gesture, which strives towards either a plane or a point. To take an example, we shall first look at the plant. In its most complete form, when it is fully grown, it consists of leaf; Goethe said: 'it is all leaf' *(alles ist Blatt),* (see Section 6.3). The planar element is obvious here, but other parts can also be understood as metamorphoses of leaves. The ovary, for example, comes into existence when one or more carpels grow together, and the flower also consists of leaves in all its components. When fully contracted into the seed, the plant has a shape which tends towards the point; when fully grown out, its physical form tends to the all-embracing plane. These two extreme manifestations of the plant are polar opposites of one another.* Phenomena of expansion and contraction also occur in numerous places of the human body. In many cases these will also have a polar relationship. Similarly, examples of the character of the plane, the line, and the point can be found in the skeleton. The parietal bone and the wing-shaped bone of the ileum are planar, the humerus and the femur are linear, and the bones of metacarpals and metatarsals are point-like in character.

The same tendencies can be recognized in the behaviour and appearance of the four elements, and also in the states of aggregation of earth substances, the physical states.

The *solid* state tends to be heavy, compact, and contracted, as seen in stones. The element of earth is *three-dimensional* in character.

In *liquids* (water) we see the shape of the *drop,* but at the same time we observe planes on the surface. So it appears to have both aspects. Since water contains the opposite characteristics of both the point and the plane, it also becomes more comprehensible why it plays such a mediating role in nature. In truth there really is only one single surface (all water surfaces on earth, lakes and seas taken together form one big drop). Thus the element of water is only *two-dimensional.*

In *air,* the gaseous state, the characteristic tendency of evaporation and expansion is evident, even though gas is still subject to gravity. The gaseous state manifests a striving away from a point to the periphery; it

---

*   This applies not only to forms, but sometimes also to processes. The fully grown plant, for example, has no potential for further growth left; the seed, by contrast, is still full of potential.

has no surfaces whatsoever, only direction. Therefore its character is *one-dimensional.*

Fire, the element of warmth, penetrates everything else. Here we are dealing with a 'substance,' which belongs to the 'all embracing plane.' Warmth can be found in space, but it is unhampered by physical boundaries. The tendency of warmth to strive outward is irrepressible; at most it can be slowed down, as is done in a thermos flask, for example.* This tendency allows us to characterize warmth as having *no dimension.*

One finds such tendencies in gesture and form not only by looking for general similarities in the sense of analogies, but by living into those tendencies with such a degree of mathematical exactness, that links to corresponding natural phenomena become obvious. When we imagine form relationships such as the ones we spoke of above not as fixed states, but as stages in everlasting processes of movement, the dimension of time enters in next to the spatial dimension. We indicated above how the sequence of cause and effect which we determined in physical space is reversed in counterspace. That means nothing less than that time runs backwards there!

Imagine the following. Lift your arm. At the same time something corresponding to your arm will move in counterspace, and it will move down!†

When we look back in the evening on all that happened during the course of the day, we are faced with a medley of causes and effects. We are subjected to those, and they can often give us the sensation that we do not live but are *being lived.* Therefore the anthroposophical path of schooling frequently recommends the so-called *Rückschau* (looking back on the day); when carried out regularly, it will counterbalance the stream of events which come to us from out of the physical world. One of the things this accomplishes is to overcome the pressure to interpret everything in terms of cause and effect. Practice of this exercise makes it noticeably easier to approach things and events openly. It is also useful to practice with other things than daily events which run their natural course in the stream of time.

As an exercise try saying the letters of the alphabet in reverse order, for example. Even more difficult would be to sing a song backwards!

---

*   The element of warmth is quite special. Even though it is spatial in that there are warmth bodies on earth, warmth also has a radiant aspect (infrared radiation), and in that respect it can be said to belong to counterspace also. Therefore we are justified in speaking of both physical warmth and etheric warmth.)

†   Note that there is an additional factor which plays a role in such an event, namely the *will.* This will (or intention) originates in an even higher realm than counterspace, in the astral world. The effect, however, shows itself in the etheric world.

Projective geometry is a path of schooling which offers the researcher new insights. When one becomes truly conversant with these newly gained insights, sensing what it is like to be a point or an expanding infinite plane, these concepts become more alive and more saturated. They will turn into something like organs of perception. This allows one to see phenomena from a different perspective than before, and to make new discoveries. It goes without saying that such a receptivity will not arise through superficial acquaintance. We can only give a fragmentary indication here. By actively drawing and constructing the figures of projective geometry one will live into the subject matter much more strongly than by looking at ready-made drawings such as those reproduced here!

5.4 Concluding remarks

In this chapter, an attempt was made to open up a different experience of space. It is possible to gain an inner sense of infinity, and of supersensory regions 'beyond' infinity. Projective geometry has an inner logic and inevitably leads to the omnipresent reality of counterspace. The two areas in which morphogenetic processes take place were introduced. The first of these areas is positive space, where the point-based forces rule;* the second, counterspace or negative space, is where the peripheral forces or cosmic forces belong. The latter is also called *sculptural space* by Rudolf Steiner. This is a very meaningful term, because it indicates where we actually should look for the origin of formative processes. It points us to the space of sculptural *planes*. We have to think first of all how shapes actually arise, for example when we shape a chunk of clay with our hands. When we do that we mainly use the palms of our hands (planar surfaces).

If we look at nature in an imaginative, creative way, we discover that spherical shapes predominate. It could be objected that trees, for example, show a pattern of branching out, and hence a more linear tendency; but closer inspection shows us that this pattern is subject to the larger striving of the tree to make a more or less spherical shape with the crown. Very clear expressions of what we mean here may be found in more primitive growth processes, clearly visible in the growth of bacteria on a culture medium in a petri dish; another clear expression can be found in a subdividing zygote. Both make a spherical shape growing from out of a central point. The sphere has its counterpart in negative space, which is also a sphere, but one that is inverted, or 'negative.' This primary mathematical

---

*   Think of the genes, which are like 'points' in the DNA sequence. They form as many focal points for the peripheral formative forces.

form is a characteristic of primitive growth. A spectacular example, of course, is the way a zygote (of lower vertebrates) develops through the morula stage into the blastula stage.

Now that we have come to recognize the differences and characteristics of two complementary spaces, we have a basis to recognize a highly dramatic event in the process of *gastrulation:* it will be immediately apparent how in one place within the spherical surface a hollow space comes into being! Does that not mean that counterspace is at work *within* the space of the central forces? We can observe repeated occurrences of this same gesture, for example in the formation of the neural tube and eye placode. Such a gesture of turning inside out does show that something from out of another world is being internalized, which in turn manifests perhaps in the behaviour of the animal or human being.* Even higher realms are at work here, namely the astral world.

In this chapter we have dealt with matters which are ostensibly far removed from everyday medical-therapeutic practice. It should be born in mind, however, that it is possible to consider changes in form and structure and physiological processes of the human body in a new way, and that is what this is about. We intentionally appealed to (mathematical) thinking, because only in thinking do we have the possibility to grasp the essence of formative processes. For thinking is *akin to* formative processes and growth processes.

> It is of the greatest importance to know that ordinary human powers of thought *are refined powers of configuration and growth* [italics added]. A spiritual principle reveals itself in the configuration and growth of the human organism. And as life progresses this principle emerges as the spiritual power of thought.†

---

* The neural tube and the eye placode are both part of the nervous system, the function of which is to take in the outer world. So here we can experience a correspondence between that function on the one side and the formative gestures on the other.

† *Es ist von der allergrössten Bedeutung zu wissen, dass die gewöhnlichen Denkkräfte des Menschen die verfeinerten Gestaltungs- und Wachstumskräfte sind. Im Gestalten und Wachsen des Menschlichen Organismus offenbart sich ein Geistiges. Denn dieses Geistige erscheint dann im Lebensverlaufe als die geistige Denkkraft.* (Rudolf Steiner and Ita Wegman: *Extending Practical Medicine,* Chapter 1, page 6.)

CHAPTER 6

Metamorphosis — Essence and Manifestation

GUUS VAN DER BIE

6.1 Introduction

The literal meaning of the word metamorphosis is 'transformation' or 'change of appearance.' An example of this is the caterpillar which pupates and becomes a butterfly. This is an example which everybody will recognize as a change of appearance. The caterpillar has disappeared and the butterfly has come into being. Another example is the shedding of wings of ants. After developing out of the larval stage, ants have wings for a short duration of time, which they lose after the initial flight. For the rest of their lives ants cannot take to the air anymore and have definitively turned into earth dwellers. The flying insect has turned into a crawling insect.

We also use the word metamorphosis in other situations. When somebody has gone through a strong inner transformation, we will speak of 'a profound metamorphosis' to indicate that this person has developed new capacities which were not apparent before. Maybe previous character traits have disappeared or changed. In the latter case, that of the human being having undergone an inner metamorphosis, it will be obvious to everybody that a big change may have occurred, but nobody will think that the actual identity of the person has altered. In the case of the caterpillar and the ant it is equally self-evident that we're dealing with a transformation of a *single* organism. This means that the human being or animal in question has changed in *appearance* but not in *identity.* Here we touch on a very old philosophical theme, one that can justifiably be called a conundrum in cultural history. We're dealing here with the question of *essence* and *manifestation,* a question which different cultures have found different answers for.

When we go back to the examples of the caterpillar and the ant we immediately find a considerable problem as far as reality or appearance is concerned. In the case of the ant, nobody will doubt that it is the *same* ant, first appearing *with* and afterwards *without* wings. That is to say, the difference can be perceived with the *senses*. The example of the caterpillar demands a different effort from us in order to come to the conclusion that the identity of the pupating creature has not changed. The kind of effort we mean lies in *digesting* the sequence of observations we have made (going from caterpillar to pupa to butterfly that is) in our *thinking*. As we are dealing with a very big change in the realm of sense-perception and the process of pupating is not so transparent, it is not immediately apparent that we are dealing here with *one* organism.

> *When we study metamorphoses we practice 'bringing to light'*
> *what is not immediately apparent to the senses. With 'bringing to*
> *light' we mean: 'making visible for our thinking.'*

6.2 Practice in observing metamorphosis

If we study how leaves of plants undergo metamorphosis, examples of which are given in Figures 6.1, 6.2, and 6.3, we encounter two aspects of the same organism. One aspect is *shape,* which is a sense-perceptible reality in space; the other aspect is its change *over time.* In order to get to the immutable aspect hiding behind the metamorphosis, we have to practice viewing the metamorphosis in its entirety, as it were. We have a clear picture of the way plants, animals and human beings appear in space. Now we have to learn to view the change in appearance over time. We can thus begin to distinguish a so-called 'time-shape,' or *Zeitgestalt,* of the organism in question. How to go about this will be indicated in a practical exercise.

6.2.1 Material and method

In Figures 6.1 through 6.5, the leaves have been portrayed next to one another in the sequence in which they came into being. The first leaf is down below on the left, the last one below on the right. The first leaf grows down below on the stem, the last one up above. Arranging them this way enables us to survey all leaves at a glance and facilitates the study of their metamorphosis. The subsequent Figures show leaves of a variety of plants.

It is most instructive to do this exercise using a real plant. For a more

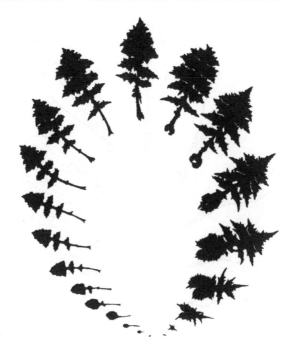

Figure 6.1. Leaves of a sow-thistle (Sonchus).

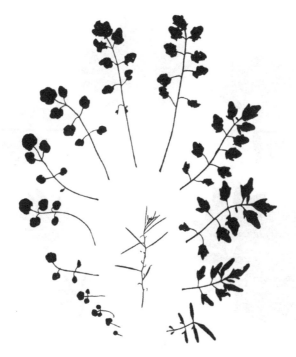

Figure 6.2. Leaves of a cuckoo flower (Cardamine pratensis).

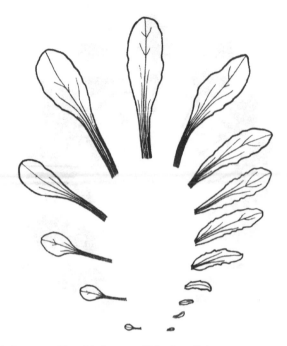

Figure 6.3. Leaves of lamb's lettuce (Valerianella).

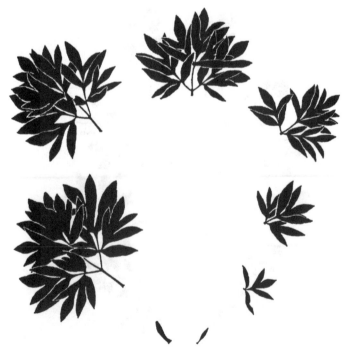

Figure 6.4. Leaves of the peony (Paeonia).

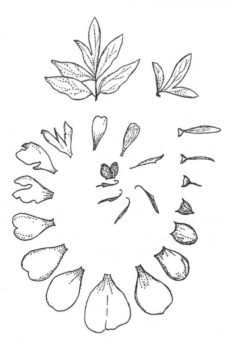

Figure 6.5. Petals of the peony (Paeonia).

elaborate description we take the peony as an example (Figure 6.4). The ubiquitous buttercup (Ranunculus) or poppy (Papaver), however, would also be highly suitable. The reader is further referred to the brilliant little book, *The Plant,* by Herbert Grohmann, which deals with the topic of metamorphosis in the plant kingdom.

In order to do our exercise we will have to 'take the plant apart,' because we need to pick all the leaves from the stem. To those who love nature, this may seem like an offense against the plant. But is a good to realize that the new insight into plants which results from our research method will also lead to a more intimate experience of the essence of plants and the way they grow. This can have healing consequences for nature itself. The closer experience of the essence of the plant, with renewed insight as a corollary, will give rise naturally to a moral feeling leading to enhanced respect for nature.

6.2.2 The peony

We will start by comparing the leaves on the stem, after which we will study the flower and the fruit. Try to first describe your own observations of what strikes you, then read on.

Letting our eyes wander along the sequence of leaves, we notice different shapes in the different leaves. Next to differences, those shapes also show a certain similarity. Let us now proceed to survey the series. To begin with, we see leaves which at this stage are mainly stalk, and which come out and *stretches,* especially in the leaf stalk. Next we see an increase in the mass of leaf substance, where the leaf surface *spreads out* in space. After that the leaf differentiates and the *indentations* become deeper. At the end we see how the leaf retreats as it were back again to the basis of the leaf, showing contraction. We experience a *pointing* movement here.

The first two directions of the growth of the leaf (stretching and spreading out) are centrifugal in their dynamics; the leaf extends into space. By contrast, the last two directions (indenting and pointing) are centripetal. In the process of stretching and spreading out, the leaf substance moves out to the periphery, then the leaf retreats from space as it were, the leaf substance moving in the direction of the leaf stalk.

Goethe studied these changes in the shapes of leaves in a variety of plants, and again and again he found a similar change in shape. He not only studied the development of the leaves on the stem, but also of the leaves of the calyx and corolla, i.e. the sepals and petals (Figures 6.4 and 6.5).

Goethe was struck by the fact that similar dynamics occur on each level. He referred to this as 'expansion and subsequent contraction.' The examples given above demonstrate this clearly. This approach allows the details to take their place within the dynamics of the whole. One could say: comparing the relationship of the shapes gives us insight into the principle underlying development. This insight becomes more acute when one repeats the described process many times in the imagination. By going through this in imagination, an intense and active inward recreation takes place of what was observed outwardly. This enhances the experience of the development in the series of leaves.

An Excursion to Goethe's Faust

At the beginning of the drama, the protagonist, Faust, comes onto the stage in a state of despair and depression. He sums up all his academic qualifications (of which there are many), but he is totally disillusioned, for he has come to realize that he has not gained any insight into the way things fit together. He concludes:

And here I am, for all my lore,
the wretched fool I was before.

*And later on, we find the following lines by Mephistopheles,
concerning 'one who would study and describe the living':*

In the palm of his hand he holds all the sections,
Lacks nothing, except the spirit's connections.[1]

*For Goethe, searching for the 'spirit's connections' was essential in
his work as a natural scientist. Studying metamorphoses, he developed
a method to make the 'invisible' visible. For Goethe, this meant that
he found the 'spirit's connections' which lend coherence to 'all the
sections.' Goethe experienced at the same time that the dynamic
connections are not of a physical, sense perceptible nature. They are
manifest to thinking, however, hence he speaks of 'spirit's
connections.' The consequences of this approach for us may be that
our insight could go as far as approaching or perhaps even entering
the realm of the supersensory. Our starting point is the level of sense
perceptible reality. But in thinking we enter the level of supersensory
reality. To put it in different words: intensive study of the sense world
leads to an ever clearer 'contour' of the essential in our
consciousness.*

6.3 Goethe, metamorphosis, and the archetypal plant

As indicated in the subtitle, studying metamorphosis leads us to the question, 'what is essence and what is appearance?' Like no one else in the history of science, Goethe practised distinguishing between manifestation and essence in actual experience. He said, 'It is not our senses which deceive us, but our judgment,' (compare this to Bacon's philosophy!) which indicates his strong awareness of the two levels of experience in the human being: of the senses and of thinking. Goethe did not limit himself to one plant, but studied many different species and compared them. In this way, by comparison and reflection, Goethe created a level of sensing by which the image of plant essence, or *the* plant, could arise for him. This should be taken as the image of the essential principles at work in the many manifestations which come to expression on the level of sense experience. Goethe called this 'visible invisible' dimension the *archetypical plant*.

Goethe saw the archetypical plant as a threefold repetition of a process of expansion followed by contraction. This principle manifests for the first time in the metamorphosis of the leaves on the stem, the second time in the sepals, petals and stamens, and the third time in the formation of fruit and seed.

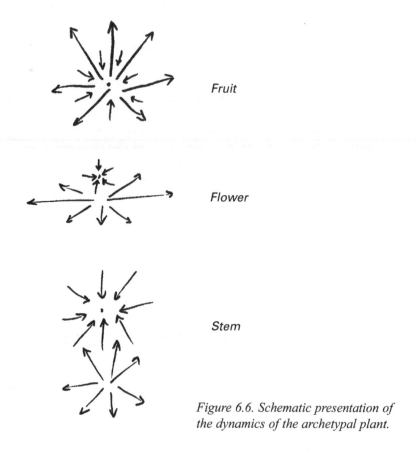

Fruit

Flower

Stem

Figure 6.6. Schematic presentation of the dynamics of the archetypal plant.

All the different manifestations in the plant world are contained within the archetypal plant, but as latent possibility, not in a fixed form. Moreover, not all aspects of the archetypal plant come to expression in every case. It is possible that only a limited part of the possibilities express themselves, as is the case with ferns. The whole process of blossoming as we know it in the *Composite,* such as chamomile or arnica, does not manifest as such in ferns. Therefore it seems as if ferns cannot blossom. That means that in ferns the archetypal plant is active on the leaf level especially. In the case of the poppy, by contrast, we will find a very short leaf metamorphosis and a highly elaborate flower development. When we look repeatedly at such differences between plants and compare them, the essential aspects of the archetypal plant will gradually arise in our consciousness.

In this respect comparison with daily life can aid us again. Are we not acutely aware of differences between the size of different people's noses, ears and necks, how they walk, etc.? It turns out that we all unconsciously carry a picture of the archetypal human being within us, even though no one has ever actually seen one. Here, too, we see how daily life furnishes us with something which can be lifted to a scientific level by a phenomenological approach and study of metamorphosis. This will give us a sense of coherence different from that gained by an analytical approach (see also Chapter 3).

6.4 Essence and manifestation

The examples given above show two different levels of experience when we study processes of metamorphosis. The first level of experience is one of perception, the second of thinking. What manifests itself to our senses lies in the realm of perception, while recognition of continuity in the plant, the human being or the animal lies in the realm of thought. In other words, grasping the personality, the identity, or essence of an organism is experienced in thinking.

When we change inwardly, we *know* all the time that it is we ourselves who experience all this. This experience of the continuity of our own essential being enables us to become aware of the continuity within another being. Thus the immediate experience, which we feel deep in the core of our being, that our human essence does not change becomes a capacity to recognize the same in another being. Despite the vicissitudes of different experiences, there lives inside us a being which remains the same. This experience of our own 'I,' which we would like to characterize as a 'sense of I,' can explain why we are able to have the experience that the archetypal plant is something essential.

In our 'sense of I' we have a direct and immediate spiritual experience. When we experience our self as 'I,' we have a purely spiritual content within our consciousness. The fact that we have this inner cognitive experience makes it possible for us to recognize the moment when we have a spiritual, essential experience of someone else. One could speak of a real meeting on the level of the 'I.' This applies not only to human beings but to all natural forms of existence.

When the experience is at the level of perception, we speak of MANIFESTATION	When the experience is at the level of thinking, we speak of ESSENCE

6.4.1 Metamorphosis in the soul and the course of life

Studying biographies of striking personalities forms an absorbing field of research into processes of metamorphosis in human life. In the course of the lives of 'those who are truly great,' we can experience the tension between that which changes and that which remains constant within the personality.

When one has woken up to these kinds of processes, it is no longer difficult to sense how patients often go through inner processes of metamorphosis in the course of illness and healing.

Assignment 1
Look for examples of patients who do not go through inner metamorphoses and show an increased tendency towards a certain illness at the same time. Give examples of patients who are clearly going through metamorphoses, either after an illness or as a change of lifestyle, with demonstrable medical preventative results.

6.5 Metamorphoses on the level of the organs

Orthodox medicine does not concern itself with questions regarding the essence of things; the reality of the world of ideas as a spiritual world is taboo. As a result, never-ending discussions continue about the exact moment when an embryo should be considered a human being. Based on the understanding we have come to in this chapter's discussions, we can put it in the following terms: whereas an embryo is a sense perceptible *manifestation,* a human being is truly a *being.* This distinction is not generally made, and therefore all regular answers to the question whether an embryo is a human *being* or not will be based on randomly chosen, subjective judgments. We have not been schooled, after all, in asking questions regarding the essence of things.

Especially since ethics committees have been appointed, doctors need not worry anymore about the moral (and hence spiritual) part of their practice of medicine. The physician practices medicine and the ethics-committee determines whether something is morally acceptable or not. We have simply not been trained to be researchers where spiritual matters are concerned.

An even greater taboo rests on using your own experience as a way to gain insight. Therefore the 'experience of I,' as we described above, would not be acceptable to regular science as a tool to research an object. By the same token, it is not considered to be the kind of experience which we can fall back on in order to gain insight regarding another human being.

This experience can now be expanded to the level of physiology, to the study of the organs for example. When we picture the total course of development of the heart, the circulatory system, the kidneys or the outer shape of the human body, the question may arise, 'what *is* the nature of *the* heart, *the* circulatory system, *the* kidney or *the* human shape as such?' If we take present-day cardiology as an example, we can be struck by the fact that the ordinary cardiologist limits his perspective of the heart to the adult heart, the children's cardiologist to the children's heart and the embryologist to the heart of the embryo. Each of the specialists only has partial contact with the other's field, limited to areas of overlap. The cardiological correspondence which the average general practitioner receives, demonstrates this unambiguously.

Since everything manifests itself in different phases and in as many different forms and functions, we would hardly be justified to speak about *the* heart in general etc. But because our thinking allows us to gather a variety of phenomena under one header, which we referred to above as 'picturing the total course of development,' we can develop a 'perception of identity,' which allows us to speak about *the* heart or, where other organs are concerned, *the* kidney, or *the* body. (Compare the text about the heart in the Appendix). In this fashion we research and experience the reality of *the* organ in general on a nonmaterial level, on the level where our thinking gives us certainty. At the same time this is the level where we experience the idea which lies at the basis of the organ. In anthroposophy, the idea is not understood in the sense of 'conceptual summary,' but as an *active principle,* which can actually be experienced. The article in the Appendix posits that the idea which lies at the basis of the heart in general is the idea of the 'reversal of poles.' In our example, this means that the reality and the actual efficacy of this idea expresses itself in every single anatomical, physiological, and pathological aspect of the heart. So to us, ideas are actual working forces. This may come as a surprise. However, we can research the effect of ideas on life. The idea of 'freedom' calls forth totally different activities in a human being than the idea of 'inequality.' People like Gandhi and Mandala are living proof of the reality of these ideas. Here we enter a level which is nonexistent for orthodox science, where idea is reality.

The study of metamorphoses forces us to reconsider our mental pictures of organs and of plants, animals, and human beings. We have to come to different inner pictures that are much richer, more mobile (meaning malleable), and comprehensive than the pictures we have acquired through conventional science. With the help of such different mental pictures of organs, however, we have a much better chance to see the coherence in a multiplicity of manifestations; otherwise there's a danger of losing sight of their interconnectedness.

The viewpoint which is adopted conventionally is one that tries to *define* organs, diseases, and diagnoses. In definitions we always find a rigid picture, which, as we saw in the example of the study of organs, is only applicable by leaving a lot of details out. Therefore definitions tend to cause problems especially where human beings are concerned, increasingly so when one takes comparative anatomy, morphology and physiology into account as well.

In the study of metamorphoses it is therefore much more important to give a good *characterization* of the research object. This will lead to a much better understanding and is preferable to attempting to define, as many things cannot be covered by a definition.

Assignment 2
Try giving a definition (that is really adequate) of pneumonia, depression, nervous exhaustion, or the liver. Then try to give a characterization of the same things. Which description gives you more of a sense of being true to reality?

6.6 What about DNA?

In present-day gene technology the argument given above would immediately meet with the objection that this is no longer valid since the discovery of DNA. After all, DNA is considered to be the determining force behind all manifestations of life. It is thought that DNA carries all information within it and hence determines physiology and morphology. This line of argument is rendered null and void by the fact that DNA as such has no power whatsoever. DNA is totally dependent on the organism it dwells in to have even the slightest effect on the shape which that organism takes. Many peripheral influences, which work in on the nucleus from the cytoplasm and determine the DNA both in form and function, wrest a certain outcome from the DNA. What would DNA be if it were not 'played upon' by the countless enzymes which determine what can come to expression, and when? It is not for nothing that one speaks of 'switching on or off, cutting out, and reading' sections of DNA. The primal moving force, therefore, does not lie *within* DNA, *but outside it,* in the organic context. All kinds of influential enzymes, which effect change, are being activated there in order to determine the possibilities of the DNA to express itself. The suggestion that DNA would be the origin of life and would contain the 'origin' of the organism, is illusory; it should be considered a basic error of thought. The German embryologist Blechschmidt put it very plainly, 'Genes never act, they react.'

6.7 Discussion

The study of metamorphosis is not practised consciously in medical school. Last remnants are still found in descriptions of older clinicians concerning the course of illnesses, the typical character of clinical phenomena such as the fever which occurs in malaria, pneumonia, measles or brucellosis and also in descriptions of changes taking place during the different stages of illnesses, as is the case in syphilis, tuberculosis, lobar pneumonia or Scheuermann's disease (an osteochondrosis).

Partly as a result of prompt therapies which work rapidly, the student no longer has the opportunity to study metamorphoses in illness directly. Another hindrance is the tendency to want to explain all phenomena on the basis of a biochemical picture of man, which can stand in the way of a macroscopic view. In medical training the world of quantifiable phenomena thus tips the balance; the whole emphasis lies on getting a handle on that world. Experiencing aspects which have to do with the essence of things is considered unimportant. Some fundamentalists even consider them non-existent. When such a view comes to determine our approach to the human being, we will come to look upon ourselves as beings without a core, which is contradicted by our daily experience in the way we sense ourselves. Referring back to what was said before about Gandhi and Mandela, we could ask ourselves what the effect would be of being 'without spirit.' What would become of us when such a concept would really take effect and to what actions would we be driven?

CHAPTER 7

Observing Nature and Studying the Elements

GUUS VAN DER BIE

A living experience of nature plays a big part in anthroposophical medicine. An inexhaustible number of observations can be made in nature concerning the natural elements, broadly speaking. By that term we do not mean the elements as we know them from the periodic chart, but the elements in a 'meteorological' sense: air, water, earth and warmth. In the four seasons, as they unfold in European latitudes, ever-changing combinations of these four elements appear. We are in a position to investigate how they work in their changing configurations through the seasons. We are never at a loss for objects of study, surrounded as we are by nature and the weather all day long. All we need to do is pay attention to them and we will notice the richness and infinite movement and development in our natural surroundings.

Our everyday language expresses relationship between processes in the human being and our natural surroundings, for instance, 'petrified with fear,' 'burning with desire,' 'losing the ground under one's feet, 'to be adrift,' and many others. These examples are a metaphor from nature applied to an inner experience, in which we obviously sense a strong relationship to the natural phenomenon. We can be fairly certain to meet with spontaneous understanding when we use such expressions in our everyday speech, which shows that there is a basis in a generally shared experience. In our experience, we find that our inner world is related to outer nature.

However exciting such an inborn sense of correspondence may be, it cannot just be taken as a basis for a scientific approach to the human being or for medicine. Yet anthroposophical medicine does make use of the elements. An attempt will be made here to describe them in such a way that their correspondence to physiological and psychological processes can be elucidated. In doing so we will therefore connect our natural experiences with a scientific methodology.

For didactic reasons we will principally describe two natural elements in their mutual relationship. As before, these descriptions serve as examples, chosen to illustrate *how* we approach phenomena. The aim is to develop an organ of perception for processes in nature, which, in a metamorphosed form, also occur in human physiology.

7.1 Water and air

As a starting point, we will consider a natural situation where we can experience open water such as a lake, sea, a large pond or a river.

We may have experienced a summer evening without a breath of wind wind, and characteristic stillness in the air. Nothing stirs. The cloudless sky arches like a cupola over the sea or the lake. Stillness all around. There are no threatening cloud banks; quiet reigns in nature. Such a nature mood must have inspired Goethe to write his poem *Über allen Gipfeln ist Ruh* [Quiet reigns over all the mountaintops]. The onlooker is likely to feel dreamy. In such a situation the water forms a mirror surface, completely smooth interrupted only by the waterbirds, fish, or perhaps a stream causing some ripples. There are no surges or waves. No movement and no sound.

The situation changes dramatically as soon as even the slightest breeze stirs. We are carressed by the air passing by, which immediately creates a sensation of movement. The direction from which the wind comes, the speed with which the air is moving, the steadiness or gustiness of the movement: we become aware of these things in a fraction of a second. They dispel the dreamy character of the moment before, making way for more 'wakefulness.' Ripples appear on the water, moving rhythmically and in a clear direction corresponding to that of the wind. The ripples are visible as long as the breeze is there. When the air becomes quiet again, the water will also show no more movements after a little while. On a large surface of water several places tend to be visible where breezes ruffled the water, incoherent patches of movement on an otherwise smooth water surface. Where these breezes ruffle the water, the surface immediately loses the capacity to mirror the surroundings. Whereas the colours of the air were mirrored in the water before, now this is broken by the movement of the water, and the colours of the air either make way for greyish tints, or their reflection is interrupted by stripes of a darker hue.

When the wind increases in strength, silence makes way for sound. First there may be a light rushing, to begin with maybe without rustling of leaves or the sound of lapping water. But when the force of the wind gradually increases, more and more sounds arise until at last, in the case of a gale, the wind roars. The movement of the air becomes so forceful that our muscles will actively react to the air currents. In extreme situations we must even take care not to lose our balance, or work hard not to be pushed off course by the wind. Everything inside us and around us is set in motion now, we are moved from the outside by the wind, from the inside we are moved by our own motor movement. And our state of consciousness will be far from dreamy! In situations such as these, staying upright, or sailing a boat home unscathed demands clear wakefulness. The water will have undergone a profound change during this process. The ripples will have been replaced by lapping undulation, which will make way for real waves in the water when the wind increases. The entire water surface, smooth to begin with, has been set in motion, there is not a place to be found without movement, and the reflection of the light and the colours on the water have turned into an ever-changing play of scintillation in a variety of colours. In due course the waves and the foam will produce their own sounds.

It is worth recalling our experience when we were *in* the water, for example at the beach in the surf when there are strong waves. Every wave which rolls towards us has the potential to push us over with its force, and we can choose to either resist it or allow it to carry us along. In the first case we will have to stand quite firm, in the second case we will be dragged along in a tumble of movement. Once the crest of the wave has passed, we will be sucked back into the trough behind it. The effects of high pressure and low pressure, which are essentially archetypal phenomena in the air, penetrate deep into the water. Playing in the surf, we are *in* the water, but feel the effects of air patterns. What we mean by this is that areas of high pressure and low pressure typically occur in the air. This can be compared to the phenomenon of the nodes and antinodes in the propagation of sound, which also travels through the air from the source of sound.

Air is preeminently the element of movement. Air can transmit
movement to water, because this is receptive to it, even though by
its own nature it does not tend to move. Thus water is permeated
by the characteristics and laws of the air.

What we have presented here applies not only applies to water, but to all liquids which are influenced in their motion by a gas. The described interaction between fluids and gases, in a wider sense includes everything that is of a fluid and a gaseous nature. As soon as water freezes, after all, it belongs to the category of 'earth,' and suddenly nothing of the above applies anymore!

Looking now to the field of medicine, the circulatory system can be viewed as the 'water' within the human being, showing phenomena based on corresponding processes. Everything that is liquid in us shows fluctuations in pressure, for example in the form of blood pressure. The way blood pressure is built up depends completely on the movement system of the cardiovascular system. The heart muscle and the musculature of the capillaries are the movement organs which achieve the way blood pressure is built up. In answer to the question 'what is a muscle?' Louis Bolk preferred, 'a component which contracts and relaxes.' Now the air is the element in which contractibility (in the sense of elasticity), compressibility and rarification are preeminently at home. So in this sense *characteristics* of the air play a major role in the muscular system, which expresses itself in tightening and stretching, corresponding to high pressure and low pressure in the air which surrounds us. Within the context chosen here it should not surprise us that the Greeks, who were vividly aware of the elements, had the word *artria* for artery, which, having pulse and contractibility, perhaps expressed the immediate effect of the element air. Building up tension in a muscle is directly related to inner experience. We are all aware of the fact that emotions will quicken the pulse, heighten blood pressure, and contract the intestines or bladder. A tense person often has hypertonic muscles, bordering on or actually causing pain, and will have a heightened consciousness in life. When we 'unwind,' we tend to relax both the striated and the smooth muscles, and we will become more dreamy again. A heightening of blood pressure is enhanced by stress, which arises especially during the waking hours, or by an increase in tension in the musculature of the heart or capillaries. In the way blood pressure is built up we always find three inextricably intertwined factors, which are movement, consciousness and tonicity. Whenever the character of the elements of air and water are more strongly connected in human physiology, these three are always to be found together. Logically, the reverse occurs during sleep in human beings and the higher animals. Consciousness decreases, tonus diminishes, and movement disappears. When we wake someone (or even a cat) up, we see those three characteristic traits return. This brings us to the characteristics of the element of air. In each of the three aspects: densification or concentration alternates with rarification or relaxation. For consciousness these consist of waking and sleeping, for movement activity and rest and for tonus a hypertonic or atonic state. That these three polarities are intimately connected could be expressed as follows: during the waking states we actively move with muscles which are balanced in tonus, during sleep we rest with relaxed muscles.

Characteristics of AIR:
consciousness — movement — tonus

Assignment 1
Comparative zoology is a captivating subject to study. We can
compare animals at their different levels of development and ask,
'What is the relationship between tonus movement and conscious-
ness within this organism?'
Do this with a worm, a fish, and a monkey.

7.2. Water and earth

Various landscapes are eminently suitable to studying the interaction between earth and water. The word earth should be understood here to comprise all mineral substance. In this respect, rock formations stand out. When one visits the same mountain region year after year, or returns to a familiar mountain massif after a period of absence, one is impressed by the immutability of the landscape. The mountains have the same profile, individual mountains have names as if they were personalities, and there are numerous mountaineering stories describing the same routes or mountain faces. The expression 'rock solid' applies not only to a single specimen; solidity and stability are essential features of all rock formations. When we find variation and change in the mountain landscape, it stems from the elements which we spoke of before, water an air. What does not change is the shape of the rocks. The naive visitor may feel questions arising such as 'how long have these rock formations existed' and 'how long will they last.' And when such questions involve a sense of time at all, they are likely to go into guesses as to placement in geological periods, and in our thinking we reach towards infinity. And thus an experience of a certain timelessness enters into our consciousness. When we are faced with folds in mountain belts with their solid undulating layers of stone, we can hardly imagine that these rocks actually moved at one time. It is not for nothing that people feel shaken to the core of their being when they experience eruptions of volcanoes or earthquakes: these create such a feeling of uncertainty, that people literally feel as if they are losing the ground under their feet! No, if water, air and fire were not to interact with rock formations, they would forever remain unchanged. Even in deserts change is only brought about by heat and wind.

7.2.1 Do rocks have an 'inside'?

The question whether rock has an inside may seem absurd. Why would one ask such a question? We posited that the characteristic feature of the element earth is contour, or boundary, or the shape of the surface. However, this implies the presence of surface, because without surface, a contour could not arise. Now suppose you have a stone in your hand, and you want to see what is inside. You chop that stone in two in order to see what is *in* it. Depending on the way you define things, you could say, 'There's stone in that stone,' or, 'I see a new surface, so that is a new out-side.' In the first case the conclusion would be that stones are the same on the inside as on the outside, both of them being stone; but in the second case the conclusion would have to be that a stone always shows its out-side: that is, a surface resulting in a boundary. This could lead to the view that rock, though appearing as a spatial body with rigid boundaries, lacks a proper inside. The reason for this discussion here is to get at a more pre-cise description of the difference between the spatial content and the inside of a thing.

The difference here seems merely philosophical, but when it comes to the study of plants, animals, or the human being, it becomes essen-tial. Only living beings can have an inner dimension next to a spatial content.

Assignment 2
Return to Figure 4.10 (mineral man), and compare it with Figures 4.15 and 4.16 (animal man) with a view to this question of spatial content or inside.

7.2.2 Beyond time

When we imagine a rock or stone in isolation, we will not expect any change to take place. As long as there are no changes in temperature, no exposure to direct sunlight or vegetation growing on top, rock will remain inert. The mountain folds show us that these rock formations have not always led a 'timeless' existence. The undulating layers in the rock reflect the movement which preceded the static state. The same goes for sedi-mentary rocks. Its layers can be read as processes in time to which the rock formation was subject. For a geologist this is all obvious, of course. Experienced phenomenologically, however, this means that the timeless phase of the substance always follows the stage during which the substance was still subject to processes. Therefore one could formulae a principal law of morphology as follows:

> Processes in time precede processes of form; form comes out of movement.

If we allow ourselves a little aside, and look at pathological processes such as arteriosclerosis and stone formation, it may become clear that a good insight into the role of time phenomena has a direct relation to the insight into physiological processes, both normal and pathological. The word 'process,' shows us the relationship to time, literally meaning 'forward motion.' This indicates going forward both in time and space. In essence everything which has 'taken on a definite form' has reached a state of earth, and has proceeded 'out of time'; with that it has fallen prey to timelessness. Developments have come to an end, there will be no changes anymore, and life will not affect it anymore.

Characteristics of EARTH
boundary — timelessness — immutability

7.3 Water as such

7.3.1 Totally selfless

Like no other fluid, water is able to transcend the rigidity of substance which has turned mineral. One of its chief characteristics is that it can *dissolve* substances within it, which thereby lose their boundary or shape. What seemed immutable and unchanging immediately enters the realm of change. Water has very specific characteristics. It is odourless, tasteless and colourless and adapts without any problem to the shape of its surroundings. The surface of the water mirrors the colours and shapes of the environs without changing them. As we saw in our description of air and water, water is able to take 'foreign' patterns and characteristics into itself and can express them. Water has the characteristic of enabling something else to reveal its own activity. Chemistry makes use of this. When two chemical substances do not react in solid form, remaining to a state of immutability, water can bring about a solution (in both senses). Dissolved, the two substances turn out to be able to react, sometimes even immediately! In a dissolved form, even latent possibilities of the substances can manifest and realize their potential.

Everyday examples are sugar in coffee and salt in soup. The sweet taste of coffee and the salt taste of soup only come to consciousness when sugar and salt have been dissolved. Thus water brings many physical and chemical characteristics to light. There is something amazing about all this. Just imagine that water would have a clearly defined odour and smell. If that were the case, one would *always* taste and smell water everywhere! Just imagine how much water vapour there is in the air, and how much water is being used by plant and animal and in our food preparation. We would be conscious of the presence of water at all times.

This brings us to a marvellous characteristic of water, which one could call *selflessness*. It is this selflessness of water, which enables it to give other elements a chance to reveal themselves in their proper dynamics, and become active.

On a large scale, water plays this role in the whole of nature as well. Substances are carried down in streams and rivers, to be deposited lower down near the estuaries, where the finer sediment benefits the vegetative life. Even the seemingly untouchable mountain contours cannot escape erosion; witness the scree slopes and landslides. Here water plays a major role, both through its power to dissolve stone and its ability to break rock apart when it freezes in the fissures.

The characteristics of water described so far could be summed up in the following concepts: *the realm of change, selflessness, and power to reveal*. The latter refers to the ability which water has to allow other substances to manifest their own dynamics. These dynamics only become active when the fixed form has been dissolved!

Looking back at our description of water and air, we can find the same dynamics, for there we indicated how the order inherent in the air (high-pressure/low-pressure, elasticity) can manifest *through* water. Water, which would never make undulating movements of itself, is able to make those under the influence of the air!

We will see how the same principle applies after the section about warmth. (The capacity of water to hold warmth is enormous.) We will explore warmth as a dynamic factor of global dimensions. Water balances warmth on a vast scale. It is due to this characteristic of water that many processes on earth can take place so that things can 'move' again.

Characteristics of WATER
change — selflessness — power to reveal

7.3.2 The uniqueness of water

Water has one characteristic which has far-reaching consequences for life on earth. We are referring here to the fact that water reaches its greatest density at 4°C. In everyday life, we are familiar with the fact that ice floats on top of water, and warm water rises in cold water. These are common phenomena which have immense consequences. Suppose water would grow denser when it is cooled below 4 degrees, like all other substances.

Then all the oceans on earth would have a layer of ice at the bottom, on which the lighter, warmer water would float. The warmer water would protect the ice below it from the warmth of the sun and would keep it from melting. Further cooling would make the colder water go down, forcing the warmer water up to be cooled. The layer of ice at the bottom of the seas would never melt.

As a result of water's unique temperature-to-density curve, we have the conditions of life on earth.

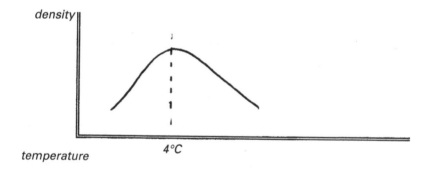

Figure 7.1.

This property of water acts as a buffer with regard to the way warmth is distributed on earth. Because of it, extreme cooling as well as extreme heating of the hydrosphere and biosphere are prevented. Through the ecological disasters of the present day we know as never before what it means when the hydro-biosphere lacks water because of erosion resulting from slash-and-burn agriculture. Water mismanagement immediately threatens vegetation, leading to desert formation to a greater or lesser degree. Water is not only the key substance for life in the oceans, but also on the earth which holds water.

Watering plants or putting bulbs in the humid earth seems like a simple everyday activity, but we need to give water more credit and contemplate it with wonder and awe.

This means that water is the *main* substance through which processes can connect with the mineral earth. Everything which can be taken again into the stream of time, which is equivalent to the stream of life, can again partake in ongoing development.

The force of water creates the 'space' within which the *vegetative principle* can manifest *in time*.

7.4 Warmth and its effect on earth, water and air

7.4.1 Form or process

The archetypal way warmth works can be demonstrated if we imagine the world in two different aggregate states. The first would arise if the earth that were to cool to absolute zero, 0°K (or –273°C). This would be a situation with a total absence of warmth. From immediate experience we know what happens when our body cools down severely. Movement becomes difficult or even impossible. When our hands are too cold we cannot open or close the buttons of our coat anymore, our limbs hardly want to move and our body threatens to stop moving altogether or even becomes rigid. In the case of real hypothermia, for instance, drowning or floating for some time in icy water, the motor movements of the internal organs slow down, and there is progressive bradycardia with direct danger to vital functions of the organism as a whole. If we imagine a world totally cooled down to absolute zero, it would be as extinguished. There would be no more chemical reactions, all substances would exist in solid form, there would be no fluids, no gases, in short, it would represent a final stage which could be indicated with the concept *inertness*. There would be a massive ice age where silence and inactivity would be present all-around. This would be a situation in which everything would be solid, and each substance would have taken on its *own form*. Water crystallizes differently from nitrogen, sulphur or phosphorus. A multiplicity of shapes in a mineralized aggregation would exist.

If, on the other hand, we were to imagine an overheated earth, we would first see how everything solid would become liquid, and having gone through that stage, would reach its boiling point. If the temperature were to increase even more, liquid substance would all boil and turn into gas. Nothing would have boundaries anymore, everything would be mixed together, everything would react with other substances, and all would be extreme *activity and movement*. We know from chemistry demonstrations in school that the speed of a reaction depends on the temperature. And creative teachers may have shown us that increased temperature ultimately leads to an explosion. In explosions we have an extreme picture of the vehement breaking of fixed boundaries. During heating everything resists crystallized form. The expansion of solids when heated can be seen in this sense.

When we think this process through to the end (is there one?), we will find everything in its most dynamic state. In that situation everything will be either invisible or, like the sun, a luminous mass. But, on closer inspection, light turns out to be invisible until it falls on the surface of a solid substance. For light to become visible it has to be reflected from a substance. A simple test will easily show us that, for when we illuminate an object with a flashlight, we will not see the light 'on its way'! The path of light becomes visible by the solid particles floating in it.

7.4.2 The sun as a source of warmth

We can attempt to imagine the state of the overheated earth, when we look at conditions on the sun. These exceed our powers of imagination: the temperatures, the size of the sun protuberances, the speed of processes, and the true nature of substance there, are all beyond us. One thing is clear, however. Everything moves; everything is activity; nothing has fixed boundaries, and inertness is unthinkable. All solids are consumed and taken into the spiralling, seething fire world of the sun.In our temperate zones we experience every year anew how everything becomes inert in winter, vegetation barely shows circulation, and hibernating animals have a radically decreased rate of metabolic activity. When spring arrives and the warmth of the sun increases, there is a fundamental change. When we notice the amount of transformation of substance taking place in a blossoming spring landscape with leaves forming, with intensive photosynthesis, with animals focused on procreation, we discern how thousands of tons of water and mineral substance are taken into the various life cycles.

The dynamic effect of warmth described above holds good equally for solids, liquids and gases. It is the temperature after all which determines the aggregate state of the substance and its visibility and activity. During heating and burning the visible manifestation disappears and the substance reappears again during cooling. So warmth has to do with coming to manifestation as such. The object of our perceptual content is not so much *what* appears, but the fact *that* something manifests.

Warmth forms the bridge between the visible world of manifestation and the invisible world of dynamic, qualitative processes.

Characteristics of the element of WARMTH
portal of manifestation — cause of processes —
connects the visible with the invisible

7.4.3 'Psychosomatics' of warmth

In human physiology, warmth is known as the origin of all phenomena. In the English language, the expression 'warming towards something or somebody' is just one example out of many. When something 'leaves us cold,' we are not likely to see any action! We cannot make the connection with something which leaves us cold. Warmth stands at the beginning of all processes. The word 'initiative' literally contains this sense. Every ideal and initiative which fires us and which we want to realize, will eventually have a visible outcome. Any disciplined self-observation easily shows the working and the importance of warmth in one's own soul. It is essential to experience that it is we ourselves who can generate warmth. When we become engaged and allow warmth and heart forces to stream out from ourselves towards other people, 'new things' can happen. This goes for any situation which we approach with warmth. In a sense, we become 'portals' through our warmth and engagement in such situations which allows new things to manifests.

Living in the ideal, the 'I' dwells in an *invisible* realm; in realizing the ideal, the I creates something *visible.* Warmth forms the connecting factor between these two levels of existence.

7.5 The dynamic relationships between the elements

In the examples given above, water, earth, air and warmth (and their interactions) were always the starting point. This approach was chosen because much can be made clear that way, as well as demonstrating that one can hardly find the elements in isolation. Both in the world around us, and within the human organism, we always find a mixture. Within that there is a *fragile balance,* with constant shifting taking place. Clear examples are shifts in temperature, altering aggregate states, and the changes in the composition of the organism. A clinical example may serve to clarify this. The human organism contains a considerable quantity of water. It is striking that water manifests in two forms during life. In a healthy situation water *defies gravity.* It moves as intracellular or extracellular liquid through the organism. In those circumstances it is totally absorbed within the organic context. In short, we could characterize this kind of water as 'living' water. Contrasting this is water which *is* subject to gravity, and which we know especially from pathological circumstances: edema. During the course of the day this water will descend into the legs in following physical laws. Due to this, the legs tend towards the shapes of drops. It is easy to move the water mechanically by bandaging the legs. By lying down the edema can also stream to another lowest point. Therefore we will find the edema localized near the sacrum in the morning. So in a sense the edema is more 'normal' in its behaviour than 'living' extracellular liquid. But this is a 'normality' in terms of the laws of inorganic nature. Therefore we could characterize edema as 'dead' water.

The study of circadian rhythms show the ups and downs which all substances and processes in an organism are subject to within a time cycle of 24 hours. These are a reflection of continual changes in the different elemental qualities in relation to one another, which determine the material composition of the organism, changes in tonicity, fluctuations in consciousness and many other physiological phenomena.

Assignment 3
Try to describe the difference in the elemental dynamics for a typical 'morning person' and an 'evening person.'
What happens in terms of the elements in the case of colic?
Why can a (warm) hot water bottle help relieve a stomach-ache?
In a pathological situation the human being can be overpowered by one of the four elements. Try to group the following list of psychiatric symptom-complexes according to the dominating element:
— mania
— depression
— stupor
— psychosis.

Since the relation of the elements is fragile, influences from outside exert a strong influence. This receptivity is the means by which disturbances actually *can* occur. Not only meteorologists have to be able to judge and assess this; the physician has to do the same thing! Being impressionable and highly sensitive are signs of a healthy organism on the one hand, but on the other hand this quality makes the organism more liable to being unsettled. Medical experience shows that constant stress is likely to seek an organic outlet in changes in blood pressure, intestinal disturbances and pathological physiological phenomena of different kinds.

7.6 Methodological remark

In this chapter, an attempt was made to practice seeing a relationship between the natural world around us and within us. We consciously chose to present this so that it could be experienced in a living way. Further acquaintance with anthroposophy will show that the elements are mentioned at several levels. Briefly summarized, what it comes down to is distinguishing between:

— the different substances of earth, water, air and fire
— the elements earth, water, air and fire
— the different kinds of ether: the life ether, the chemical ether, the light ether and the warmth ether.

It would go too far here to go into further detail, but it is good to bear in mind that a conscious choice was made to avoid various nuances for the time being.

CHAPTER 8

The Anthroposophical View of the Human Being

ARIE BOS AND GUUS VAN DER BIE

If one holds the view that the human being is an incarnated spiritual being, as held in the previous chapters, the question arises what concepts will help to bridge the Cartesian gap (see Section 2.2.2) between matter and spirit. This chapter will deal with this question. The importance of the answer to this question goes beyond mere philosophical satisfaction: in anthroposophical medicine it forms the basis of diagnosis, pathology and therapy. The question regarding the connection between spirit and matter will be the subject of this chapter about the fourfold view of the human being. The question of how spirit expresses itself in the body is the subject of the threefold view of the human being. But first a 'little apology of the spirit.'

8.1 A little apology of the spirit

We are used to identifying ourselves with our bodies. This is obvious, because that's how we know ourselves primarily. And science, as taught in universities in this day and age, supports the idea that we *are* body, and *have* spirit. Brain cells are thought to produce consciousness. In such a way of thinking, consciousness and spirit are the same thing. This is one of the ideas which is a starting point for present-day culture. It is the logical consequence of the Darwinian evolutionary theory, which assumes that life arose spontaneously in the course of earth evolution, and that consciousness also arose spontaneously as a result of the ever-increasing complexity of organisms.[1]

In spite of this, we consider ourselves responsible for our deeds as human beings. This brings us into conflict with the above hypothesis. If our thoughts, and with them our behaviour, were determined by bodily processes, we would be unable to help it if that behaviour were antisocial. Responsibility presupposes that we can rise above these processes with our consciousness. That would be hard to do if these processes themselves determined our consciousness. We meet with yet another problem when we identify ourselves with our bodies. The body does not remain the same: the proteins, including those of our brains, do not live more than a few days and are therefore being exchanged continually. All the molecules of our body are changed so that we have a completely new body every seven years, viewed materially. In addition, the body changes by aging, illness and accidents. Psychologically, we will also change during the course of our life, if all goes well. Except on the molecular level we can perceive all these changes in ourselves. And this is what is important: we are not only able to perceive our own bodies, but our own behaviour, feelings and thoughts as well. And furthermore we can also influence them. For that reason, we can call on one another with respect to our responsibilities, which demonstrates the presence of self-awareness. Our culture definitely starts from the premise that we have the freedom to observe our thoughts, feelings, and behaviour and to direct them. We can even be punished when we exhibit undesirable behaviour. (Of course conceiving consciousness as a product of the brain leads to a corresponding hypothesis regarding responsible behaviour: we learn such behaviour by reward and punishment. But then again, it would be pretty inhumane to keep punishing criminals only because they're bad at learning). So in our culture we implicitly presuppose something which stands above thoughts, inclinations and feelings. In our faculty of self-awareness we can surmise the manifestation of spirit. After all, self-awareness cannot be explained from the body, and does not metamorphose along with the body.

8.2 The fourfold view

Using our observations of everyday reality and common sense, let us now attempt an exercise in thought, and imagine how matter and spirit can become linked. We will not find an answer when we stick to dead matter. It is hard to imagine, for example, how spirit can manifest in a stone. Dead matter is too inert for that; at least we need to be presented with the potential for something dynamic. The first prerequisite is a metamorphosis of matter into a dynamic substance, which we find in living nature. Plants meet this requirement, but in them we do not expect to find consciousness. Being alive is obviously not enough. The organism has to be brought to a higher level. The possibility for consciousness has to be present in it, which we find in the animal kingdom. Yet, however intelligent animals can be, we do not expect them to be conscious of themselves. (Animals cannot be held responsible for their behaviour, at least not to the same degree as human beings. They themselves cannot be brought to justice, only their owners can.) This point of view necessarily leads to the conclusion that only human organisms meet the requirements which enable them to make a connection with the spirit: they are both material, alive and conscious, just like the animals. Below we will return to the difference between the human and the animal organism. We will first concentrate on a discussion of the metamorphoses of matter as caused by life, consciousness and self-awareness.

8.3 Matter

8.3.1 The physical body

In medicine, only the pathologist is concerned with the physical body. That is to say, the body insofar as it is determined by the natural laws of dead nature described in physics and chemistry. It takes up space, is subject to gravity, forces of cohesion, capillary forces, laws of mechanics and thermodynamics, chemical reactions etc. Theoretically, we are familiar with this reality so that we do not have to go into this further.

8.3.2 Earth

We can bring dead nature into connection with the element of earth, as was done in Chapter 7. However, the characteristics of the element of earth, listed in that chapter as contour, timelessness, and immutability, turns out to be not applicable to the body in post-mortem state. The body decomposes; it disintegrates into its separate substances, and loses its shape and structure. It is subject to the second law of thermodynamics, the increase of entropy.[2] This entropy is the result of the aforementioned natural laws. Apparently those were not the only ones governing during the time that the body was still alive. What, then, distinguishes the living world from the dead, physical world?

Characteristics of the physical body:
The area within the human organism in which inorganic forces of
physics and chemistry are at work.

8.4 Life

8.4.1 The etheric body

Living nature can be seen as comprising the domain where the natural forces of dead matter do not have free play.

Assignment 1
Suppose somebody who is out walking suffers from a heart attack.
Why will bystanders immediately notice that something is the matter?

A striking characteristic of both plants, animals and human beings is that they all have the inclination to overcome gravity. But apparently there is more. The living organism presents a paradox for physics: even though it consists of many different substances which can react with one another and have the ability to make the organism disintegrate, the capacity to preserve itself wins out during life; the organism remains intact. As long as we are alive, we will not spontaneously disintegrate. Why is that? We are accustomed to describe this as a cybernetic problem. The body contains many regulatory systems. Here, however, we meet the same paradox which we discussed before when we talked about the primacy of the spirit. Matter, which is characterized by entropy, supposedly would have to take care of its own more complex coherence. Life is not the product of matter, nor is it the result of physical laws, but, as was suggested in previous chapters, it is a cosmic given, it is 'God-given.' The regulatory systems are subject to a higher, cosmic principle. We call this principle the *ether body* in anthroposophy.

We cannot see this principle; its kernel does not reside in the brain. We can only see the results of its presence. (It should be remarked here that people with clairvoyant capacities claim that it is visible for them. It is then spoken about as the aura. More is at play in this, which will be discussed later.) Because the results are visible to the eye, we can also study the characteristics of this ether body. The plant kingdom can help us in this, because the picture is not further complicated by the presence of consciousness or self-awareness. What are the characteristics of the plant kingdom, which cannot be found in dead nature?

Form
A first feature of the plants is that they have an individual shape, in contrast to dead nature. Granite, limestone or iron do not have their own shape but are shaped by natural forces from the outside. Crystalline forms arise out of

a combination of inner natural forces, the molecular structure, and outer circumstances. (Antimonite crystals from Japan look different from European ones, and pyrite crystals have an even greater diversity of form, depending on where they are found.) Every plant species has its own shape, with variations depending on its location. So this shape is a characteristic of being alive. It is a trait of the ether body of that particular plant. But where does DNA come in? In *A New Science of Life,* the English biologist Rupert Sheldrake writes about the problem that DNA only contains the code of a sequence of amino acids in proteins. How are we to imagine that it also contains a design for the shape of the organism, especially since every cell is equipped with the same 'genetic code,' which implies that every new cell would have to look like the old one? That would result in a shapeless lump. Of course regulatory mechanisms such as the suppressing or the activating of genes play a role, but here we are faced with the same paradox again: how does matter know it has to do one thing in one place and something else in another place? There are no natural laws on which these mechanisms would be based (see Section 6.6). Formulated in this way, it is a spatial problem. Therefore Sheldrake postulates his morphogenetic fields theory, which shows striking similarities to the anthroposophical concept of the ether body. The ether body is also conceived as being morphogenetic. Steiner used to speak of 'the body of formative forces' at times.*

Not only does the ether body determine the shape, it also maintains this as much as possible. Think of what happens after mowing or pruning. The plants will continue growing as much as possible in the same shape. The plant (the ether body) strives to maintain and preserve form.

Metamorphosis in time
The metamorphosis of plants was discussed in Chapter 6. We should add here that plants not only change shape, but that a new aspect of the total form is continually being added in the course of growth. It is striking to

---

*   Note that there is a semantic trap here: the Latin word *genetivus* (synonymous with *genitivus)* means 'born with,' from the verb *generare,* to generate. Since Mendel, a monk, formulated his laws of heredity, we have become used to seeing everything which the organism contains in the way of inborn traits, as coming from its forebears. As a result, 'genetically determined' has come to mean 'inherited.' Thanks to the work of Watson and Crick, the structure of DNA and RNA has been unravelled in the meantime, and with it the mechanisms by which clusters of these structures codify the production of proteins. These clusters were named genes after the same Latin stem. A shift in meaning has taken place, therefore, which has gone unnoticed. Genetic has come to mean 'determined by genes.' As a result, three concepts are now being used interchangeably: inherited, genetic, determined by genes.

note that this changing of form implies that a form can no longer be defined in three dimensions, as can be done in the case of dead nature. The changes in shape can only take place in time. Thus time enters into the realm of life as a new dimension. Therefore the ether body is also referred to as 'time body.'

Growth

This metamorphosis is only possible due to another characteristic of life: growth or building up. In contrast to the physical world, where a crystal can also be said to grow because more and more material is being added from the outside, the plant grows from the inside out.

Reproduction

Obviously life, being finite, must guarantee its continuation by means of some form of reproduction.

Open to the cosmos

Next to the autonomous characteristics mentioned above, the plant is actually at the mercy of the influences coming from the surroundings. Light and warmth determine the quality of its growing shape. That is to say, the sun is the determining factor here. Even the activity of the sunspots, which have a rhythm of about 11 years, is reflected in plant growth. We see it for example in tree rings, or the germination percentage of plants.[3] The evening primrose, for example, has a germination percentage which varies from 5 to 95 percent, depending on the phase in sun activity.[4] The moon likewise influences the plant world: the amount of water a bean can absorb during the phase in which it absorbs moisture before germination corresponds exactly to the quarter moon phases.[5] Interesting research is currently in process to gauge the influence of the plants and even the constellations, but no scientific publications are available as yet.

Vitality

Compared to humans and animals, the plant world is distinguished by an incredible surplus of vitality. Despite being subject to the aforementioned pruning and mowing, climatic influence, consumption by animals, and clear-cutting by human beings, the plant continually tries to secure its continued existence by new growth. And when the plant dies, other plants try to restore plant coverage. This only comes to an end when the most important condition of life is no longer met: the presence of water.

8.4.2 Water

Without water there is no life. The characteristics of water (Section 7.3.1) show how water can play its mediating role in physiology, without interfering itself. Water is the carrier of life processes. In the plant world, water lends turgor and shine to tissue. It is not clear whether sap's streaming can be explained purely mechanically, but it takes care of the transportation of nutrients and waste products, thereby enabling the dynamics of building up and growth to take place. The ether body derives its dynamic potential in the body from the element of water.

Assignment 2
The first phenomenon which alerts us to vitality in living beings is shininess. This applies equally to the leaf of a tree, the fur of a cat, the feathers of a chicken, or the scales of a fish. What does this point to? Pay special attention to this for a period of time.

8.4.3 Characteristics of the ether body

Even though the ether body is invisible (except to someone who has developed clairvoyant capacities), we can definitely characterize the ether body by looking at phenomena of life. (Even the skeptic should not be deterred by this invisibility: Many accepted phenomena in physics are invisible. The black holes in astronomy are even defined as being invisible!) We are concerned with a 'body' or field which is to be imagined spatially, and which determines the shape of the physical body and its changing forms in the course of time. Spatially, it coincides with the physical body. Hence one can speak of 'the etheric arm or 'the etheric liver.' It has the tendency to swell up (growth and upbuilding) and it has a streaming nature (sap streams). It is open to influences from the cosmos and is able to organize earthly substances into organic structures (see Section 7.3.1). It influences the physical body and brings it to a higher plane.

8.5 Consciousness

8.5.1 The astral body

In the animal world we are dealing for the first time with the ability to move freely and autnomously. This would be unthinkable without consciousness, because autonomous movement is always directed. This presupposes preference or aversion. Sympathy and antipathy, like and dislike: these play a decisive role; why else would we want to move at all?

In the section concerning the ether body we could still generalize about the plant world as a whole, even though it is differentiated into higher and lower plants; we could do this because it is impossible to say that one plant is more alive than another one, even though there are differences in vitality. Such a generalization is no longer possible when we are discussing consciousness in relation to phenomena in the animal world. After all, animals differ significantly in their level of consciousness. Additionally, the presence of consciousness in an animal can vary according to the time of day, as in sleeping and waking.

8.5.2 Evolution

Again, it must be stated that consciousness cannot be taken to be the product of matter. As higher plants get more and more complex in their structure, we do not find that consciousness arises spontaneously at a certain point. When we come to animals, we meet a totally new principle, which, seen as a stage in evolution, starts all over again with the most primitive life forms. So consciousness also is a God-given thing. Even though people maintain that intelligence and behaviour are also determined by genes, we immediately run into the same problem we met in discussing the ether body, something which Sheldrake also argues. It is obvious that genes have been discovered which can be connected with certain qualities of behaviour or intelligence. Consciousness can only manifest on earth through incarnation. For this, there has to be substance and that substance is codified by the genes. Their task, however, is to serve, not to initiate (see Section 6.6).

Being endowed with consciousness therefore has consequences for the way incarnation takes place. Even though one can speak of a certain automatic movement in the plant kingdom (such as turning towards the sun, opening and closing in response to the light, the closing of 'meat eating' plants, and the snapping shut of the Touch-me-not, the *Mimosa pudica),* plants do not change location. Bacteria do not move of their own accord, but by virtue of Brownian motion. Only amoebas display a certain form of independent movement, which depends on the presence of a substratum against which the pseudopodia can react. But in that case we meet with a new phenomenon: other single cell organisms are engulfed (phagocytosis), whereby the cell membrane is turned in and functions as a primitive stomach. This development continues with flagellates, ciliates, and multiple cell organisms. As far as the latter are concerned, note that the movements are initiated by a process of contraction and expansion taking place in the whole of the organism. The most notable differences between the physiology of plants and animals, however, is to be found in the exchange of gases. In plants this happens by means of diffusion, whereby carbon dioxide is the main element which is consumed, and oxygen is produced. When we come to animals, diffusion no longer suffices, so that different means of breathing are introduced. In their case it is oxygen which is consumed and carbon dioxide which is produced. It used to be that the characterizations which were given for the animal world were 'all that breathes' or 'ensouled nature.' The new principle found here is called the astral body in anthroposophy.

8.5.3 The influence of the astral on the ether body

When we want to discuss the presence of consciousness in organisms somewhat more systematically, we have to begin with the observation that the ether body no longer has free rein in the animal world, just as the laws of physics no longer had free rein in the plant world. The overwhelming vitality which is to be observed in the way that a lawn continues to grow in spite of frequent mowing, the ease with which cuttings can be taken from plants, and the way growth is stimulated after trees have been pruned: all this is unthinkable in the animal world. In this respect it is also interesting to note that the ability of the ether body to restore the physical body is less restricted in lower animals (such as molluscs) than in more highly developed animals. Animals at a lower stage of development have retained more 'plant characteristics' than higher animals have. Other examples of this phenomenon are the way the two halves of a worm, which has been cut through in the middle wiggle away from the accident and continue their lives separately, and lizards can leave their tails in someone's hands and grow a new one which is somewhat smaller. Many more examples can be found to show that the degree of consciousness is inversely proportional to this form of regenerative vitality. Trees, perennial plants and bushes grow on and on, in principle that is. Animals and human beings are 'grown-up' at a certain moment, and will grow no further. Apparently the ether body has completed its formative task at that point. What happens with these creative forces? It would seem that consciousness uses up vitality and these forces will be used in another form for consciousness. Another thing which can be observed in lower animals, especially in the usually hermaphroditic molluscs, is the cosmic influence on the reproductive cycle, which is totally oriented to the rhythms of the moon.[6] In that case reproduction somewhat resembles that of plants, even though we can now talk of a form of mutual attraction, a trait of higher animals behaviour. In higher animals there are more and more signs of sexuality for the sake of procreation, in the form of instincts, drives, and desires.

Thus we can distinguish the following characteristics of the astral body:

Consciousness
From behaviour we can conclude whether organisms have consciousness, and to what degree. We call the behaviour of amoebas still automatic; for animals of a slightly higher order we use the term instinctual. In animals of a still higher order we also recognize like and dislike, we therefore in addition speak of feeling. When we surmise that a process of combining and deducing underlies behaviour, we speak of intelligence. Higher animals can display impressive forms of intelligence. We have seen that these forms of consciousness cannot be separated from bodily characteristics.

Movement
Various specific structures are necessary for outer movement. These progress from pseudopodia to flagella, cilia and real limbs with muscles. These structures need increasingly more energy, necessitating a more active metabolism by means of inner organs. These develop a form of inner movement, which is not found in plants.

Organs
These organs grow in the course of time and change shape. However, this metamorphosis takes place in a fundamentally different way from that of plants. Plant metamorphosis can be called sequential: after one leaf-form another one comes into existence above the previous one; in animals the organ itself changes form, either in the course of embryonic development, or through maturing and aging.

Formation of inner hollow space
This metamorphosis starts early in embryonic development (gastrulation) and makes possible the hollow space which many organs need. This means that animals have a real 'inside,' in contrast to plants which are basically always 'solid.' This throws an interesting light on the bodily

basis of consciousness: in order to be conscious of an outer world there first has to be an inner world.

Breaking down

This type of metamorphosis is only possible when there is not only building up, as with plants, but also breaking down. We speak of planned cell death: apoptosis. The astral body introduces destruction in order to make development possible!

Excretion

The animal therefore excretes not only residues of the metabolic processes, but also residues of its own organism: organic material. This rots, and smells, it is a kind of waste product that the plant does not produce during its life.

Sexuality

Human beings and animals have all the bodily and psychological characteristics which prepare them for autonomous sexual procreation. Even though so-called monoecious plants exist, one cannot really speak of sexuality in plants. Fructification (pollination) is taken care of by animals or the air. It is only human beings and animals which have all the prerequisites which enable them to procreate sexually.

Death

Of course plants die, but sometimes it can be avoided. taking cuttings from a plant can basically be repeated ad infinitum. (This was known in ancient times, e.g. Job 14:7–12.) There are plants which become incredibly old. The Macrozamia tree from Queensland, Australia can reach an age of 12,000 to 15,000 years. The oldest known animal, on the other hand, was a tortoise from the Seychelles, reported to have lived in captivity in Mauritius for 152 years. It must have been 20 years old when it arrived there, so therefore it must have reached the ripe old age of 172 years.[7] In 1968, L. Hayflick wrote that animal and human diploid cells went through a finite and constant quantity of divisions in cell cultivation, in contrast to plant cells and also cancer cells.[8] This means that there is an end to the life of an animal or human being, and that this is 'built in.' It can only be continued when reproduction takes place or by combining two haploid cells. The astral body not only introduces destruction but also planned or rather built in death.

The nervous system

It will be obvious that the presence of consciousness goes together with the presence and increasing complexity of a nervous system. This is one of the structures through which the astral body can penetrate a body.

Pain

Pain deserves special consideration in this medical book. Of course pain is a sensation and as such it forms part of the many facets of consciousness. Neurology teaches us that pain signals are carried along afferent nerve tracks to the central nervous system. What happens centrally so that pain comes to consciousness is a riddle. It is interesting that we have no trouble talking in terms of pain in the soul realm either: 'soul pain.' In most (maybe all) languages the same concept is used for these two phenomena, which are very different neurologically speaking. The soul, an obsolete concept for many people, is now usually designated as consciousness. Consciousness is thought to be located in the brain. Of course no afferent tracks of the soul or consciousness are known. Grey or white matter itself, by the way, has no sensation. When the astral body, also called *sense body,* is seen as the locus where conscious experience arises, it is obvious that pain of both body and soul are experienced in a related fashion.

8.5.4 Air

We first encounter breathing when we come to the animal kingdom. It is interesting that we see increasing complexity in the respiratory organs, the higher the animal is on the ladder of consciousness. We should distinguish between 'gas exchange' and 'breathing.' Animals can both breathe and exchange gas; plants can only exchange gas.

Assignment 3
Think of some examples of the different respiratory organs mentioned above, increasing in complexity. Which phenomena do you recognize which illustrate the connection between breathing and consciousness? The connection between breathing and the life of feeling is well-known. Try closing your eyes and concentrating on a thought while you hold your breath; then try doing the same having just breathed out.

It is striking that the movements in breathing are inborn even in the most primitive of animal organisms, but there they serve locomotion.

Assignment 4
Try to characterize the inner movement which comes about through the opposite feelings of happiness and sadness, laughing and crying, love and fear: in short, sympathy and antipathy.

The movement between sympathy and antipathy comes down to expansion and contraction, tension and relaxation. It forms the basis of primitive locomotion, breathing, and also of the movement of the heart.

Assignment 5
Trace the connection between the heart and the life of feeling.

In contrast to earth and water, the element of air can be compressed and it can also expand: this corresponds to the movement of the astral body. If in addition we recapitulate the characteristics of air (Section 7.1), it will be clear what the link is between the astral body and this element.

Characterization of the Astral Body.
The astral body can also be conceived of as a 'field.' We characterize its movement as contraction and expansion. It would be more precise to speak of contraction/shrinking/cramping on the one hand and getting out of a cramp or tension/relaxation on the other. When the astral body relaxes, the expansion happens of its own accord. The ether body then gets the chance to do that, because swelling is its natural tendency. The exercise made clear that feelings of antipathy go together with shrinking/cramping. We are familiar with this from psychosomatic phenomena. The astral body is experienced by a clairvoyant not so much spatially as qualitatively. It is experienced more as a play of colours in the aura; at least it makes an impression which is akin to the one which colours make in the ordinary sense world.

8.6 Self-awareness

8.6.1 The I

It is easy to observe the moment in which awareness of the self lights up in a child. That is the moment that Annie no longer says, 'Annie wants ice cream,' but, 'I want ice cream.' With the word 'I' we can only designate ourselves. That cannot happen until we perceive ourselves.

The following consideration can tell us something of the nature of the *I*. In the case of the ether body and the astral body we could still draw the conclusion that we owe those to the cosmos (they are 'God-given'). The same goes for the material out of which our physical body is made. Astronomers will confirm that we 'are made of star matter.' In view of the introduction to this chapter we can say that we partake of a spiritual reality in our I nature. This, of course, does not exclude the possibility that our I can also be 'God-given.'

Assignment 6

In the context of the members of the human being as they are described here, the following questions are interesting to pursue:
— Can the spirit (the I) be ill?
— How should we understand mental illnesses in terms of the dynamics of the members of the human being?

An American 'enlightened Master,' Ram Days, tells a striking story about this. A woman called him in the middle of the night, who told him she had taken LSD, was going insane and wanted to commit suicide. He lived in New York, and she was calling from California. Not yet quite awake, he first answered like a therapist from the school of Rogers would, in this vein, 'OK, you have taken LSD, you think you're going insane and now you want to commit suicide.' Suddenly, something dawned on him and he said: 'Listen, you're obviously in no state to talk. Could I talk to the person who picked up the telephone and dialled the seven numbers with the area code in order to reach me? Whoever that was obviously could think straight, so I would like to talk to that person.' Twelve people who have been through a psychosis can often describe afterwards that they can still recall every single thing they did. They say they could observe everything, but had no way of intervening. So a characteristic trait of a healthy, fully present I it is not only self-awareness, but also the ability to 'steer' the self. With the word self, we here mean everything which *can* be perceived and directed. So that includes personality, character, temperament and whatever other individual traits. Therefore those aspects do not form part of the I.

We can distinguish the following qualities of the I:

Will and the course of life

Giving direction ('steering') is a function of *will* and manifests in the deeds we perform in life. The fact that we have an individual course of life, in contrast to the animals, is the result of the fact that a part of the spirit really incarnates in our body and dwells there, in the form of our I. This is echoed in the greeting *Namaste* which people use in India and Nepal, meaning 'I greet the God in you.'

Uprightness

Does the presence of an I also result in different physical properties, in the same way that animals are really different from plants? There is a striking fact which distinguishes us from animals: uprightness. Owing to this, our hands are free and it seems to give us the necessary distance from the world, which we must have in order to have a rudimentary degree of self-awareness.

In both Chapters 3 and 4, extensive mention was made of the uniqueness of the upright posture of the human being in comparison with the animal, and a link was also made there with the influence of the I.

Is it a coincidence that the most intelligent ape we know, the Bonobo, comes closest to the human being in uprightness? When great efforts are made by people, this ape is even able to learn a simple symbol language (though unable to learn to speak), so that a form of communication has become possible with the human researcher, whose language he understands. He even seems to show a kind of shame when he is being reprimanded, which could mean the beginning of self reflection. Of course it is interesting to note that these capacities remain dormant unless they're called to life by a human being, and that they are only used when a human being is present.

Holding back

It is fascinating to note the specializations which different animal species show in their relationship to the world. Hawks drop-down on their prey, cats pounce, mice gnaw, beavers build, weaver birds weave, wasps make paper, moles dig, and so on and so forth. Immediately after birth, physical development serves this particular adaptation. Human beings, however, are not physically equipped for anything in particular. All possible ways of relating to the world are still open by virtue of the fact that there is no particular physical specialization. Our time of playing and learning is relatively long, and during that period a basis is laid for an individual biography. In the case of animals, adulthood can be equated with sexual maturity. Human beings, however, reach sexual maturity long before adulthood. Later on, after that period of sexual maturity, which for animals means the end of their lives, human beings still have a whole creative phase of life ahead of them.

8.6.2 The influence of the I on the astral body

The influence of the astral body on the ether body was described before, in Section 8.5.3. In line with the previous discussion it becomes clear that the astral body is in turn dominated by the I. This is seen especially in that the human soul is lacking in instincts and that bodily specialization is held back. Therefore the human organism cannot be regarded as 'a specific instrument for a specific instinct.' The human body is the *instrument of freedom,* as meant in the 'little apology of the spirit' with which this chapter began. And this is based on the effect of the I. The I makes sure that the astral body is held in check (see also Sections 3.4 and 4.5.7, where this influence of the I is approached more from the angle of morphology).

8.6.3 Warmth

Shame was mentioned above, and this is preeminently an aspect of self-awareness. Whoever still knows this human feeling, knows that warmth is generated in conjunction with it, which can even be visible as blushing. Something similar can occur when the will is involved: warming towards something. Warmth is the element with which the I can penetrate into the body. The blood is the 'organ' which can help warmth reach all areas of the body. Of the four elements warmth is also the only one which can permeate the other elements. It was not for nothing that warmth was called the bridge between the visible world of manifestations and the invisible world of dynamic, qualitative processes in Chapter 7.

We experience the I in our consciousness, which means in the astral body. With the astral body the ego can work down into the ether body and thus into the physical body. In this way the I individualizes the astral body into our individual personality, the ether body as time body into the carrier of individual memory, and the etheric-physical complex (the living body) into our individual shape (think of fingerprints!) and physiology (the immune system which distinguishes between what is I and not I on a biological level).

Some linguistic confusion exists regarding the I. There are philosophical schools which maintain that the human being does not have one I but many. For one's partner, one is somebody totally different than for the greengrocer or one's neighbour's son. This argument is undoubtedly true, but here we are dealing not with a changing I, but with different sides of the personality, *chosen by* the I. Because of our ability to choose, we have the theatre, in which the actor chooses a 'persona,' a mask. The 'theatre' of everyday life does not mean the multiplication of the I, nor does it have to be a sign of a weak I, but it can be a social attitude, in which the I directs. We speak of a weakness of the I when somebody's behaviour is directed much more by personality traits, drives, temperament, character, wishes and desires than by the moral direction given by the I.

Assignment 7
One could say that this chapter describes the human being during the waking state. How would the relationship be between physical, etheric, astral and I during sleep? And what would happen when the human being dies?

Waking and sleeping, dying and what comes after

During life, the physical and etheric body have great affinity towards one another (the 'physical-etheric complex'), and then we have the astral body and I, the combination which we could call soul-spiritual. During sleep the latter disengages from the former and exists not in the physical world but in the spiritual world. Unfortunately, we do not know anything about this sojourn when we come back in the next morning, because a perception has to be imprinted into the ether body (time body) in order to be fixed in memory. The connection between physical and ether body is severed at death, and henceforth the soul-spiritual being can therefore no longer connect to the body. In the spiritual world there is a corresponding slow severance of the connection between the astral body and ego of the old personality.

Do we come back again?

When a child is born, spirit connects with a physical entity (that is to say the combination of physical, etheric, and astral body). After death, it returns to the spiritual world. Therefore, to say with Voltaire, it is 'not all that much more amazing to be born twice than once.' It would be amazing, however, if the *same* Voltaire appeared here again. That personality will never return. By this reasoning, however, his spiritual entity, his individuality, does have the possibility to return. There's no reason to assume that the spiritual world is less rich and differentiated than our earthly world. In the spiritual world we can meet one characteristic of spiritual beings which we know very well, because we ourselves are spiritual beings: they can create. On earth we human beings are the ones who create new things: *culture,* to be distinguished from the world which has been created: *nature* (see Section 9.5)

8.6.4 The members of the human being in a coherent worldview?

The physical, etheric, astral body and the I are sometimes called the four members of the human being.

Since Aristotle, the word 'body' has been the scientific term to indicate an entity of matter or forces. Examples are solid or fluid bodies, regular and irregular bodies, antibodies and so on. Perhaps Sheldrake's introduction of a much more up-to-date term, 'field,' offers possibilities of making the anthroposophical concept of the members of the human being more accessible. In using the term, it is important to distinguish sharply when it denotes a refined materialistic concept of 'field,' and when it has a spiritual connotation.

Of course these bodies have not been invented by Rudolf Steiner. They have been in existence since time immemorial, even though there is reason to assume that the balance between the different members has shifted in the course of the millennia. The Chinese concept of *Chi,* the Japanese *Ki,* the old Egyptian *Ka,* the Greek *Entelecheia,* Paracelsus' *Archaeus:* all these concepts indicate something of what we have sketched here as the ether body. What we have sketched here as the astral body is less defined in antiquity, but still to be recognized in the *Ying* of the Chinese, the *Ba* of the Egyptians and the *Pneuma* of the Greeks. Our concept of the conscious I cannot be found as such, but the Chinese do have the eternal and immortal principle of the *Shen,* the Egyptians have the *Khu,* and the Greeks the *Nous.*

This enumeration could create the impression that we are dealing with absolute concepts. But ever since J.O. de la Mettrie published his *Traité de l'Ame* in 1745, we can no longer talk of 'speculations' concerning a nonmaterial source of the manifestations of life or the soul. Some theologians, impressed by the accomplishments of science and the corresponding conceptions of (neo) positivism, feel compelled to drop the monotheistic God of creation. Probably this was a logical step in the history of theology, which, like all history, is generally viewed as progress, going from pantheism through polytheism to monotheism. It should be noted, however, that even though there was no place for other gods in monotheism, the spiritual world for a long time remained populated with choirs of angels and other hierarchical beings. This was outlined by Karen Armstrong in her *History of God.* In her work as in so many others, what remains of God is the subject of poetry and personal mysticism. It is surprising that scientists especially, when not too strongly imprinted (not too rigidly moulded) by their own discipline, arrive at conclusions similar to Rudolf Steiner's around the turn of the last century. Independent of any tradition (or acquaintance with anthroposophy), they achieve this through a process of logical thinking, based on known physical and biological facts. Thus Rupert Sheldrake arrived at the concept of 'morphogenetic fields,' 'motoric fields' (in which he includes behaviour and consciousness), a 'conscious I,' a 'creative universe' and a transcendent reality. Another Englishman, Paul Davis, a professor in theoretical physics, also comes to the conclusion that higher creative forces must be at work in nature. The Dutch scientist Arie van den Beukel, a physics professor in Delft, makes it clear that physical laws can never explain the whole of reality.

8.7 Threefoldness

A similar history cannot be given of threefoldness, which was indicated in Chapter 4. The trinity of body, soul and spirit is of course not new. Threefoldness as in upper pole (nerve sense system), middle (rhythmic system), and lower pole (metabolic-limb system), was elaborated in this way for the first time by Rudolf Steiner. Yet Plato already distinguished three parts of the human soul. He was the first to make distinctions between the thinking soul *(logistikon)*, the emotional soul, and the soul of desires. He locates the first in the head, the second in the chest and the third below the midriff. In addition to this, threefoldness can especially be recognized by considering where people in the course of history located the centre of the human being. For the Chinese, it was the point of *Chi-Chung* or *Tan-tien,* 'the palace of energy,' located in the navel. The Japanese called it *Hara,* located in the belly below the navel, recognized as a source of energy and will. Later on, in biblical times, the area of the heart became the most important, which still lives on in the genius of our language. Now, in our time, everything is located between the ears. Thus we find the awareness that successively willing, feeling and thinking are related to different bodily locations.*

8.8 Pathology

The physician's view of pathology determines how a therapy is arrived at. If we are of the opinion that the origin of a carcinoma lies in the 'first' malignant cell, we will strive to detect that cell as early as possible and to remove it. Continuing logically, we will think that the cause of this change in cell form lies in defective information within the physiology of the cell; our search for the cause thus seems to be satisfied definitively, because we found the cause of the carcinoma on the cellular level. Our therapy will then consists of finding defects and their causes in the information within the physiology of the cell, and in preventing or removing of this false

---

*   A different description of the members of the human being can be found in the Appendix, in 'The Different Members of the Human Being.'

information. In this line of reasoning, we can equate curing with removing of the 'first' malignant cell, or false information. This way of thinking is characterized by searching for causes within physical, sense-perceptible reality, and a treatment on that level. Orthodox medicine has no pathological/physiological model for a possible psychological constitution which could cause the pathological condition. Even if we would assume that the psyche could cause the disease, we would not be able to see how such a thing would work.

Another question should be considered as well, how it is possible that the patient experiences something. It could be that an organic/chemical situation *is experienced* as a depression. Of course chemistry cannot explain the *nature of a patient's experience!* It remains a riddle why a patient feels depressed, and why a person will register *a change in mood* rather than say, 'something is the matter with my serotonin.' The disturbance in the metabolism of the serotonin demands a separate explanation.

> *It seems that every pathological/physiological process taking place at the physical level demands a causal explanation. If this explanation were to stay within the physical level, this would signify that the long rejected* generatio spontanea *(the coming into being of biological phenomena without a specific reason) would once again be re-established, which is unacceptable. Here orthodox medicine comes to a limit!*

8.8.1 The hierarchal relationship between the four members

Earlier in Chapter 8 the four members of the human being and their mutual relationships were described. In Chapter 7 the way the elements interact was described with an indication how the elements in nature *outside* the human being, correlate with the members *within* the human being.

For Paracelsus, studying nature and meteorology *outside* the human being was a very important schooling to learn how the same things are at work *inside* the human being in a metamorphosed form. Steiner attached great value to the process of learning to see how the members of the human being are related to the elements working *inside* the human being. There is a dynamic balance between the interrelationship of the members themselves, and also between the members and the elements in the form in which they function inside the human being. This dynamic balance implies the *possibility* of the genesis of pathological processes. This also contains an aspect of *causality* founded in the interaction and hierarchical relationship between the different members. What we mean to indicate with this is the following *general* principle: *The higher member determines the one below.*

8.8.2 The psychosomatic direction

We can see a fine example of this general law when we look at sleeping and waking (see Section 8.6.3), or at pregnancy, both in their healthy form, and study the pertinent phenomena. In the case of pregnancy the following physiological changes occur: lower blood pressure, diminished peristalsis in the intestines and urinary tracts, weaker muscles, varicose veins; the patient tires easily, has trouble concentrating and needs more sleep; in addition there will be a decrease in haemoglobin, partly because the non-cellular part of the blood increases in volume, an increased tendency to accumulate fluids, alcohol intolerance, increased risk of diabetes mellitus, and hypersensitivity to influences from the immediate surroundings. One can interpret these phenomena as results of a 'retracting' astral body; due to this, the ether body is not toned properly and shows the qualities of a watery metabolism; it becomes too plant-like, as it were. This means that the working of the ether body is weakened. As a result, the ether body cannot 'master' physical substance anymore. The pregnant woman becomes too 'heavy.' Because of this 'heaviness,' the extracellular fluid comes under the influence of gravity again, and edema can form as a result.

When a person is psychologically overtaxed, the opposite appears of what happens during pregnancy. Blood pressure will rise, there will be increased peristalsis in the intestines, frequency, tachycardia, increased muscle tone, pain in tendons, ligaments and muscles, hyper-alertness, difficulty going to sleep and/or insomnia, inability to let go of mental pictures or thoughts, fear, increased desire for alcohol and nicotine (to numb the misery). The astral body penetrates too deeply into the ether body. Hence the forces of consciousness, which break things down, are directly in touch with the physical body, especially the nervous system. People who are suffering from too much stress often will say, 'I cannot let go of things.' This letting go signifies letting the astral body release from the physical and etheric. In other situations, the same dynamics can lead to ailments such as ulcers, hypertension, asthma or irritable bowel syndrome.

Assignment 8
Study the following two illnesses: Cushing's disease and Addison's disease. Can you discover for yourself what the interrelationship between the astral and the etheric body is in these two diseases?

When you compare the examples given here with what was said in Chapters 7 and 8, you can begin to experience the reality of the members of the human being. At the same time you will experience that the concepts presented regarding the different members allow you to comprehend a whole series of phenomena from one point of view and things fall into place.

The interaction of the members also has consequences for *morphology.* In order to see how the different members affect morphology, look again at Chapters 3 and 4.

In the paragraphs above the pathological results of the higher members penetrating too much into the lower ones was discussed; we could call this *the psychosomatic direction.* The phenomena on the physical/functional level were explained out of the working of the higher members. They were seen as manifestations of 'psychological' functions.

8.8.3 The reverse direction

Can the direction be turned around? Do the lower members affect the higher members as well? The higher members with their psychological functions have created their specific organs in the organism during embryonic development, enabling the lower members to influence the higher ones. Thus our nervous system is a central organ of the astral body. On the one hand, the astral body can make use of the nervous system in order to manifest itself (examples are conscious perception and movement), on the other hand the astral body can be directly 'manipulated' via the nervous system. The alarm clock is a nice example of this; owing to the presence of organs of hearing it can force us to wake up every morning. Our (conscious) astral functioning is woken out of its unconscious state by means of the body. Another example is the sense of satisfaction we get from drinking water when we are thirsty; this process begins at the physical level and affects us psychologically so the process goes from physical to psychological. We could call it 'somato-psychological.'

In pathology we are especially familiar with psychiatric diseases which have a strong somato-psychological dynamic, and in which the chemistry within the organism determines what is being experienced on the higher levels. An example of this is metabolic disturbances in depression. Another instructive example is obsessive-compulsive disorder. The symptoms of compulsiveness can be recognized in characteristics of the physical body and the element of earth: inability to change, halting of time, and immutability of form are essential characteristics of compulsion.

Within the human astral body we can distinguish three psychological functions, namely *thinking, feeling* and *action*. What works in the physical body has the possibility to 'wrongly' affect these astral functions.

When *thinking* is 'gripped' by a pathological shift of what should work on the physical level, *obsessions* or *compulsive thoughts* arise.

When *feeling* is affected, *phobia* arises.

When *action* and *will* are affected, *compulsive actions* result such as checking doors, tightening taps etc.

It goes without saying that many phenomena can only be understood as a combination of things. It is known, for example, that compulsive washing often goes together with a phobia for dirt and obsessions about infection and bacteria.

The side effects of drugs are numerous, and a considerable part of them are psychological in nature, even though the drugs are supposed to work purely on the somatic level. Think, for example, of prednisone and allergy medications. Painkillers as such are a textbook case of the somato-psychological direction, and the effects of beta-blockers, thyroxine and insulin also extend to the psychological level. In every single case, these are examples of effects that start in the body, and end up on the level of perception.

8.8.4 Summary

In order to understand pathological processes, starting from the different members of the human being has proven to be fruitful. During embryonic development, these members have started to create an organism from the top down in psychosomatic fashion, thereby creating their 'organs of choice.' After this has taken place the somato-psychological path 'back up' can be taken via these organs of choice. Examples of this have been given above. The latter insight prompted the German embryologist Blechschmidt to say, 'What has not been taken *in* during embryonic life on the physical level, cannot be brought *out* later on the psychological level.' [*Was im Embryonalleben nicht physisch eingeübt wird, kann später nicht psychisch* ausgeübt *werden.*]

Assignment 9

Try to imagine how somatic illnesses are physical manifestations of the higher members (peptic ulcer, hypertension), and how psychiatric diseases are astral manifestations of physical/etheric processes (depressions, psychoses).

Learning to think in terms of interactions of members thus opens up new vistas. One can look at certain pathologies from a new angle, and this view offers new starting points for a rational therapy.

8.9 Therapy

Within the framework of this training manual it is not possible to give a detailed survey of all the therapeutic possibilities which anthroposophical medicine offers. We can, however, give a general idea of the range of anthroposophical diagnostic tools and therapies. There are several reasons why a complete survey is not feasible.

To begin with, there are many different therapies. Listing them immediately demonstrates what we mean: medicines from the various realms of nature are used, which are often prepared in a special way; conversation and psychotherapy are of fundamental importance in treatment; and apart from that there is a rich palette of therapies such as artistic therapy, eurythmy therapy, hydrotherapy, rhythmical massage, external applications, music therapy, speech as therapy; there are institutions for curative education and social therapy. All therapies are administered by trained therapists, though not every therapeutic centre can offer all therapies. New therapies are constantly being developed, such as movement therapy, chiro-phonetics and meridian therapy. One therapy is not more important than another, even though listing them this way might give that impression; the individual situation determines the choice of therapy.

Secondly, there can be a variety of therapeutic approaches in any given situation, which is nothing new in itself. In standard medical practice, there can be a variety of therapeutic options in any given case, as well. In the case of deficiency states, we have the option to prescribe supplements; in the case of undesired cell growth we can operate and/or prescribe cytostatics or radiation; in the case of bacterial infections we can treat the bacteria and not the sick person, etc. Within anthroposophical medicine too, several therapeutic viewpoints are possible, which have one point in common, however: the treatment aims to call forth a reaction in the organism. The point is that the sick person or organism *does* something with the treatment offered, so that changes occur within the total organism or between the different members and their relationships, changes which have a correcting effect. We will confine ourselves to a few examples out of medical practice.

8.9.1 Asthma

In the anthroposophical medical view, bronchial asthma occurs when the astral body enters too deeply into the middle realm of the human being, specifically in the bronchial system. We are faced with the following symptoms: in-breathing, spasms and consciousness (an experience of constriction), which are called forth by the astral body. In the healthy situation, the ether body 'pushes' the astral body out again after every in-breath, and this pushing out forms the out-breath. That can no longer take place in the case of asthma. This results in a cramped in-breath of the lungs, increased FRC (functional residual capacity), whereby gas exchange becomes insufficient. At the alveolar level, the air comes to standstill, a situation which is normal in the paranasal cavities. On a microsopic level, inflammations practically always play an important role.

8.9.2 Therapy with medication

Therapy by means of medication aims to lead the astral body 'back up' and to rein in the inflammatory process. Three plants can be used therapeutically to achieve this.

Nicotiana tabacum (the tobacco plant) is a plant which belongs to the nightshade family, which all excel in alkaloid formation and have an antispasmodic effect (Belladonna!); administered as injection.

Prunus spinosa (sloe) is a very vital plant which will grow anywhere it gets a chance to, by the side of the road, in hedgerows and along streams. It belongs to the Rosaceae family which is already strikingly vital in its own right. Despite a strong astral penetration, prunus can maintain this vitality. We can read this strong astral influence in the phenomena of thorn formation and high acidity of the fruit, and also from the leathery leaf of the tree. Prunus spinosa shows us how vitality can be maintained in spite of a strong astral imprint. This is something which the asthma patient does not quite succeed in. Therefore prunus is very good to generally *strengthen the ether body* and thereby strengthen the process of breathing out. It is also administered as subcutaneous injection.

Gencydo is prepared from a combination of the rind of Citrus medica (lemon) and Cydonia (quince). Both plants are exceptionally good at protecting and maintaining their moisture content. In both cases the rind gives excellent protection against influences from the environment. Because of that, the moisture content of the fruit remains intact for a long time, and also keeps its structure well. Gencydo offers an example, as it were, showing the vulnerable bronchial mucous membrane, which produces mucus too readily, how to control and regulate its own moisture content. It is a tried and true preparation for all cases of allergies and hyper-reactive bronchi. It can be prescribed either as an injection or it can be inhaled.

Why administer the injections subcutaneously? The organism has developed out of three germinal disks (see Figures 4.12, 4.15 and 4.17). The ectoderm led to the formation of the nerve-sense system and the skin; the mesoderm led to the internal organs such as the heart and the blood vessels, the kidneys and (relevant to our example) the mesodermal components of the respiratory tract in the form of connective tissue, muscle tissue and cartilage. Lastly, we owe to the endoderm our digestive system with corresponding glands and organs (liver). In the respiratory system, the tissue which has a metabolic character (mucous membrane and alveolar coating) stems from the endoderm. This is not without meaning for therapy. The organism, after all, offers us 'places of application' for medication which show a certain predilection for one of the three systems of the threefold human being. Asthma is primarily a disturbance of the rhythmical system, of the functions of the middle. Therefore the best route of access for treating asthma is that particular area in the organism which belongs intrinsically to the domain of the middle. Those are: the circulatory system and the subcutaneous lymph channels (injections), and the airways themselves (inhalation). In a comparable fashion the skin can be used when we want to link in to the nervous system, or we can prescribe medicine to be taken orally when we want to link in to the metabolic system.

Nicotiana tabacum, Prunus spinosa and Gencydo are effective medicines in the case of asthma to help counteract the spasms, to strengthen the etheric body (strengthen out-breathing) and to make the mucus membranes less vulnerable (reduce inflammation).

8.9.3 Rhythmical massage

Another way to achieve the same results is the application of so-called *rhythmical massage,* either with or without a medicinal oil. In this type of massage, which, as the name already indicates, has *rhythm as its starting point,* the therapist uses specific hand movements and holds the hands in specific ways which have a direct effect on the different members. Different manipulations are used, for example, depending on whether one wants to bring about a better tonus, stimulate vitality, enhance consciousness or promote elimination. When the therapist is familiar with the working of the different members, and knows where and how he can work on them through the organism, he can bring the 'derailed' members back into a proper relationship, using different kinds of manipulation.

The diagnosis of the masseur is of special importance. The warmth-relationships within the organism and how that warmth-organism allows itself to be manipulated can give important information for the therapeutic strategy to be followed. The quality of the patient's breathing, the muscle tone and a sense of the vitality of the organism can be assessed by the therapist by means of massage. The diagnoses of the therapist and the physician together will result in the criteria for treatment. It would be possible to give a 'technical treatise' about the specifics of the massage, albeit not in a strictly prescriptive way, as every therapy is in fact always individually adapted to each patient.

8.9.4 Artistic therapy

The colours of the visible spectrum of light (the rainbow) are related to various physiological processes in the organism. The warm colours work on everything connected to metabolic processes in physiology; different shades of blue and purple correspond more to nerve-sense processes. Green connects these areas with one another and is related to the quality of the middle.

In the asthma patient, the astral body works too deeply from the head into the breathing. The 'stagnation of the air' in the bronchial tree and the alveoli is a picture of this. In the pneumatized parts of the skull (the sinuses, the mastoid, the tympanic cavity) the air is naturally stagnant. One could speak in this case of 'nerve-sense air,' because the functioning of our senses and consciousness (smell, vision, hearing, and conscious functioning in general) is determined to a large degree by the aeration of the skull. Studying or solving a problem with a bad sinusitis is therefore not likely to succeed very well! In the barrel form of the thorax and the increase in functional residual capacity we see a morphological expression of the tendency of the thorax to 'become a nasal cavity.' Among other things through the effect of colour we have a way to influence and correct this relationship of the different members. In the case of asthma, the patient 'has become too blue in the middle.' If we succeed in leading the patient from cooler colours to warmer ones, the metabolic forces should, through the etheric body, be able to regain ground where they had lost it, namely in the thorax. We thus support the lower man (metabolic-limb system), in its struggle with upper man (nerve sense system). The lower man can thereby develop greater capacity to regain a breathing relationship to the upper man.

8.9.5 Other therapies

Since we are only giving an orientation with regard to the various possible anthroposophical treatments, we will only give a summary of other therapies. One thing all therapies have in common is that they aim to influence the relationship between the various members of the human being.

Eurythmy therapy
By means of specific movement exercises, the different members are purposely steered in a direction which can either be harmonizing, strengthening or dampening. When one realizes how much is 'in movement in a living organism — especially in the case of an ensouled organism — it should not be all that difficult to grasp that movement has the potential to heal.

Speech as therapy
Vowels and consonants, the breath, and the force of speech in which the whole organism partakes, all deeply influence the organism. A speech exercise, directed by the I, works via the astral body down into the lower members. The relationship of the word to the I is evidenced by the fact that only the human being has the capacity for speech. The relationship to the astral body shows in the fact that we are able to emit countless sounds proceeding from basic, primary emotions or deliberations.

Music therapy
Music influences the organism in a variety of ways: different categories of instruments (percussion, wind instruments, or strings); the different keys; the intervals; beat, rhythm and melody: all these facets work in a specific way and have a different effect on the organism. A military march stimulates the will, gives courage and stirs us up; a Viennese waltz invites more of an artistic, aesthetic art of motion induced by the feelings; a hymn, especially one sung unaccompanied is more likely to stimulate our perception of the spiritual dimension of life. These seemingly trivial examples indicate superficially the deep relationship which the human being has to music. In music therapy this relationship has been deepened to promote health.

CHAPTER 9

Working with the Texts of Rudolf Steiner

ANTON DEKKERS

9.1 Studying anthroposophical literature

Studying the work of Rudolf Steiner demands careful consideration of the method of study. Steiner himself often points out that an anthroposophical book cannot be read for its content only, but needs to be studied differently. In his first truly anthroposophical book, *Theosophy* (GA 9, 1904), he emphasizes that it is necessary to bring every word to life first, if the real content of what is written is to begin to speak to us inwardly. He then goes on to say that this way of bringing the text to life presupposes a heightened spiritual activity, which has been taken into account in the writing of the book. In a certain sense this also goes for the lectures which are published. One also has to take into account that Steiner held these lectures for a specific audience in a specific location, so that each lecture received its own special nuances.

Here we will focus on one specific method of study, as used in the Dutch doctors' course. We will reflect on the physiological basis of this particular method, in order to make clear that it was not chosen randomly, but corresponds to our own bodily and spiritual nature.

Each person has an individual way of studying in order to read and digest a text. We are often not totally conscious of our own specific way of doing that. Let us take a look at the way we read a professional medical journal. We will usually check the table of content first in order to find what is important or interesting. This is of fundamental importance; without *interest,* any article one reads or studies would be boring and dry. Who does not remember the laborious process when, as a student, we had to study things which either were of no interest to us or even made us wonder whether we would ever need to know them in the future. Interest is therefore the first activity which is required.

When we now proceed to read an article, we take in the information and compare it to what we already know about the subject; we organize the information and try to get at the essence, and also try to gauge what the consequences are for daily practice. When we have studied the article well we will either understand the subject better or better understand where the problems lie, and we will have a better sense of the practical application.

In order to remember an article, we will have to read a summary or the essence of the piece a few more times or reflect on it.

These are general ways to come to an understanding of the text. It will be clear that our depth of understanding of the text will depend on the intensity of such activities. Our interest is decisive here and stimulates the other activities. Even a text which is very dry and boring to most, will not be dry at all for one who is highly interested in the subject, because he can place the article in the total context of problems and could recognize, say, the brilliance of a certain treatise on a small aspect within a larger complex of problems.

All this applies also to the study of texts by Steiner. When Steiner writes that every word of the text needs to be brought to life, it becomes clear that the intensity of the aforementioned activities needs to be increased, especially the factor of interest. As a consequence, texts will begin to live more vividly and more deeply for a reader. This aspect of inner life however, also points to a totally different quality. This is a quality we will not meet so easily when we study professional medical literature, because this quality has to do with how the text originated. In the case of spiritual texts, one can experience strongly that these spring from a totally different sphere than articles in, for example, *The Lancet*. There are, of course, varying degrees.

What Steiner seems to point at in the passage quoted above from the book *Theosophy* is that his work was derived from concrete scientific research into the spiritual world. The results of this research were translated into concepts of such a nature that people who are less conscious of the spiritual world can nevertheless consciously partake in it, albeit in a form which is conceptual to begin with. To this end, however, the strengthening of intensity is needed in order to bring the concepts to life. And when these concepts then begin to live inside us, this will have consequences for our whole inner life, not only the life of thought, but also for our feeling, intuitive capacities, imagination etc. We find plenty of indications of these things in ordinary life. A sailor will have a much more comprehensive and living concept of the sea than a landlubber who has never seen the sea. Not only the outer life but also the inner life of the sailor will have been shaped by the sea to a high degree. He will be able to place all kinds of things which have to do with the sea directly; he knows how to interpret them and he knows the consequences. You could say that a sailor has created an inner sense organ for everything which concerns the sea.

Even though this may not always be so in individual cases, this does not detract from the principle meant here, and only shows that many other factors are of importance. In analogy, we could say that when the text begins to live in us long and intensively, it will create an inner organ for the spiritual world. And the above consideration will also make clear that not every text is suitable for this. When we speak about consequences for our whole life of soul, this has considerable consequences for medical work: for example our empathy with the patient, and an increased sense of what a patient needs at a particular moment, etc.

Summing up, we can recognize two aspects in the way Steiner speaks of a different way of studying anthroposophical literature.

— Normal study habits still apply, but with enhanced activity.
— A spiritual scientific text is rooted in conscious experience of the spiritual world. When we allow this text to live *inside* us, this will have consequences for our whole life of soul in the sense that we will live more concretely out of our connection to the spiritual world and act correspondingly. Our lives will change, both inwardly and outwardly.

It is therefore not surprising that Steiner, in discussing the inner meditative path, calls the study of spiritual scientific literature a first step on this path. He does so in *Theosophy,* and also mentions it explicitly in *Esoteric Science.*

9.2 Physiological basis of the study method

We would now like to enter more deeply into the physiological basis of the above-mentioned method of study. In the third part of this chapter the method will be discussed in detail. When we study, we take something from the outside, namely information, and introduce it into ourselves. We are familiar with the process of taking something in and digesting it, in a different way, in that we eat, drink and breathe (we will come back later to the question whether this comparison of the process of study with nutrition is a real one). We eat bread, that is to say we *absorb* something from the outer world. We experience, however, direct changes: our stomach begins to rumble, our mouth begins to water, etc.; that is to say: we *receive* and *adapt* our food in a very special way. If we were not to do that, bread would remain a foreign body inside of us. We chew it, warm it, we liquefy it and, not to forget: we taste it. The receiving of this food is followed by all that comprises the *digestive* processes. For even though the process of receiving it has made a certain degree of adaptation to our bodily condition possible, bread remains bread and my body remains my body. The bread has to be digested completely, that is to say: it must be stripped of its non-human qualities. Only then we can absorb it and process it further. This digesting is made possible by a process of *secretion* by several glands, beginning with the salivary glands. In a more comprehensive sense, the whole endocrine system partakes in this.

Thus we have met four processes that have to do with making food our own: *1) absorption; 2) adaptation; 3) digestion; 4) secretion.* Every day anew, we have to eat and drink in order to maintain life in us and to *regenerate* ourselves, that is to say to build up again what we have broken down during the day. So that is the next process: food becomes our own bodily substance and goes to all locations where it is needed. In youth there is also a sixth process: *growth,* and during the reproductive phase a seventh: *reproduction.* Both processes spring from a certain surplus of forces, something which is not directly required for ordinary life. Yet they are real life processes. Just imagine what would happen if these last two processes were not there. So the last three are: *5) regeneration; 6) growth; 7) reproduction.*

9.3 The life processes as an organism

These seven processes, which Steiner calls *life processes,* enable us to live. We could also say they are the seven processes which constitute our *ether body.* This ether body, however, also forms an entity in itself, it is also a unity. Among other things this means that these seven processes not only occur after one another, but that they have a meaningful relationship to one another in other ways. They rely on one another and are all dependent on one another. We can experience the meaningful coherence if we not only place them in the sequence as before, but place them in opposition to one another, the first opposed to the last, the second opposed to the sixth, etc.

With *absorption* something foreign enters us, yet it is not so foreign that we cannot do anything with it. Food has a certain relationship to us. In *reproduction* something which we have formed separates out from us. It acquires life independent from us, yet it is also related to us. So with process 1 the direction is from outside to inside, and with process 7 the direction is from inside to outside.

In the case of *adaptation* something foreign which enters us is adapted to our bodily environment. When we take *growth* only in a quantitative sense, we do not get very far. A baby still has to be taken care of, receives its mother's milk, clothes, warmth, etc. The small child is not adapted to the world to such a degree that it can function independently. In a quantitative sense, growth is in many respects the constant adaptation of the individual to the environment. It is an active process of adaptation, even though it is often unconscious. In the case of the second process we thus see that the small adapts to the large (our body). With the sixth process we see that the small (the infant) adapts to the large (the world).

In the case of *digestion* we find that the foreign substance is totally destroyed. What comes from the outside is broken down. The opposite happens in *regeneration,* where our own substance is built up again.

The process of *secretion* is subdivided into different parts. On the one hand there is the secretion described above which has to do with enabling digestion (i.e. the processes which take in the foreign substance and break them down). On the other hand there is the secretion which is directed inwards, namely the movement from lymph to blood to organs. This secretion which is directed inwards forms the basis of the last three processes.

There are many ways in which we can place these seven processes next to and opposite one another, which enables us to see more and more how they form an organism together. We can only give an introductory description here, but they warrant further deepening.

9.4 Two questions

We described these bodily processes here in order to clarify, or rather 'substantiate,' the process of taking in and digesting study content. Exploring the process of studying further now, we will have to answer two questions: 1) Is the comparison with the process of nutrition only a metaphor, or does it have a reality based in human nature? 2) What is the meaning of the last two processes, described as growth and reproduction, in the case of the process of studying?

9.5 The transformation of our ether body

In many places in his work, Rudolf Steiner describes how the etheric body undergoes an important change around the sixth or seventh year. He does so amongst other places in *The Education of the Child in the Light of Anthroposophy,* which constitutes an elaboration of an early lecture, but also in his very last book, *Extending Practical Medicine.* He describes this process from various points of view, which we cannot go into further. In *Extending Practical Medicine* he describes it as follows: having introduced the importance of the ether body, with special emphasis on the importance of growth, regeneration and so forth, he sketches how around the time of the change of teeth a part of the ether body emancipates itself from these bodily tasks and becomes the basis for our life of soul, especially our thinking. Just as our capacity for thought is based in an independent physical body, which in turn has its centre in a well formed brain, thinking also needs to be based in an independent ether body, which has more or less emancipated from the task of caring for the physical body. The onset of the change of teeth is an expression of the fact that this emancipation has taken place. All this means that we can distinguish two corresponding aspects in the ether body: one as a basis for the care of our body, and the other as a basis for our capacity for thought. We could also call these two aspects of our ether bodies *nature* and *culture.* They are corresponding because the one, so to speak, gives birth to the other.

9.6 Our thinking as a gateway to the life processes

The previous deliberations form the basis for answering the two questions posed in Section 9.4. Now that we have found seven life processes which constitute our ether body in its function of shaping the body, we are likely to also find these seven processes in the part of our ether body which is turned towards our capacity of thought. And because these two aspects of the ether body are connected, we will be able to find an entry to the seven life processes in our thinking capacity. This is surprising because we usually do not find the life processes easily accessible for research. We can research the body in its outer appearance with the help of the senses or ever more refined equipment, and we can likewise research the lives of our souls by turning inward, or do that research with someone else in reflection. Manifestations of life in us can be perceived first of all in their physical form or as they appear in the soul. When one realizes, however, that the inner nature of our thinking is closely connected to our etheric body, the same laws which are to be found in the ether body can be recognized in thinking. As a consequence, the comparison of the process of taking in nourishment with the process of studying is not an empty one, but is founded in human nature.

9.7 The seven processes of our thinking organism

When we look at the process of studying more closely we shall quickly be able to find the first life processes. We *take in* something by reading, for example. After that we imprint the text into the *memory*. By doing that we bring the text into a closer connection with ourselves. We then go on to make *distinctions,* we *analyse,* we determine what is of relevance to us and what is not, and to what things we have more or less affinity. All this corresponds to digestion. As we have seen, *interest* is of paramount importance in this whole process, and this manifests especially in *asking questions*. That corresponds to secretion. We have seen how there are outward and inward secretions. This is also the case with a questioning interest, namely in that there is an analysing and a synthesizing side to it. The questions concerning synthesis thus form the basis of the last three processes. *Synthesis* comes into being as the fifth process. We can characterize this with another name: finding the thread, or seeing the overall picture, the main line. Just as we look at the detail or the particular when we analyse, we here look at the larger overview. We usually look upon these five processes as our general method of study, with all kinds of individual variants.

When we look for *growth* and *reproduction* in our method of study, closer scrutiny will show us examples of this as well in our daily lives. In this case we have to take growth in an inner sense and reproduction will have to be something which has grown within us and then is brought out of us. We all know about growth in the form of accumulating life experience. That partly happens to us in a passive way, simply by what we live through, but it is possible to actively bring this growth about. We digest our experiences and deep within us life experience grows. What has ripened through inner experience is brought forth and ends up outside of us, in our work, in our community, or in an artistic area. In the process something proceeds from us which remains inwardly connected to us, even though the results go their own way.

9.8 Meditation

Where studying a text is concerned, this means that the text will have to start living in us in such a way that we grow and ripen inwardly. This ripening has to be of such a nature, that we gradually grow into the spiritual substance which lies at the basis of the text. *Unconsciously* one is already connected to the spiritual world in all its aspects, including that which forms the basis of the text. By enhanced activity such as we discussed above, the spiritual substance of the text can bring it about that an inner organ will grow in us, through which we learn to behold spiritual reality *consciously.* In essence this path is one of meditation, of living intensively with a thought. Out of this beholding of a spiritual reality something can be born which one subsequently brings out, as has been described: in work, community and so on. This last process could also be called *shaping.*

We have thus described the seven processes which, when applied consciously, can become a method in the study of anthroposophical texts. In summary:

1. Taking in = reading, observing
2. Remembering
3. Distinguishing, analysing
4. Interest = asking questions
5. Synthesis
6. Becoming an organ
7. Shaping

Assignment
Study the first chapter of Fundamentals of Therapy *in this way (see Appendix).*

CHAPTER 10

The Anthroposophical Path of Inner Development

MARION VAN BREE, GUUS VAN DER BIE,
MACHTELD HUBER

This chapter presupposes familiarity with Rudolf Steiner's *How to Know Higher Worlds.*

In the previous chapter we have dealt with subjects of a more historical, philosophical, or medical/phenomenological character. In this last chapter we will go deeper into the inner aspects, both with regards to the professional practice of the physician and to personal life. There are definite reasons for this. In the present age, we risk becoming estranged from the visible and invisible worlds around us, and it is the very task of anthroposophy to bring about a new, conscious connection to these worlds. The path of inner development allows this connection to grow.

10.1 Development of consciousness

In his lectures, *The Gospel According to St Luke,* Rudolf Steiner describes the course of development of humanity at large as one in which, starting in a far distant past, consciousness increasingly became removed from contact with the 'invisible' spiritual world, and became more and more filled with content of the visible, material world instead. In recent centuries this is recognizable among other things in the mechanization of our worldview. This also can be seen in the development of medicine, as described in Chapter 1. In the present time, including the nineteenth century with the culmination of materialism, and also the twentieth century, human consciousness is furthest removed from a direct experience of the spiritual world and has become most 'earthly.' The molecular and biochemical approaches to the human being and nature have brought about an estrangement from visible nature. Yet Rudolf Steiner maintains that the development of consciousness will return of its own accord to an experience of the spiritual world. On the other hand, the human being also faces a task and a challenge, namely to consciously shape this return. The point is that spiritual *experience* can become spiritual *insight,* and also that it can become a capacity to 'read' the visible world as a picture of spiritual reality.

In a diagram, the development of human consciousness between past and future can be represented as follows:

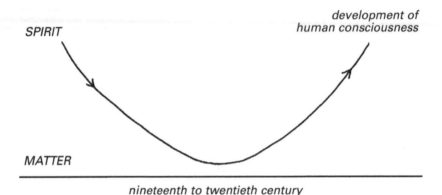

nineteenth to twentieth century

Figure 10.1

The initial 'descent' of consciousness serves a purpose, according to Rudolf Steiner. By virtue of the fact that humanity is going through the present materialistic phase, the new connection to the spiritual world which is to come about in the future can become much more awake and conscious in character than was possible in former times. This new consciousness is growing and becoming increasingly stronger. Our readiness to work on shaping and schooling our consciousness will be a decisive factor in bringing this about, as will the method we choose for this.

Anthroposophy offers a way to develop consciousness which honours the valuable fruits of the present materialistic phase of development. In addition, it adds new possibilities for developing both warmth of heart and knowledge of spiritual realities. This particular way is called the anthroposophical path of inner development.

10.1.1 The context of the path of development

It is a characteristic trait of the anthroposophical path that this schooling is not only for the benefit of personal life, but aims to promote further development and renewal in practical life, i.e. in different professions. In schooling ourselves we can therefore distinguish between a more general, individual path and a path meant more specifically for professional development. Both will be introduced in this chapter, although this can in no way replace Steiner's works in these areas. We will now concentrate on the personal path, and then go on to the one specifically oriented towards a profession.

10.2 The general path of development

More and more people sense that they can bring about inner change by their own activity, which brings about a change in the way they view both themselves and the world. Participation in group work to achieve personal growth and following diverse training in inner development has become a normal cultural phenomenon, and we place the general anthroposophical path of schooling in this context.

What types of change can happen inwardly when one follows such a general path? As these changes differ depending on the individual, we can only give examples from experiences people have made on this path.

Characteristically, people will wake up to the possibility of the existence of the spiritual world because of certain experiences in their personal lives. Such experiences often arise spontaneously when many different and seemingly unrelated events *coincide* in life, which on closer inspection *fit together like pieces in a puzzle.* It can often happen that people meet adverse events or things which befall them with a reaction such as 'this is typically something that would happen to me.' This shows that they experience a spiritual coherence in the events. If such a perception does not arise, such events will tend to be interpreted either as good luck, bad luck or pure chance. Experience teaches us that the one or the other interpretation of events can have a significant influence on the way one stands in life.

At a later stage, this experience of the likelihood of the existence of the spiritual world can grow into certainty; a nonphysical cause 'behind' things becomes a tangible and even identifiable experience.

10.2.1 Inner and outer effects

This development often has *two directions.* On the one hand one can experience a spiritual centre within, in which existence is no longer felt as a purely physical thing; on the other hand one can experience living beings or life connections *in surrounding nature,* which — expressed in philosophical terms — demonstrate independent 'levels of being.' This applies first to other people, but can also begin to extend to other realms of nature. When we direct our gaze inward, we will have the experience that the richness and scope of *inner experiences increase,* with regard to both positive and negative experiences. At the same time one will perceive how confused, chaotic and colourfully mixed ordinary soul-reactions often are. One will recognize that mental images and feelings tend to live a life of their own: emotions come and go, often unbidden and unchecked, sometimes unwanted, too. Hence the need can arise to bring a certain order into this, in order to maintain dependability and stability. By inner exercises one gradually gets more of a handle on one's own character, both in its positive and negative aspects. Apart from that a heightened sensitivity to different nuances will be apparent. To our senses, the world around us becomes more and more differentiated and rich in nuances.

Such experiences arise because slumbering spiritual capacities within the developing human being begin to unfold. Similar effects can be brought about by numerous other paths of schooling practised in this day and age. It is important to realize that the anthroposophical path differs in a number of respects from other paths which are popular at this time. Anthroposophy consciously advises a 'slow' path. When one goes on a path of inner development, new capacities within a human being must be allowed to be 'born,' as it were. This comparison is an exact one. Every birth is preceded by a fructification, followed by phases of gestation and development. Only after these processes have occurred can a timely birth take place. Enough is known in biology about the harmful effects of a birth which comes either too early or too late. A *good* birth is one that takes place at the right time. This is no different for our inner growth. For years, no appreciable results may be noticed when one practices specific exercises. Other exercises can actually lead to results sooner than expected, which may be due to an innate maturity of the soul in a certain area.

Much importance is attached to this in anthroposophy, because the eventual aim is to acquire insight into the spiritual world. This differs from having only *experiences* of the spiritual world. In the latter case it may be that there is a real experience of something spiritual without knowledge of what the particular experience means or what its nature and quality actually is. The anthroposophical path aims to train the capacity to *distinguish* what is what in spiritual reality. Especially when one seeks to have spiritual experiences, one may find the anthroposophical path cumbersome, not effective enough and too indirect. After all, one can go much faster, something which many other methods aim for.

Developing a certain degree of inner equanimity is an important prerequisite for a good capacity of judgment regarding spiritual experiences. For when the soul is very unbalanced, or one-sided, the capacity of judgment will be influenced unfavourably. This development of inner balance in particular can be taken in hand in a specific way through the general anthroposophical path of schooling.

10.3 General rules, subsidiary exercises, meditation

When one intends to tread the anthroposophical path, one does well to keep to the primary literature. Both the contents and the way in which Rudolf Steiner describes things make reading these a schooling in itself. Steiner's way of writing demands inner effort in the reading process which works in a specific way and has a formative effect on the soul life. Therefore studying anthroposophical literature can be regarded as a first step on the anthroposophical path of development.

10.3.1 General rules

First there are those exercises which could be called conditional, in that they create the conditions for development. By this we mean that the *conditions* for the initial development and ripening of the soul life come into being by doing the exercises concerned. If experience and insight of something spiritual is to 'be allowed to be born' in our consciousness (for example in meditation), the practice of these conditional exercises will help with the 'conception,' 'ripening' and 'growth' of that which will be born within. We are talking here of the exercises of *reverence, inner quiet,* and *patience.* The books which are mentioned at the beginning of the chapter elaborate how these exercises need to be carried out, why they are done, and to what purpose. (See specifically *How to Know Higher Worlds,* Chapter 1).

10.3.2 Subsidiary exercises

Of the many existing exercises we select here the subsidiary exercises which Steiner describes in several places in his books. He always stressed that doing these kinds of exercises needs to be part of the daily inner hygiene of the soul. These exercises strengthen the inner structure of the soul, so that it is prepared to stand the often impressive, real spiritual experiences properly. The exercises keep the soul 'healthy.' They are:

— *Control of thinking:* through this one learns to create moments during which one determines the course of one's thoughts in total autonomy.
— *Control of will:* this exercise enables one to 'orchestrate' and plan the course of events much more frequently and adequately in life.
— *Equanimity:* this exercise makes it possible to inwardly remain upright during moments of intense experiences, while allowing their intensity to exist at the same time.
— *Positivity* teaches us to experience the positive aspects in events which by their nature call forth a negative judgment.
— *Open-mindedness:* it is not easy to be free of norms, conventions and social influences in one's interaction with the world. When one makes progress in this respect (or even succeeds), a multitude of new experiences will be the result.

The next exercise concerns combining the previous exercises: *Equilibrium.* By this Rudolf Steiner means a harmonious combination of the five previously described exercises, so that the inner structure of the psyche is made healthy and resilient.*

10.3.3 Meditation

In anthroposophy, meditation is always meant in the sense of meditation through *concentration.* That is to say that the contents of the meditation is always placed in the centre of consciousness by means of inner effort, and kept there. In that process concentrated attention on the feelings which arise from the meditated content is important. This is different from drifting away in one's feelings, and being carried by a certain atmosphere. Some of the meditations have the character of *imagination.* For example one can picture inwardly how a seed sprouts, begins to grow, flourishes, forms seeds and wilts. Another example of an image in meditation described by Rudolf Steiner is the rose-cross meditation. Other meditations are given in the form of words as mantra and have more of the character of *sound (inspiration).* The latter form the most direct entry to the contents of the spiritual world and work like a window which is formed in the soul and through which the spirit can enter.

The different parts of the path of schooling stand in a concentric relationship to one another. This is expressed in Figure 10.2 below.

---

*   See also the section on the subsidiary exercises in Appendix 5.

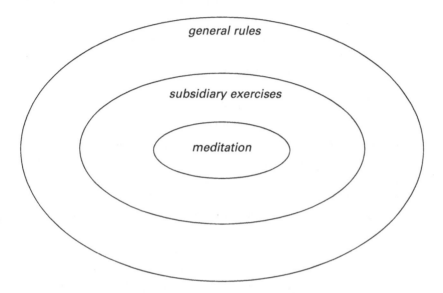

Figure 10.2.

10.4 The professional path of development

As indicated in the introduction, the first chapters of this book contain a large number of components of the specific professional path of the anthroposophical physician. For every education is a form of discipline leading to a specific inner development. In schools like the ones we have all been educated in, schooling first took place under the guidance of one teacher, and later, when specific skills needed to be learned, we came in contact with different teachers for different subjects such as mathematics or physical education. Studying medicine is no exception to this. The student will meet teachers who will coach him into an understanding of the human being through physiology and pathology. Thus one gathers a large quantity of knowledge *of a specific kind,* namely natural scientific knowledge. Such knowledge continues to work inside of us, where feelings exist next to knowledge and impulses for action. Our feelings and will impulses will be coloured by the kind of knowledge at our disposal, and will take on a corresponding character. Thus the way in which we think about the human being influences our own life of soul. Because this is the case, the kind of knowledge which we carry within ourselves influences the way we meet our patients. Therefore the kind of knowledge which we acquire, and also the way in which we acquire it, is of great importance for our social interactions and therapeutic work as physicians.

An example of the influence of a way of thinking on the personality, extreme yet helpful in order to clarify the point we are making, is to be found in the autobiography of Charles Darwin.

> In one respect my mind has changed during the last twenty or thirty years. Up to the age of thirty, or beyond it, poetry of many kinds, such as the works of Milton, Gray, Byron, Wordsworth, Coleridge, and Shelly, gave me great pleasure ... Formerly pictures gave me considerable, and music very great delight. But now for many years I cannot endure to read a line of poetry ... I have also almost lost any taste for pictures or music ... [Darwin calls this a] curious and lamentable loss of the higher aesthetic tastes.
>
> My mind seems to have become a kind of machine for grinding general laws out of large collections of facts, but why this should have caused the atrophy of that part of the brain alone, on which the higher tastes depend, I cannot conceive ... The loss of these tastes is a loss of happiness, and may possibly be injurious to the intellect, and more probably to the moral character, by enfeebling the emotional part of our nature.[1]

Even though the average physician will not be influenced to the degree Darwin was, anthroposophical medical schooling does aim to work differently on the total personality than standard study of medicine does. Not only the development of thinking is addressed, but also the development of feeling and willing. Such a training will gradually make a different kind of physician out of a person and it is this total complex of changes which is of importance to patients and their treatment. This book makes a start in this direction.

10.5 Elements of schooling contained in this manual

We will review briefly in order to survey the elements of schooling/inner development which are contained in each chapter.

In **Chapter 1** the *history of medicine* was described in a number of principal streams since the time before Hippocrates. This showed where anthroposophical medicine stands. It both is and is not new; it integrates modern achievements with valuable older, but metamorphosed, visions on processes of life and healing.

It is important for doctors to know where they stand in their choice of a certain form of practising medicine. Knowledge of history shows that anthroposophical medicine is not an unrelated 'alternative' to orthodox medicine, but an extension of it. It presents a possible next step in the development of modern medicine. By studying the history of medicine it becomes possible to place anthroposophical medicine *in a larger perspective.* In fact, this achieves the same thing as placing a patient's illness within the larger perspective of that patient's biography. The result will be a deeper understanding and perhaps increased enthusiasm for the approach chosen.

This was followed in **Chapter 2** by a *philosophical orientation* of anthroposophical medicine. While conceding that anthroposophical doctors are nice people who spend a lot of time with their patients, regular colleagues often voice the reproach that 'anthroposophy is a belief system which has nothing to do with science.' Because medical philosophy is usually missing from the curriculum, many physicians do not realize that philosophers see the natural scientific paradigm as only one possible vision of reality, which entails many limitations. Blinkers can therefore cause pretentiousness. Familiarity with philosophy can give a doctor the self-confidence that it is not irresponsible or, if you like, unscientific to explore different points of view. In addition, philosophy offers practice in thinking and feeling which can foster inner certainty. Such practice builds a different and stronger basis for practising medicine than can be offered by most regular medical theories and guidelines in the way of outer certainty. In anthroposophy, the whole point is to find *inner anchoring and certainty.*

Chapter 3 introduced *observation* as a fundamental and necessary skill to arrive at *insights for renewal* in medicine. The point is to learn to observe forms as a whole and to get to know the dynamics of the formative forces by inwardly *moving along* and taking all aspects into account. This discipline is called *'phenomenological observation.'* It is inevitable that the observer is 'touched' in this process; thereby the *life of feeling* is developed into an instrument of cognition, through which valuable information can be gained. This phenomenological approach is partly new in medicine; it does play a role in the 'diagnostic glance,' by which we mean the capacity which older, more experienced doctors have to come to a diagnosis in an instant. Present-day medical study, on the other hand, focuses very little on the 'character' of diseases but turns towards details and facts to such degree that this capacity does not receive much attention. Anthroposophical medicine does make use of phenomenological observation as a starting point to discover connections. Connections between the human being and nature, but also between symptoms of a disease and medicinal substances found in nature. All this must take place in a very exact way and not in a loosely associative manner. This means that things are a little bit more complicated than thinking that walnuts are good for the brain because they show a similarity in form, or that carrots and intestines are related because of their shape. In this chapter and the one that followed it the foundations of phenomenological observation and thinking were discussed in order to lay a basis for the development of important inner 'instruments' with which anthroposophical physicians work.

In **Chapter 4** more of the phenomenological method was demonstrated by applying it to aspects of human physiology and embryology. Through observations such as these, it can gradually become clear that the body's shape cannot be viewed in isolation, but that its whole formation is directly connected to psychological functions. A very concrete form of psychosomatics begins to emerge. In this way materialistic knowledge is essentially metamorphosed.

By means of *projective geometry,* **Chapter 5** made a strong demand on *sense-free imagination and thinking,* and also exercised the mobility of those two functions. Those who enjoyed this aspect of mathematics in school will relish this. The purpose of this chapter in the context of this book is that it forms an introduction to the world of the etheric, i.e. the world of the formative life forces. Life forces are often viewed now as a form of 'energy' which permeates the body. This view is problematic in that it is an extension of materialistic thinking and materialistic concepts of reality. According to Rudolf Steiner, the etheric is not to be found in ordinary space, but in *counterspace.* Whereas the force of gravity 'pulls,' the etheric brings 'suction,' and in addition to that, one has to imagine this as a polar process turned inside out! Practice in projective geometry helps to grasp the laws which are at work here. And it has the potential to make spiritual realities tangible; by exercising thinking, they can be known.

Chapter 6 introduced a way of working with *metamorphoses* (both temporal and spatial) in the study of forms and functions of plant and animal organisms. This makes a strong demand on the capacity to form inner pictures and appeals to an artistic ability to inwardly move along with what has been observed. By this process, the principles of formative forces can be discovered. The capacity to *metamorphose* is an archetypal phenomenon of living nature.

In **Chapter 7** we proceeded another step into the world behind the phenomena of nature, the *dynamics of the elements* were introduced. So the relationship between the human being and the environment is not seen as a purely material/molecular one, but as one in which there are corresponding *qualities*. More thorough studying of anthroposophy will acquaint one with the creative beings which are behind the elements, both in nature and in the human being. It is a question of learning to distinguish those qualities not only objectively, outside oneself, but also in one's own inner world of experience.

Chapter 8 links up with this and forms an introduction to the world of the *elements* as they exist in the human being: the anthroposophical picture of man and the concepts prerequisite for its understanding. Here one finds descriptions of the healthy human being, examples of pathological processes, and therapeutic options to treat them. The examples given are a first introduction to practical applications of anthroposophical medicine.

Chapter 9 deals with a totally new subject, namely the way to *study texts* and lectures by *Rudolf Steiner.* Steiner is often hard to follow and *seems* to contradict himself now and then. What can be done towards a better *understanding?* In addition, Steiner appeals to us to not just take his word for it, but to put his pronouncements to the test. Understanding Steiner demands a 'digestive process' on a conceptual level. How does one do that? This can only be done by treading a path of inner development, and by independently taking the first steps in *spiritual scientific research.* Such steps are indicated in this chapter.

This training manual offered an introduction to a number of *fundamental components* necessary to become an anthroposophical doctor. But of course a book such as this can only form part of the training. As stated before, this book can in no way replace study of Steiner's texts concerning the inner path of development. An important part of any training for anthroposophical doctors will be living contact with experienced colleagues, as many things which are discussed in this book are hard to put into words, and might be easier to grasp in conversation, where different words can be found to convey the experiences intended to be conveyed here. After all, anthroposophy is not a theory, but the living reality of a tangible spiritual world, which is a differentiated world of living beings.

The professional path of schooling is described in *Extending Practical Medicine,* the fundamental book on anthroposophical medicine, and in *Meditative Contemplations and Indications on How to Deepen the Art of Healing,* the so-called *Course for Young Doctors.* In this last book especially Steiner speaks repeatedly about the inner attitude of the physician, the will and the courage to heal and the being of illness. Why does the human being fall ill? The book also contains several meditations by means of which the doctor can establish a relationship to the essence of illness and healing forces.

APPENDIX 1:

Lecture from *Introducing Anthroposophical Medicine*

RUDOLF STEINER

It is quite evident that this course will be able to touch on only a very small portion of your probable expectations with regard to the future of medicine, since you will all agree with me that any real, enduring work in this field depends on reforms in the actual education of physicians. What can be communicated in a course of lectures cannot instigate such reforms, even in the remotest way, except possibly by imbuing a number of people with the urge to participate in the reform process. Any medical subject discussed today, however, always has as its other pole and background the way people are prepared to work in the field of medicine through their studies in anatomy, physiology, and general biology. This preparation gives the thinking of medical students a particular slant from the very beginning, and this slant, above all else, is what we must get away from.

I hope to achieve the educational purpose of these lectures by making the following programmatic divisions in our subject matter: First of all, I would like to give you a few indications of the obstacles that the modern, conventional study of medicine presents to a truly objective grasp of the nature of illness as such. Second, I would like to indicate where we must look in our search for an understanding of the human being that is capable of providing a true foundation for work in the field of medicine. Third, I would like use an understanding of human connections to the rest of the world to suggest the possibilities of a rational system of healing. In this third section, I would like to answer the question of whether healing is altogether possible and conceivable.

Fourth — and I think this may perhaps be the most important component

Taken from *Introducing Anthroposophical Medicine:* Lecture 1, March 21, 1920. Reprinted with kind permission of Anthroposophic Press.

of our studies, although it will have to be intertwined with the other three viewpoints — I would like each of you to jot down your special wishes for me on a piece of paper and give it to me by tomorrow or the next day. Please write down whatever you would like to hear about in this course. These wishes can extend to all sorts of topics. What I hope to accomplish through this fourth aspect of the program — which, as I said, will be worked into the other three — is to avoid having you leave this course with the feeling that you have not heard something you particularly wanted to hear. For this reason, I will structure the course in such a way as to work in all the questions you have jotted down. So please give me your requests by tomorrow, or — if that is not possible — by this time the day after tomorrow. I think this is the best way to achieve some sort of completeness in the context of this conference.

Today I would like to give only an introduction of sorts, a few observations for purposes of orientation. Above all, I have been making an effort to assemble everything that can be made known to physicians as a result of spiritual scientific research, and I would like to take this as my starting point. I do not want what I am going to attempt here to be confused with a medical course as such, although in fact it is one. We will focus on anything that can possibly be important to physicians, regardless of its origin. A true science or art of medicine, if I may put it this way, can be built up only by taking into account everything considered in the sense I have indicated.

I will begin today with a few observations for the sake of orientation. If you have reflected on your task as physicians, you will probably have stumbled frequently over the question of what illness actually is, what a sick human being is. Although explanations of illness and the sick person may be disguised by one or the other seemingly objective insertions, they are rarely anything other than this: that disease processes are deviations from the normal processes of life; that certain phenomena, which work on an individual and to which his or her normal life processes are not adapted, produce changes in these normal life processes and in the person's bodily organization; and that illness consists of these change-related functional impairments of parts of the body. You will have to admit, however, that this is nothing more than a negative definition of illness. It is nothing that can help you when you are dealing with actual diseases. This missing practical aspect is what I want to work toward here. To arrive at a definitive view on this subject, I think we would do well to look at certain views on disease that have arisen over the course of time — not so much because I find this absolutely essential for a modern understanding of disease symptoms, but because we will be able to orient ourselves more easily if we are able to consider the older views that have led to current ones.

You all know that when we consider the origins of modern medicine, we usually point to ancient Greece in the fifth and fourth centuries BC, to Hippocrates. It can be said — or at least we have the feeling — that the view that first appeared with Hippocrates and later led to what is known as humoral pathology (which basically continued to play a role right into the nineteenth century) was the beginning of the development of Western medicine. The influence of this belief, which is actually fundamentally erroneous, persists even today and prevents us from achieving an unbiased view of the nature of disease. The first thing we have to do is to eliminate this fundamental error.

To an unbiased student, Hippocrates' views — which, as you may already have noticed, continue to play a role right into the nineteenth century, right up to Rokitansky — constitute not only a new beginning but also, to a very significant extent, the end of ancient views on medicine.[1] In what comes down to us from Hippocrates, we encounter the last filtered remnant, so to speak, of very ancient views on medicine that were acquired by means of atavistic clairvoyance rather than by taking the anatomical route, as is done today. The relative position of Hippocratic medicine might be characterized best by saying that it was the point in time when ancient medicine based on atavistic clairvoyance came to an end. Speaking superficially — but only superficially — we can say that Hippocratic physicians sought the origin of all disease states in an imbalance among the fluid bodies that work together in the human organism. They pointed out that in a normal organism, these fluid bodies must stand in a definite relationship and that in a diseased body, their proportions deviate from the norm. Correct proportions were called crasis and incorrect proportions *dyscrasy*. Of course, these physicians looked for ways to influence the imbalance and reestablish the correct proportions. Four components in the outer world were seen as constituting all physical existence: earth, water, air, and fire (although fire was the same as what we now simply call warmth). As far as human and also animal bodies were concerned, these four elements were seen as being specialized into black gall, yellow gall, mucus, and blood. It was thought that the human organism needed the right mixture of blood, mucus, and black and yellow gall in order to function.

If modern, scientifically educated individuals approach a subject like this, their first thought is that when blood, mucus, and yellow and black gall mingle, they do so in accordance with intrinsic properties that can be determined by means of elementary or advanced chemistry. Seeing it in this light, people imagine this to be the origin of humoral pathology, as if the Hippocratic physicians had seen blood, mucus, and so on only in this way. This was not the case, or rather, it was true of only one of these components, namely black gall, which seems most typically Hippocratic to modern observers. As far as black gall was concerned, Hippocratic physicians did indeed think that its ordinary chemical properties were the active factors. But with regard to all the rest — white or yellow gall, mucus, and blood — they were not thinking only of the properties that can be determined through chemical reactions. They thought that these other fluid constituents of the human organism — for the present, I will always restrict myself to the human organism, without considering the animal organism — possessed certain intrinsic properties in the form of forces or energies lying outside our earthly existence. Thus, just as they saw water, air, and warmth as being dependent on the forces of the cosmos beyond Earth, they also saw these constituents of the human organism as being imbued with forces coming from outside the Earth.

In the course of the evolution of Western science, we have completely ceased looking toward forces that come from outside the Earth. Today's scientists would find it downright peculiar if they were expected to think that water, when it influences the human organism, supposedly possesses not only those properties that can be confirmed through chemistry, but also others it possesses by virtue of belonging to the supra-earthly cosmos. But according to ancient views, the effects of forces originating in the cosmos itself are introduced into the human organism through its fluid constituents. Although the effects of these cosmic forces gradually ceased to be taken into account, medical thought into the fifteenth century continued to be based on remnants of the filtered view we encounter in Hippocrates. This is why it is so difficult for modern scientists to understand medical texts written before the fifteenth century, for it must be said that most of the authors of that time did not have any real understanding of what they were writing. They talked about the four basic constituents of the human organism, but their reasons for describing these constituents in one way or another were derived from a knowledge that had died with Hippocrates. In talking about the properties of the fluids that build up the human organism, people were simply talking about the aftereffects of Hippocratic knowledge.

Galen then contributed a compilation of old traditions that worked on into the fifteenth century, although they were becoming more and more incomprehensible.[2] But there were always single individuals capable of recognizing and pointing to the existence of something whose possibilities are not exhausted by the purely earthly element, by what can be ascertained chemically or physically. These individuals acknowledged the need to point to something in the human organism that makes its fluid substances work in ways other than those that can be confirmed through chemistry. These opponents of the prevailing school of humoral pathology included Paracelsus and van Helmont, although others could also be

mentioned.[3] They brought a new quality into medical thought in the six-
teenth and seventeenth centuries simply by trying to formulate a concept
that others were no longer formulating. Their formulation, however, contained thoughts that could be followed only by those who were still
somewhat clairvoyant, as Paracelsus and van Helmont very definitely
were. If we are not clear about all these matters, we will not be able to
communicate understandably with each other about certain remnants that
still cling to modern medical terminology, although their origins are no
longer recognizable. Thus Paracelsus — and later others who were influenced by him — assumed the *archeus* to be the basis of the action of fluids within the organism. He assumed the *archeus* to be similar to what we
speak of as the human ether body.

The terms '*archeus*' as Paracelsus uses it and 'human ether body' as we
use it actually sum up something that does indeed exist, but without tracing its actual origins. Doing so would oblige us to proceed as follows: we
would have to say that the human being has both a physical organism [see
drawing], which consists essentially of forces that work out of the Earth,
and an etheric organism [drawing, 'red'], which consists essentially of
forces that work out of the periphery of the cosmos. Our physical organism is a portion of the entire organization of the Earth, as it were. Our
ether body, and also Paracelsus's *archeus*, is a portion of something that
does not belong to the Earth, something that therefore works into the
earthly element from the cosmos from all directions. Thus, in his view of
an etheric organism underlying the physical organism, Paracelsus
summed up everything that had been described earlier as simply the cosmic aspect of the human being — a concept that came to an end in
Hippocratic medicine. Although he indicated details here and there, he did
not investigate further into the supra-earthly forces connected to what was
at work in the *archeus*.

We might say that Paracelsus's meaning has become ever more incomprehensible. This is especially evident if we jump forward into the seventeenth and eighteenth centuries, where we encounter Stahl's school of
medical thought, which no longer understood anything of how the cosmic
aspect works into the terrestrial.[4] Stahl's school of medicine enlisted the
help of all sorts of unfounded concepts — concepts of a life force, of life
spirits, and so forth. Whereas Paracelsus and van Helmont still spoke with
some degree of consciousness about what lay between the soul/spirit and
the physical organization of the human being, Stahl and his followers
spoke as if it were simply a matter of another form of the conscious soul
playing into the structuring of the human body. Of course, Stahl's view
elicited a strong reaction, because anyone who carries on in this way,
hypothesizing about some sort of vitalism, is entering the realm of purely

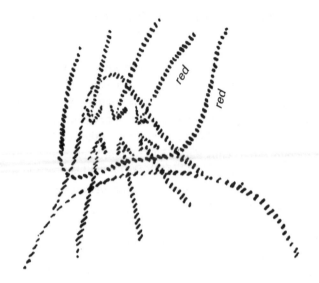

arbitrary constructs. And, as you know, the nineteenth century then rose up in arms against these arbitrary constructs. It can be said that only very great minds like Johannes Muller, who died in 1858 and was the teacher of Ernst Haeckel, managed to overcome some of the harm that resulted from this unclear way of speaking that addressed life forces as if they were soul forces at work in the human organism but had no clear idea of how they were supposed to work.[5]

At the same time, however, a totally different trend was emerging. We have traced the declining trend to its last vestiges. But more recent times saw the dawning of an idea that then became definitive in a different way in terms of the formulation of medical concepts, especially in the nineteenth century. Basically, this idea was derived from a single, unusually authoritative eighteenth century work, *De sedibus et causis morborum per anatomen indagatis* (1761, 'On the Bases and Causes of Diseases through Anatomical Investigation'), by the Paduan physician Morgagni.[6] This book saw the emergence of a totally new view that essentially introduced the materialistic trend into medicine. We need to characterize these things completely objectively, without sympathy or antipathy, because what came to light in this book directed people's attention to the consequences of disease in the human organism. The autopsy became definitive. Only from this time onward can it be said that the autopsy became definitive. It was possible to tell from the corpse that if a certain illness — regardless of what it was called — was present, a particular organ must have undergone a specific change. These changes began to be studied during postmortem examinations. This practice constitutes the actual beginnings of pathological anatomy, while everything that had previously existed in the field of medicine was based on certain persistent effects of ancient clairvoyance.

It is interesting to note how this great shift finally took place in one fell swoop. Interestingly enough, it is possible to point precisely to the two decades in which this transformation came about, when any remainders of the ancient legacy were abandoned and the atomistic and materialistic view of modern medicine was established. If you take the trouble to read through Rokitansky's handbook on pathological anatomy, published in 1842, you will still find traces of the old humoral pathology, remnants of the view that disease is based on the abnormal interaction of fluids. Rokitansky very ingeniously incorporated this view — which can be maintained only by legatees of the old view of the supra-earthly qualities of fluids — into his observations of changes in organs. Thus his book, although based on postmortem observations of organ changes, also suggests that particular organ changes came about under the influence of abnormal fluid mixtures. There you have, in 1842, the final appearance of the legacy of ancient humoral pathology. In the next few days we will talk about how forward-looking attempts (such as Hahnemann's) to consider more comprehensive concepts of disease were introduced into the decline of the old humoral pathology.[7] Hahnemann's and similar attempts are too important to be presented in a mere introduction and will have to be discussed later in greater detail.

At this point, however, I would like to draw your attention to the fact that in the two decades following the publication of Rokitanksy's book on pathological anatomy, the foundations were laid for the atomistic, materialistic view of medicine. In a very strange way, old views still played into the ideas that developed in the first half of the nineteenth century. It is interesting to observe that Schwann, for example, who might be said to have discovered that plants have cells, was still of the opinion that cell formation was underlain by the development of some sort of shapeless fluid (which he called 'blastema') and that the cell nucleus condensed out of this fluid formation, gathering cell protoplasm around it.[8] It is interesting to note that Schwann still posits an underlying fluid element possessing attributes whose tendency to differentiate brings about the cells as such. It is also interesting to trace the gradual subsequent development of a view that can be summed up in these words: The human organism builds itself up out of cells. This idea approximates today's customary view that the cell is a type of building-block for organisms and that the human organism is built up out of cells.

At heart, the view that was still evident between the lines (or even more pervasively) in Schwann's work is the final remnant of the old system of

medicine, because it does not lead to atomism. It sees an atomistic phenomenon — cells — as emerging from something that, if considered
rightly, can never be thought of as atomistic, namely, a preexisting fluid
essence that possesses inherent forces and gives rise to the atomistic element through differentiation. Thus, in the two decades of the 1840s and
1850s the older, more universal view was coming to an end and the atomistic view of medicine was dawning. It was fully present by the time
Virchow published his book on cellular pathology in 1858.[9] We must recognize that an enormous leap, an enormous shift in the direction of modern medical thinking, took place between the publication of Rokitansky's
book in 1842 and Virchow's in 1858. Virchow's book deduces all pathological phenomena in the human being from changes in cellular functioning. Ever since its publication, the ideal official view has been to study
changes in cells in organ tissue and to understand all illness as resulting
from such cellular changes. This atomistic view simplifies matters
because it makes them very clear and lays them out in a way that is easy
to understand. And more recent science, in spite of all its advances, always
aims to understand everything in the simplest possible terms, without considering that it is the character of nature and the cosmos to be extremely
complicated.

It is very easy to demonstrate experimentally, for example, that an
amoeba in water changes its shape, extending and retracting its armlike
processes. Then, if you warm the liquid it is floating in, you will see that
its processes extend and retract more quickly, at least until the temperature
reaches a certain point. Then the amoeba contracts and is no longer able
to respond to changes in the surrounding medium. You can also introduce
an electric current into the liquid and observe how the amoeba assumes a
spherical shape. It eventually bursts if the current running through the liquid becomes too strong. In this way, the changes an individual cell undergoes under the influence of its environment can be studied and used as the
basis of a theory of how disease gradually develops through alterations in
the character of the cell.

What is the essence of the results of that great shift that took place
within two decades? What emerged then lives on and now permeates all
of official medical science. It is none other than the general tendency that
has developed in the age of materialism — the tendency to grasp the world
in atomistic terms.

Please take note of the following. I began by drawing your attention to
the fact that anyone working in the medical field today is absolutely
obliged to consider the question of what diseases are. What kind of
processes are they, and how do they differ from the human organism's so
called normal processes? We need a positive conception of this deviation

in order to be able to work with it at all, but the usual descriptions supplied by official science are exclusively negative and serve only to point out that such deviations exist. Then attempts are made to eliminate the deviations. But there is still no comprehensive view of the nature of the human being, and our entire philosophy of medicine suffers from the absence of such a comprehensive view.

What are disease processes, really? You will not be able to avoid calling them natural processes. Suppose you trace the consequences of some external process in nature. It is not so easy to make an abstract distinction between that process and a disease process. You call the natural process 'normal' and the disease process 'abnormal' without pointing out why the process taking place within the human organism is an abnormal one. You cannot develop practical applications until you can at least explain to yourself why the process is abnormal. Only then can you investigate how to do away with it, because only then will you be able to discover which corner of the cosmos makes it possible to eliminate such a process. Ultimately, even calling something abnormal is an obstacle, for why should any process in the human being be considered abnormal? Even if I cut my finger, that is only abnormal as it relates to the human being, because if I cut a piece of wood into a particular shape, that is a normal process. But if it is my finger that gets cut, I call that an abnormal process. The mere fact that we customarily engage in processes other than finger-cutting tells us nothing; it is merely playing with words. From a certain perspective, what happens when I cut my finger follows a course similar to that of other processes and is just as normal as any other natural process.

Our task is to discover the real difference between those processes within the human organism that we call disease processes — which are basically quite normal natural processes, even though specific causes must precipitate them — and the everyday processes that we usually call 'healthy.' We must discover this radical distinction, but we will not be able to do so if we cannot take up a way of looking at human beings that really leads us to their essential nature. In this introduction, I would like to sketch for you at least the first elements of this way of looking at the human being, with the intention of elaborating on them later.

I am sure you understand that in these lectures, which are necessarily limited in number, I will be giving you primarily what you will not find in books or other lectures, and I will assume a knowledge on your part of what is available elsewhere. I do not think it would be especially valuable to present a theory to you in constructs that you could also find somewhere else. For this reason, let us turn now to what you can discover by simply comparing what you can see in a human skeleton and the skeleton of one of the so-called higher apes — a gorilla, for example. If

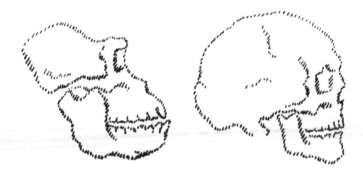

you compare these two skeletons on a purely superficial level, the main thing you will notice in the gorilla is the exceptional development of the entire lower jaw, simply in terms of mass. The lower jaw weighs heavily on the skull. When you look at the head of a gorilla with its massive lower jaw, you get the feeling that the lower jaw weighs heavily on the entire skeleton in some way, pushing it forward, and that the gorilla makes a considerable effort to remain upright in spite of this burden.

You will find the same distribution of weight, in contrast to the human skeleton, when you look at the gorilla's forearms and the lower part of the hands. They seem heavy. In the gorilla, everything is massive. In contrast, everything is refined and delicately jointed in the human being; weight moves into the background here. In these particular parts of the body — the lower jaw and the forearms and fingers — the element of weight moves into the background in the human being, while it is prominent in the gorilla. Anyone who has cultivated a sharp eye for these pro-

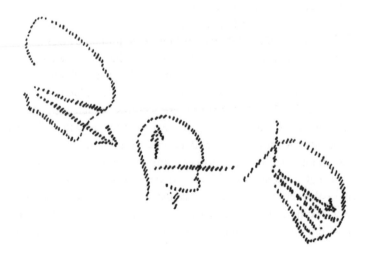

portions will be able to find them again in the bones of the feet and legs. There, too, an element of weight is present in the gorilla, pushing in a certain direction.

I would like to use this line [arrows] as a schematic indication of the force that can be seen in the gorilla's lower jaw, arms, and legs. In the human being, this force is counteracted by an upward-striving element. This conclusion is inevitable if you observe a human lower jaw, which no longer weighs down the skeleton, and the delicate shaping of human arms and fingers. The difference between a gorilla skeleton and a human skeleton is evident to the naked eye. You will have to deduce the form-creating element in the human being from a kind of parallelogram of forces, which

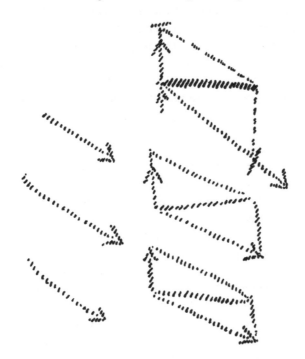

results from the same upward force to which gorillas adapt only outwardly, as you can tell by the effort required for them to maintain uprightness. Here is the resulting parallelogram with its lines of force:

The very strange thing about this is that nowadays we usually restrict ourselves to simply comparing the bones or muscles of higher animals to those of humans and fail to place enough emphasis on this morphological transformation. In observing it, we must look for one essential aspect. You see, in the human being the forces that counteract those determining a gorilla's form must actually be present. Those forces must exist; they must be at work. If we look for them, we will rediscover the aspect of ancient medicine that was abandoned or filtered out by the Hippocratic system. We will rediscover that the original forces in the parallelogram are earthly in character. The other forces, however, must be sought outside the Earth. They unite with the original forces, and the resultant owes its origin to supra-earthly, extraterrestrial forces rather than to earthly ones.

We must look for forces that pull human beings into the upright position. This is not the same as the upright position higher animals assume from time to time, because the forces active in bringing about human uprightness are also formative forces. It makes a difference whether we are dealing with apes, who walk upright but still possess forces that weigh them down in the other direction, or with humans, whose skeletal development works in the direction of forces that are non-earthly in origin. If we simply look at the form of the human skeleton in the right way, tracing the dynamics at work in building it up instead of restricting ourselves to describing the individual bones and comparing them to animal bones, we will realize that what we see there is not to be found anywhere in the other kingdoms of nature. We must unite the specifically human forces with the original forces in the parallelogram. The resultant cannot be accounted for by considering only forces that exist outside the human being. It will be important for us make a careful study of this leap from the animal to the human. When we do, we will be able to discover the origin of disease in both humans and animals. I can show only these elements to you little by little, but when we pursue them further we will be able to make many discoveries.

In connection with what I have just presented to you, I would like to mention the following. If we move on from the skeletal system to the muscular system, we discover significant differences in the character of muscles. A muscle at rest is alkaline in reaction, if we take its typical chemical effect into account. But we can actually say only that its reaction is alkaline-like, because in a resting muscle the reaction is not as clear-cut as alkaline reactions otherwise are. Similarly, in an active muscle a somewhat indefinite acid reaction occurs.

As you recall, in a metabolic sense muscles are composed, of course, of what human beings ingest. Therefore, in a certain respect, they are a result of the forces present in earthly substances. But when human beings become active, it becomes increasingly evident that what their muscle tissue contains as a result of being subject only to ordinary metabolism is being overcome. The changes appearing in active muscle tissue stand in contrast to ordinary metabolic changes and can ultimately be compared only to the forces bringing about the formation of the human skeletal system. These latter forces, which transcend what humans acquire from outside, imbue themselves with terrestrial forces, uniting with them to bring about a resultant force. Similarly, we must also see muscle metabolism as containing something chemically active that is working into the Earth's chemistry. You might say that in the skeleton, something we can no longer find within the earthly element is working into earthly mechanics and dynamics. Similarly, in our metabolism we have non-earthly chemistry working into earthly chemistry to produce effects different from those that can appear under the influence of earthly chemistry alone.

These observations about morphology on the one hand and quality on the other will have to constitute our point of departure if we want to discover what actually lies within the human being. This approach will reopen the way back to something that has been lost but is obviously still needed if we are not willing to accept a mere formal definition of disease that is useless in actual practice. You see, a very important question is emerging. Earthly remedies from our surroundings are all we have available to work on the human organism when it undergoes changes. Non-earthly forces, however, are at work in us — or at least forces that turn our processes into non-earthly processes. This gives rise to the question of how we can bring about an interaction between the sick human organism and its physical earthly environment, an interaction that leads from illness to health. How can we call forth a reciprocal relationship of this sort that will really also be able to influence those forces active in the human organism that are not encompassed by the realm of processes from which we select our medicines, even if these processes are dietary prescriptions and so forth?

You see that what can ultimately lead to a specific therapy is intimately related to an appropriate understanding of the essential nature of the human being. These first rudimentary elements of what is intended to enable us to rise to a solution to this problem have been derived from distinctions between humans and animals. I am fully aware of the very facile objection that animals and even plants can also become ill (lately there has even been talk of diseases in minerals!) and that therefore no distinction should be made between humans and animals as far as illness is concerned. We will deal with this objection later. These distinctions will become evident once you see how little physicians stand to gain in the long run from investigating the animal kingdom with the goal of making headway in human medicine. To be sure, animal experimentation does have something to offer with regard to human healing — and we will find out later why this is so — but only if the radical difference between animals and humans, a difference that persists right into the details of their organization, is fundamentally clear to us. For this reason, it will be important to find appropriate ways to continue to clarify the significance of animal experimentation for the development of the field of human medicine.

As we continue, I would like to draw your attention to the fact that when we are obliged to point to such supra-earthly forces, the personality of the individual is involved to a much greater extent than it is if we can always point to so-called objective rules or objective laws of nature. Admittedly, it will be important to work toward the intuitive element to a much greater extent in the field of medicine. We need to realize that an intuition trained to observe forms — the gift of drawing conclusions from morphological phenomena about the character of an individual human organism that may be sick. or healthy in some respect — must play an ever greater role in the future development of medicine.

As I said, these things were intended to serve only as an introduction and orientation of sorts, because the important point for today is to show that medicine must once again turn its attention to something that cannot be accomplished through either chemistry or conventional comparative anatomy, something that can be achieved only if we move on to consider the facts from a spiritual scientific viewpoint. Several errors are still prevalent in this regard. The main issue in the spiritualization of medicine is thought to be replacing material remedies with spiritual ones. This approach may be totally justified in particular areas, but it is totally unjustified on the whole, because what is most needed is a spiritual recognition of the healing value that may be present in a material remedy — that is, using spiritual science to evaluate material remedies. That will be the task of the portion of this course that I described as searching for healing possibilities by recognizing the connection between the human being and the rest of the world.

I want all the things I will say about specific therapeutic processes to be as well founded as possible and to help in acquiring a view, in each single illness, of the connection between the so-called abnormal process, which is of necessity a natural process, and so-called normal processes, which are also nothing other than natural processes. I would merely like to add a brief postscript: Whenever the fundamental question has arisen of how to come to terms with the fact that disease processes are also natural processes, attempts have always been made to evade the issue. For example, I was interested to learn that already in the first half of the nineteenth century, Troxler, who taught in Bern, was very emphatically pointing out that illness needed to be investigated as a normal phenomenon.[10] He claimed that this view would ultimately lead us to acknowledge the existence of a certain world that is connected to our world but forces its way into it through illegitimate channels, as it were, and that the results of such an investigation could have something to do with disease symptoms.

I want to touch on this only superficially at this point. Just imagine, however, a world existing in the background whose governing principles are very justified processes that happen to bring about disease symptoms in our world. If that were the case, if these laws that are totally justified in a different world were to break through into our world through certain gaps, they could cause all kinds of damage. This was what Troxler was aiming at. In spite of the fact that he expressed himself without clarity in some respects, it is still possible to see that he was on a path that was leading toward a certain healing for medical science.

Since Troxler had lectured at the university in Bern, a friend there once helped me investigate how he was regarded by his colleagues and what came of his suggestions. In the encyclopedia that documents many incidents in the history of the university, we were able to find only that Troxler had been the cause of a great many arguments! We found nothing in particular about his importance to science.

As I said, my intention today was only to point out these things. Please do write down all of your wishes for me by tomorrow or the next day so that I can weave them into what I myself intend to present. The form that these lectures will take will be based on these wishes of yours. I think this will be the best way to proceed, so please make extensive requests.

Excerpts from the *Corpus Hippocraticum*

The human body contains of *blood, phlegm, yellow bile* and *black bile*; they form the nature of this body, and it is because of these that we feel pain or enjoy health. Now the body will enjoy the most perfect health when these elements have the right relationship to one another in terms of consistency, strength and size, and when they are *mixed perfectly*. Pain is felt when there is too much or too little of one of these elements, or when one of them is isolated without being in communication with the others. For when an element is isolated and stands on its own, *not only the place which it has left will become ill, but also the place where it has gone to and where it forms an excess* must cause hurt and distress because there is too much of it in one spot.

(From *The Nature of Man* Chapter 4, Περι Φυσειος Ανθρωπου)

Here we find a short description of the four humors, *the* krasis *and the* diskrasis *(good and bad mixture), and also the viewpoint that health consists of a specific relationship of substances and forces. It explains in a very simple way how imbalance works: when there's too much in one place, there will be too little in another. In a modified form, we will often encounter this view of disease again in anthroposophical medicine.* (Anton Dekkers).

When one wants to practice the science of medicine correctly, one has to proceed as follows: first of all one must consider the effects produced by each season of the year; because the seasons are not the same at all, but they differ to a high degree, both viewed by themselves and with respect to their changes. The next point to consider is this: the warm and dry winds, specifically those which are general, but also those which are specific to a separate region. But one also needs to weigh the qualities of different waters: because to the degree that they differ in taste and weight, they also differ in their relationship to one another. Therefore a physician who visits a town he doesn't know needs to check out the position of that town in relationship to the winds, and in relationship to the places where the sun rises. Because a north, south, east and a west aspects each have their individual character. All these things need to the weighed with the greatest care: how the inhabitants acquire their water, whether they use marshy, soft water, or hard water coming from rocky heights, or brackish and unpalatable water. The consistency of the ground must be considered: whether it is bare and dry or forested and wet, low and hot or high and cold.

One must also take into consideration how the inhabitants live. Do they drink a lot? Do they eat lunch? Are they inactive or do they lead athletic and energetic lives? Do they eat much and drink little?

Using these indications, the physician must investigate the various problems which arise. When he knows these things well, preferably all of them, but at least most, then he will not be ignorant with regard to local diseases or the nature of those diseases which usually occur there when he arrives in an unknown town. All this to prevent that he is clueless in the treatment of diseases or makes blunders, which will be the case when he lacks this knowledge before considering the various problems. According to the time and the passing of the year, he will be able to say which epidemics will attack the state both in summer and in winter. Also which diseases are likely to occur for individual people as a result of a change in lifestyle. For knowledge of the changes of the seasons, the ascent and descent of stars, and of the circumstances belonging to these phenomena, will prepare him in advance for the nature of the coming year. By considerations such as these and perceiving the times in advance he will have a full knowledge of each specific case and is likely to succeed best in guaranteeing health and will have the greatest success in practicing his art...

(From: *Airs, Waters, Places*, Chapter 1&2)

We see here how the physician looks at the environment, taken in a larger sense, which includes the stars. The approach to the surroundings is a qualitative one, and conclusions are drawn with regard to epidemics but also with regard to individual illnesses. It is interesting to contrast this with the way we work in our surgeries. Do we take the position of the stars into account, do we consider the weather (in a long-term perspective, not only today), the quality of the wind, the quality of the water, etc.? (Anton Dekkers).

APPENDIX 3

Heart and 'Turning Point in Time'

GUUS VAN DER BIE

Present day cardiology pictures the working of the heart as an occurrence which has two phases. In the first phase a very rapid contraction of all muscle tissue takes place. One has to imagine that after a period of 'inactivity' a certain sudden activation of the heart muscle occurs. Even though we can distinguish a sequence in the activity of the separate parts of the heart, separated by fractions of seconds, we can only view it macroscopically as something involving the heart as a whole. The contracting heart looks as if it is being hit. This phase of contraction is called systole. The impulse to this systole comes from heart muscle tissue which has gone through massive transformation. As a result of this transformation, the function of this tissue is strongly akin to the characteristics of nerve tissue. In this '*heart-nerve*' electrical/biological phenomena occur which can be better understood as a function of the nervous system than as a function of muscle tissue. The beat character of the systole is determined to a large degree by this 'heart nerve.' Through this nerve tissue the contraction impulse can be conducted at great speed. Compared to the heart muscle, a normal muscle contracts much more gradually; it pulls gradually together as it were, until a state of maximum contraction has been reached.

During systole, the heart's own blood vessels (coronary arteries) are not being filled, in contrast to the other blood vessels in the body. As a result, a certain *bloodlessness* of the heart muscle tissue occurs, persisting for the duration of the systole. In principle, this is a life-threatening situation for the heart itself, for the vitality of our organs is directly dependent on oxygen-rich blood streaming through. Proper functioning of muscles

Originally published as 'Hart en Zeitenwende,' *Mededelingen van de Anthroposofische Vereniging in Nederland,* 1986, No.12.

always depends on blood circulation. In this sense the heart is not a normal muscle. The heart simultaneously contracts and becomes bloodless. Even though our skeletal muscles show a comparable process, this total contraction of the heart during the systole makes the situation as it were precarious for the heart. No part of the heart can avoid going through systole, whereas contraction all at once only occurs as an exception in skeletal muscles.

Seen in terms of the contrast of blood and nerve, systole is decidedly 'nerve-determined'. The biochemical changes occurring in the heart during systole correspond to this. During systole the heart muscle becomes more acidic. Acidity in an organism is generally an expression of 'astralization'. During periods of waking and intensive work the organism becomes relatively more acidic than during periods of sleep or rest. Our nervous system plays an indispensable role in processes taking place when we are awake and working. During waking hours, the force of systole increases therefore, as our blood pressure shows. On waking up, our blood pressure is usually lowest, and will increase during the course of the day as we are taxed more through wakefulness and work. A second phenomenon which should be mentioned here is the chemical salinization of the heart during the systole. Especially saline enters into the heart muscle cells in great quantities, which are thereby being 'impregnated' with saline. In radical terms, the nervous system is a 'saline system.' For it to function properly, it depends completely on saline processes.

Systole can be registered on an electrocardiogram. This electrocardiogram shows a definite pattern. The character of systole is such that the process can be registered down to the finest details. The form is so clear that the normal shape which is registered can clearly be distinguished from an abnormal one, as is the case with disturbances of heart rhythm. The *pattern of contraction* threatens to get lost when there are deviations. In such cases, form deviations arise as it were in the systolic phase of the heart. Every human being will at one point have a conscious experience of the activity of the heart, when heart palpitations are felt. What are these heart palpitations? They are conscious experiences of one or more systoles. In whatever form they may occur, only the systole will come to consciousness. Insofar as waking consciousness can extend to the organs in the breast, the heart will only be felt in the systolic moments.

Systole is followed by diastole, whereby the heart relaxes. Let us keep the same order as we did for systole when we now study diastole. Following systole, the 'nerve of the heart' is completely 'spent.' The same paralyzed situation occurs in the heart nerve when we compare it for example to the eye. When we have caught an image in the eye, the eye is blind for $^{1}/_{16}$ of a second; for one moment we can see nothing, not even the harshest flash of light. It is the same with the heart-nerve. For a short duration the heart-nerve *cannot be stimulated* and a renewed contraction is not possible at that point. During diastole, the coronary arteries fill with oxygen-rich blood which is nourishing for the heart. The preceding blood-lessness is suddenly changed into the opposite situation: diastole is characteristically *rich in blood*. Due to this better circulation the existing acidity and salinization can be neutralized in a very short time. The heart recovers as it were from the harm caused by esystole.

Here, the electrocardiogram shows nothing at all; that is to say, it shows no recognizable pattern formation. During diastole a *form dissolution* predominates in the functioning of the heart. This form dissolution should be seen in contrast with what was mentioned before as pattern formation during systole. Let us round off by considering the relationship to our waking consciousness. Whereas systole can be consciously perceived, diastole never can. We know of no situation, including illness, in which the human being can be conscious of diastole. It always remains hidden from our consciousness. One could say that the kind of consciousness which characterizes diastole is the *consciousness of sleep*.

When we survey the above, we can confine ourselves to listing the key-words which give us a sense of the incompatibility of systole with diastole. Faced with two processes which are the polar opposite of one another and have two totally different effects in the heart, what are we to say about the function of the heart as a whole? After all, it is apparent that the description given above of the functioning of the heart in systole and diastole does not describe the total function very well. It seems safe to put it this way: in systole we can see the nerve sense pole of the human being at work. Systole is not the working of the heart, but it is the upper pole of the human being at work in the heart. By the same token one can take diastole as the manifestation of the blood pole working in the human being. Diastole is a function of the lower pole in the heart.

Having established this, we can begin to see how the heart works. We can see it in the space created between systole and diastole. Shouldn't the place where one process is carried over into its polar opposite be regarded as the central function of the heart?

Having come this far, we could also propose a way to describe this particular working of the heart and we would like to call it '*transpolation*.' A transpolation which works either from systole into diastole, or from diastole into systole. The heart has to conquer the immediate threat of polarisation many, many times a minute. *The heart achieves this in its capacity as an organ of transpolation.* In essence this means that all life 'wells up 'in our hearts, not in the extremities of systole or diastole, but in between, in the process of tranpolation. And it is from a point which can no longer be registered physically and to which we will give the name 'point of transpolation,' that life streams into the organism by the minute. In this way we can view the heart as a supremely concentrated organ of three-foldness. It appears that the polarity of the human being reaches a culmination in the heart, and the quality of the heart itself elevates this into threefoldness.

The point between systole and diastole, the 'transpolation-point,' merits closer study. For in the physiology of the heart this point seems of eminent importance. Yet at the same time this moment escapes registration. We will have a hard time finding a way to study this moment more closely if we confine ourselves to the physical. In order to experience what we are after, we need the help of a musical analogy. For it is in music that we also find quantities which can be registered: on the one hand there is beat (which can be compared to systole), on the other hand there is the melody with its succession of different intervals. Music creatively employs beat and melody, but in no way is it just a melody played by keeping time. If one rigidly beats time, playing the music measure by measure, no melody will come to life. Yet the sequence of intervals which forms the melody can dissolve the measure, so to speak, or at least break the rigidity. In making music, the musician creates from a point which is poised between melody and beat in a realm which (once again) cannot be registered. Out of this point the musician creates the rhythm of the interpretation; the music 'comes to life'. The greater the artists, the greater is the capacity of 'empathy with' that which lives in the musical creation and bring that to expression. At that moment, the musician is not in the physical world, but in a realm of experience which is of a higher plane. What is experienced at this higher plane, comes to life with the aid of beat and melody on the earthly level. This example can help us realize that there are other realms where rhythmical processes are at work which are essentially not of a physical nature, but of a higher order directly adjacent to the physical world. Therefore every rhythmical process is a trinity-process which, in the middle phase, transcends the physical. In that phase it is never totally physical. In this sense our heart connects us in the most striking way with the world beyond the physical. Even though biology has long known that all organs function through rhythmical processes, no organ demonstrates that (this) as clearly as the heart. The 'transpolation point' in the heart has features which are of existential importance for the human being. Out of this central point in the working of the heart, life streams out and reaches all the way into our physical existence. It is a constant source of renewal, boundless in intensity. When one experiences systole as a working of the upper pole, one is immediately struck by the pathological tendency at work there, manifesting in coldness, cramps, sclerosis, which are all hardening processes terminating in 'death in form.' The healing impulse which the heart places over against this is the warmth impulse. This warmth impulse doesn't spring from the physical level in the working of the heart; it is a warmth-stream from beyond the physical, originating in spiritual warmth. In diastole, in which the lower pole is at work, another tendency to illness can be recognized. It is a tendency to a loss of structure, dissolution of form; 'death in chaos' is the threat we meet there. The healing tendency which the heart places over against this is a light impulse. The light in this impulse is spiritual in origin, penetrating into physical processes, giving form, bestowing structure.

Viewed in this way one can experience the heart as the organ of the turning point in time; it is preeminently the place where the spiritual world can reach the human being, and where the human being can carry the spiritual world within.

APPENDIX 4

Fundamentals of Therapy

RUDOLF STEINER & ITA WEGMAN

PREFACE TO THE FIRST EDITION BY ITA WEGMAN

Rudolf Steiner, the teacher, guide and friend, is no longer among the living on the Earth. A severe illness, beginning in sheer physical exhaustion, tore him away. In the very midst of his work he had to lie down on the bed of sickness. The powers he had devoted so copiously, so unstintingly, to the work of the Anthroposophical Society no longer sufficed to overcome his own illness. With untold grief and pain, all those who loved and honoured him had to stand by and witness how he who was loved by so many, who had been able to help so many others, had to allow fate to take its appointed course when his own illness came, well-knowing that higher powers were guiding these events.

In this small volume the fruits of our united work are recorded. The teaching of Anthroposophy is for medical science a veritable mine of inspiration. From my knowledge and experience as a doctor, I was able to confirm it without reserve. I found in it a fount of wisdom from which it was possible untiringly to draw, and which was able to solve and illumine many a problem as yet unsolved in Medicine. Thus there arose between Rudolf Steiner and myself a living co-operation in the field of medical discovery. Our co-operation gradually deepened, especially in the last two years, so that the united authorship of a book became a possibility and an achievement. It had always been Rudolf Steiner's endeavour — and in this I could meet him with fullest sympathy of understanding to renew the life of the ancient Mysteries and cause it to flow once more into the sphere of Medicine. From time immemorial, the Mysteries were most intimately united with the art of healing, and the attainment of spiritual knowledge was brought into connection with the healing of the sick. We had no

Taken from *Fundamentals of Therapy*. Reprinted by kind permission of Mercury Press.

thought, after the style of quacks and dilettanti, of underrating the scientific Medicine of our time. We recognized it fully. Our aim was to supplement the science already in existence by the illumination that can flow from a true knowledge of the Spirit, towards a living grasp of the processes of illness and of healing. Needless to say, our purpose was to bring into new life, not the instinctive habit of the soul which still existed in the Mysteries of ancient time, but a method of research corresponding to the fully evolved consciousness of modern man, which can be lifted into spiritual regions.

Thus the first beginnings of our work were made. In the Clinical and Therapeutic Institute founded by myself at Arlesheim. in Switzerland, a basis was given in practice for the theories set forth in this book. And we endeavoured to unfold new ways in the art of healing to those who were seeking, in the sense here indicated, for a widening of their medical knowledge.

We had intended to follow up this small volume with further productions of our united work. This, alas, was no longer possible. It is, however, still my purpose, from the many notes and fruitful indications I received, to publish a second volume and possibly a third. As to this first volume, the manuscript of which was corrected with inner joy and satisfaction by Rudolf Steiner only three days before his death, may it find its way to those for whom it is intended those who are striving to reach out from life's deep riddles to an understanding of life in its true greatness and glory.

CHAPTER I

True Knowledge of the Human Being as a Foundation for the Art of Medicine

This book will indicate new possibilities for the science and art of Medicine. It will only be possible to form an accurate view of what is described if the reader is willing to accept the points of view that predominated at that time when the medical approach outlined here came into being.

It is not a question of opposition to modern [homogenic] medicine which is working with scientific methods. We take full cognizance of the value of its principles. It is also our opinion that what we are offering should only be used in medical work by those individuals who can be fully active as qualified physicians in the sense of those principles.

On the other hand, to all that can be known about the human being with the scientific methods that are recognized today, we add a further knowledge, whose discoveries are made by different methods. And out of this deeper knowledge of the World and Man, we find ourselves compelled to work for an extension of the art of medicine.

Fundamentally speaking, the [homogenic] medicine of today can offer no objection to what we have to say, seeing that we on our side do not deny its principles. He alone could reject our efforts a priori who would require us not only to affirm his science but to adduce no further knowledge extending beyond the limits of his own. We see this extension of our knowledge of the World and Man in Anthroposophy, which was founded by Rudolf Steiner. To the knowledge of the physical man which alone is accessible to the natural-scientific methods of today, Anthroposophy adds that of spiritual man. Nor does it merely proceed by dint of reflective thought from knowledge of the physical to knowledge of the spiritual. On such a path, one only finds oneself face to face with more or less well conceived hypotheses, of which no one can prove that there is anything in reality to correspond to them. Before making statements about the spiritual, Anthroposophy evolves the methods which give it the right to make such statements. Some insight will be gained into the nature of these methods if the following be considered: all the results of the accepted science of our time are derived in the last resort from the impressions of the human senses. However far man may extend the sphere of what is yielded by his senses, in experiment or in observation with the help of instruments, nothing essentially new is added by these means to his experience of the world in which the senses place him. His thinking, too, in as much as he applies it in his researches of the physical world, can add nothing new to what is given through the senses. In thought he combines and analyses the sense-impressions in order to discover laws (the laws of nature), and yet, as a researcher of the material world he must admit: this thinking that wells up from within me adds nothing real to what is already real in the material world of sense.

All this immediately changes if we no longer stop short at that thinking which man acquires through his experience of ordinary life and education. This thinking can be strengthened and reinforced within ourselves. We place some simple, easily encompassed idea in the centre of consciousness and, to the exclusion of all other thoughts, concentrate all the power of the soul on such representations. As a muscle grows strong when exerted again and again in the direction of the same force, so our force of soul grows strong when exercised in this way with respect to that sphere of existence which otherwise holds sway in thought. It should again be emphasized that these exercises must be based on simple, easily encompassed thoughts. For in carrying out the exercises the soul must not be exposed to any kind of influences from the subconscious or unconscious. (Here we can but indicate the principle of such exercises; a fuller description, and directions showing how such exercises should be done in individual cases, will be found in the books, such as Knowledge of the Higher Worlds and Occult Science, and other anthroposophical works.

It is tempting to object that anyone who thus gives himself up with all his strength to certain thoughts placed in the focus of consciousness will thereby expose himself to all manner of auto-suggestion and the like, and that he will simply enter a realm of fantasy. But Anthroposophy shows how the exercises should be done from the outset, so that this objection loses its validity. It shows the way to advance within the sphere of consciousness, step by step and fully wide-awake in carrying out the exercises, as in the solving of an arithmetical or geometrical problem. At no point in solving a problem of arithmetic or geometry can our consciousness veer off into unconscious regions; nor can it do so during the practices here indicated, provided always that the anthroposophical suggestions are properly observed.

In the course of such practice we attain a strengthening of a power of thought, of which we had not the remotest idea before. Like a new content of our human being we feel this power of thought holding sway within us. And with this new content of our own human being there is revealed at the same time a world-content which, though we may perhaps have divined its existence before, was unknown to us by actual experience until now. If in moments of introspection we consider our everyday activity of thought, we find that the thoughts are pale and shadow-like beside the impressions that our senses give us.

What we experience in the now strengthened capacity of thought is not pale or shadow-like by any means. It is full of inner content, vividly real and graphic; it is, indeed, of a reality far more intense than the contents of our sense perceptions. A new world begins to dawn for the man who has thus enhanced the force of his perceptive faculty.

He, who until now was only able to perceive in the world of the senses, learns to apperceive in this new world; and as he does so he discovers that all the laws of nature known to him before hold good in the physical world only; it is of the intrinsic nature of the world he has now entered that its laws are different, in fact, the very opposite to those of the physical world. In this world for instance the earthly force of gravity does not apply, on the contrary, another force emerges, working not from the centre of the earth outwards but in the reverse direction, from the circumference of the universe towards the centre of the earth. And so it is in like manner with the other forces of the physical world. Man's faculty to perceive in this world, attainable as it is by exercise and practice, is called, in Anthroposophy, the imaginative faculty of knowledge. Imaginative not for the reason that one is dealing with 'fantasies,' the word is used because the content of consciousness is filled with pictures, instead of the mere shadows of thought. And as in sense perception we feel as an immediate experience that we are in a world of reality, so it is in the activity of soul, which is here called imaginative knowledge. The world to which this knowledge relates is called in Anthroposophy the etheric world. This is not to suggest the hypothetical ether of modern physics, it is something really seen in the spirit. The name is used in keeping with older, instinctive presentiments with regard to that world. Against what can now be known with full clarity, these old presentiments no longer have a scientific value; but if we wish to designate a thing we have to choose some name. Within the etheric world an etheric bodily nature of man is perceptible, existing in addition to the physical bodily nature. This etheric body is also to be found in its essential nature in the plant-world. Plants too have their etheric body. The physical laws really only hold good for the world of lifeless mineral nature. The plant-world is possible on earth because there are substances in the earthly realm which do not remain enclosed within, or limited to the physical laws, but can lay aside the whole complex of physical law and assume one which opposes it. The physical laws work streaming from the earth; the etheric work from all sides of the universe streaming to the earth. It is not possible for man to understand how the plant world comes into being, till he sees in it the interplay of the earthly and physical with the cosmic-etheric. So it is with the etheric body of man himself. Through the etheric body something is taking place in man which is not a straightforward continuation of the laws and workings of the physical body with its forces, but rests on a quite different foundation: in effect the physical substances, as they pour into the etheric realm, divest themselves to begin with of their physical forces. The forces that prevail in the etheric body are active at the beginning of man's life on earth, and most distinctly during the embryonic period; they are the forces of growth and formative development. During the course of earthly life a part of these forces emancipates itself from this formative and growth activity and becomes the forces of thought, just those forces which, for the ordinary consciousness, bring forth the shadow-like world of man's thoughts.

It is of the greatest importance to know that man's ordinary forces of thought are refined formative and growth forces. Something spiritual reveals itself in the formation and growth of the human organism. The spiritual element then appears during the course of life as the spiritual force of thought. And this force of thought is only a part of the human formative and growth force that works in the etheric.

The other part remains true to the purpose it fulfilled in the beginning of man's life. But because the human being continues to evolve even when his growth and formation have reached an advanced stage, that is, when they are to a certain degree completed, the etheric spiritual force, which lives and works in the organism, is able to emerge in later life as the capacity for thought. Thus the formative or sculptural force, appearing from the one side in the soul-content of our thought, is revealed to the imaginative spiritual vision from the other side as an etheric-spiritual reality.

If we now follow the material substance of the earth into the etheric formative process we find wherever they enter this formative process these substances assume a form of being which estranges them from physical nature. While they are thus estranged, they enter into a world where the spiritual comes to meet them transforming them into its own being.

The way of ascending to the etherically living nature of man as described here is a very different thing from the unscientific postulation of a 'vital force' which was customary even up to the middle of the nineteenth century in order to explain the living entities. Here it is a question of the actual seeing — that is to say, the spiritual perception — of a reality which, like the physical body, is present in man and in everything that lives. To bring about spiritual perception of the etheric we do not merely continue ordinary thinking nor do we invent another world through fantasy. Rather we extend the human powers of cognition in an exact way; and this extension yields experience of an extended universe. The exercises leading to higher perception can be carried further. Just as we exert an enhanced power in concentrating on thoughts placed deliberately in the centre of our consciousness, so we can now apply such an enhanced power in order to suppress the imaginations — (pictures of a spiritual-etheric reality) — achieved by the former process. We then reach a state of completely emptied consciousness. We are awake and aware, but our wakefulness to begin with has no content. (Further details are to be found in the above-mentioned books.) But this wakefulness does not remain without content. Our consciousness, emptied as it is of any physical or etheric pictorial impressions, becomes filled with a content that pours into it from a real spiritual world, even as the impressions from the physical world pour into the physical senses. By imaginative knowledge we have come to know a second member of the human being; by the emptied consciousness becoming filled with spiritual content we learn to know a third. Anthroposophy calls the knowledge that comes about in this way knowledge by inspiration. (The reader should not let these terms confuse him, they are borrowed from the instinctive ways of looking into spiritual worlds which belonged to more primitive ages, but the sense in which they are here used is stated exactly.) The world to which man gains entry by 'inspiration' is called the 'astral world'. When one is speaking in the sense explained here of an 'etheric world,' we mean those influences that work from the circumference of the universe towards the earth. If we speak of the 'astral world,' we proceed, as is seen by the perception of inspired consciousness, from the influences of the cosmos towards certain spiritual beings which reveal themselves in these influences, just as the materials of the earth reveal themselves in the forces that radiate out from the earth. We speak of real spiritual beings working from the distant universe just as we speak of the stars and constellations when we look out physically into the heavens at nighttime. Hence the expression 'astral world'. In this astral world man bears the third member of his human nature, namely his astral body.

The earth's substances must also flow into this astral body. Through this it is estranged from its physical nature. — Just as man has the etheric body in common with the world of plants, so he has his astral body in common with the world of animals. What essentially raises the human being above the animal world can be recognized through a form of cognition still higher than inspiration. At this point Anthroposophy speaks of intuition. In inspiration a world of spiritual beings manifests itself; in intuition, the relationship of the discerning human being to the world grows more intimate. He now brings to fullest consciousness within himself that which is purely spiritual, and in the conscious experience of it, he realises immediately that it has nothing to do with experience from bodily nature. Through this he transplants himself into a life which can only be described as a life of the human spirit among other spirit-beings. In inspiration the spiritual beings of the world reveal themselves; through intuition we ourselves live with these beings.

Through this we come to acknowledge the fourth member of the human being, the essential 'I'. Once again we become aware of how the material of the earth, in adapting to the life and being of the 'I,' estranges itself yet further from its physical nature. The nature which this material assumes as 'ego organization' is, to begin with, that form of earthly substance in which it is farthest estranged from its earthly physical character.

In the human organization, that which we thus learn to know as the 'astral body' and 'I' is not bound to the physical body in the same way as the etheric body. Inspiration and intuition show how in sleep the 'astral body' and the 'I' separate from the physical and etheric, and that it is only in the waking state that there is the full mutual permeation of the four members of man's nature to form a human entity.

In sleep the physical and the etheric human body are left behind in the physical and etheric world. Yet they are not in the same position as the physical and the etheric body of a plant or plant-like being. For they bear within them the after-effects of the astral and the Ego-nature. Indeed, in the very moment when they would no longer bear these aftereffects within them, the human being must awaken. A human physical body must never be subjected to the merely physical, nor a human etheric body to the merely etheric effects. Through this they would disintegrate. Inspiration and intuition however also show something else. Physical substance experiences further development of its nature in its transition to living and moving in the etheric. It is a condition of life that the organic body is snatched out of the earthly state to be built up by the extraterrestrial cosmos. This building activity however brings about life, but not consciousness, and not self-consciousness.

The astral body must build up its organization within the physical and the etheric; the ego must do the same with regard to the ego organization. But in this building there is no conscious development of the soul life. For this to occur a process of destruction must oppose the process of building. The astral body builds up its organs; it destroys them by allowing the soul to develop an activity of feeling within consciousness; the ego builds up its 'ego-organization'; it destroys this, in that will-activity becomes active in self-consciousness.

The spirit within the human being does not unfold on the basis of constructive material activity but on the basis of what it destroys. Wherever the spirit is to work in man, matter must withdraw from its activity.

Even the origin of thought in the etheric body depends not on a further development but, on the contrary, on a destruction of etheric being. Conscious thinking does not take place in the processes of growth and formation, but in the processes of deformation, fading, dying which are continually interwoven with the etheric events.

In conscious thinking, the thoughts liberate themselves out of the physical form and become human experiences as soul formations. If we consider the human being on the basis of such a knowledge of man, we become aware that the nature of the whole man, or of any single organ, is only seen with clarity if one knows how the physical, the etheric, the astral body and the ego work in him. There are organs in which the chief agent is the ego; in others the ego works but little, and the physical organization is predominant. Just as the healthy man can only be understood by recognizing how the higher members of man's being take possession of the earthly substance, compelling it into their service, and in this connection also recognizing how the earthly substance becomes transformed when it enters the sphere of action of the higher members of man's nature; so we can only understand the unhealthy man if we understand the situation in which the organism as a whole, or a certain organ or series of organs, find themselves when the mode of action of the higher members falls into irregularity. We shall only be able to think of therapeutic substances when we evolve a knowledge of how some earthly substance or earthly process is related to the etheric, to the astral and to the ego. Only then shall we be able to achieve the desired result, by introducing an earthly substance into the human organism or by treatment with an earthly process of activity, enabling the higher members of the human being to unfold again unhindered, or by the earthly substance (of the physical body) finding, in what has been added, the necessary support to bring it into the path where it becomes a basis for the earthly working of the spiritual.

Man is what he is by virtue of physical body, etheric body, soul (astral body) and ego (spirit). He must, in health, be seen and understood from the aspect of these his members; in disease he must be observed in the disturbance of their equilibrium, and for his healing we must find the therapeutic substances that can restore the balance.

A medical approach built on such a basis is to be suggested in this book.

APPENDIX 5:

Extract from
An Outline of Esoteric Science

Rudolf Steiner

Objectivity is what our thinking needs most of all for spiritual training. In the physical world of the senses, life is the great teacher of the human I as far as objectivity is concerned. If the soul chose to allow its thoughts to wander aimlessly, it would have to be immediately corrected by life so as not to come into conflict with it. The soul's thinking must correspond to the actual course of life's realities. When we turn our attention away from the physical world of the senses, we are no longer subject to its automatic correction, so our thinking will go astray if it is not able to self-correct. This is why students of the spirit must train their thinking so that it can set its own direction and goals. Their thinking must teach itself inner stability and the ability to stick strictly to one subject. For this reason, the appropriate 'thought exercises' we undertake should not deal with unfamiliar and complicated objects, but with ones that are simple and familiar.

Over a matter of months, if we can overcome ourselves to the point of being able to focus our thoughts for at least five minutes a day on some ordinary object (for example, a pin, a pencil, or the like), and if, during this time, we exclude all thoughts unrelated to this object, we will have made a big step in the right direction. (We can consider a new object each day or stay with the same one for several days.) Even those who consider themselves thinkers because of their scientific education should not scorn this means of preparing themselves for spiritual training, because if we fix our thoughts on something very familiar for a certain period of time, we can be certain that we are thinking objectively. If we ask: What is a

Taken from *An Outline of Esoteric Science:* Knowledge of Higher Worlds – Initiation, pp.320ff. Reprinted by kind permission of Anthroposophic Press.

pencil made of? How are these materials prepared? How are they put together to make pencils? When were pencils invented? and so on, our thoughts correspond to reality much more closely than they do if we think about the origin of human beings or the nature of life. Simple thought exercises are better for developing objective thinking about the Saturn, Sun, and Moon phases of evolution than any complicated scholarly ideas, because what we think about is not the point, at least initially. The point is to think objectively, using our own inner strength. Once we have taught ourselves objectivity by practicing on sense-perceptible physical processes that are easily surveyed, our thinking becomes accustomed to striving for objectivity even when it does not feel constrained by the physical world of the senses and its laws. We break ourselves of the habit of allowing our thoughts to wander without regard for the facts.

The soul must become a ruler in the domain of the will just as it is in the world of thoughts. Here again, life itself appears as the controlling element in the physical world of the senses. It makes us need certain things, and our will feels roused to satisfy these needs. For the sake of higher training, we must get used to strictly obeying our own commands. If we do this, we will become less and less inclined to desire nonessentials. Dissatisfaction and instability in our life of will, however, are based on desiring things without having any clear concept of realizing these desires. This dissatisfaction can disrupt our entire mental life when a higher I is trying to emerge from the soul.

A good exercise is to tell ourselves to do something daily at a specific time, over a number of months: Today at this particular time I will do *this*. We then gradually become able to determine what to do and when to do it in a way that makes it possible to carry out the action in question with great precision. In this way, we rise above damaging thoughts, such as: 'I'd like this, I want to do that,' which disregard totally the feasibility of what we want. A very great man put these words into the mouth of a seer: 'I love whomever longs for the impossible.'[1] This great man himself said, 'Living in ideas means treating the impossible as if it were possible.'[2] These statements, however, should not be used as objections to what has been presented here, because what Goethe and his seeress Manto ask can only be accomplished by those who have trained themselves in desiring what is possible in order to then be able to apply their strong will to 'impossibilities' in a way that transforms them into possibilities.

For the sake of spiritual training, the soul should also acquire a certain degree of composure with regard to the domain of feeling. For this to happen, the soul must master its expressions of joy and sorrow, pleasure and pain. There are many prejudices that become evident with regard to acquiring this particular quality. We might imagine that we would become dull and unreceptive to the world around us if we are not meant to empathize with rejoicing or pain. However, that is not the point. The soul should indeed rejoice when there is reason to rejoice, and it should feel pain when something sad happens. It is only meant to master its *expressions* of joy and sorrow, of pleasure and displeasure. With this as our goal, we will soon notice that rather than becoming dulled to pleasurable and painful events in our surroundings, the opposite is true.

We are becoming more receptive to these things than we were previously. Admittedly, acquiring this character trait requires strict self-observation over a long period of time. We must make sure that we are able to empathize fully with joy and sorrow without losing ourselves and expressing our feelings involuntarily. What we are meant to suppress is not our justified pain, but involuntary weeping; not our abhorrence of a misdeed, but blind rage; not alertness to danger, but fruitless fear, and so on.

Exercises like this are the only way for students of the spirit to acquire the mental tranquillity that is needed to prevent the soul from leading a second, unhealthy life, like a shadowy double, alongside the higher I when this I is born and especially when it begins to be active. Especially with regard to these things, it is important not to succumb to self-deception. It can easily seem to people that they already possess a certain equilibrium in ordinary life and that they therefore do not need this exercise, but in fact it is doubly necessary for people like this. It's quite possible to be calm and composed in confronting things in ordinary life and yet have our suppressed lack of equilibrium assert itself all the more when we ascend into a higher world. It is essential to realize that for purposes of spiritual training, what we seem to possess already is much less important than systematically practicing what we need to acquire. This sentence is quite correct, regardless of how contradictory it may seem. No matter what life may have taught us, *what we teach ourselves* is what serves the purposes of spiritual training. If life has taught us excitability we need to break that habit, but if it has taught us complacency we need to shake ourselves up through self-education so that our souls' reactions correspond to the impressions they receive. People who cannot laugh at anything have as little control over their lives as people who are constantly provoked to uncontrollable laughter.

An additional way of training our thinking and feeling is by acquiring a quality we can call 'positivity.' There is a beautiful legend that tells of Christ Jesus and several other people walking past a dead dog.[3] The others all turned away from the ugly sight, but Christ Jesus spoke admiringly of the animal's beautiful teeth. We can practice maintaining the soul-attitude toward the world that this legend exemplifies. The erroneous, the bad, and the ugly must not prevent the soul from finding the true, the good, and the beautiful wherever they are present. We must not confuse this positivity with being artificially uncritical or arbitrarily closing our eyes to things that are bad, false, or inferior. It is possible to admire a dead animal's 'beautiful teeth' and still see the decaying corpse; the corpse does not prevent us from seeing the beautiful teeth. We cannot consider bad things good and false things true, but we can reach the point where the bad does not prevent us from seeing the good and errors do not keep us from seeing the truth.

Our thinking undergoes a certain maturing process in connection with the will when we attempt never to allow anything we have experienced to deprive us of our unbiased receptivity to new experiences. For students of the spirit, the thought: 'I've never heard of that; I don't believe it,' should totally lose its meaning. During specific periods of time, we should be intent on using every opportunity to learn something new concerning every thing and every being. If we are ready and willing to take previously unaccustomed points of view, we can learn from every current of air, every leaf, every babbling baby. Admittedly, it is easy to go too far with regard to this ability. At any given stage in life, we should not disregard all our previous experiences. We should indeed judge what we are experiencing in the present on the basis of past experiences. This belongs on one side of the scales; on the other, however, students of the spirit must place their inclination to constantly experience new things and especially their faith in the possibility that new experiences will contradict old ones.

We have now listed five soul qualities that students in a genuine spiritual training need to acquire: control of one's train of thought, control of one's will impulses, composure in the face of joy and sorrow, positivity in judging the world, and receptivity in one's attitude toward life. Having spent certain periods of time practicing these qualities consecutively, we will then need to bring them into harmony with each other in our souls. We will need to practice them in pairs, or in combinations of three and one at the same time, and so on, in order to bring about this harmony.

Methods of spiritual training recommend these exercises because if conscientiously carried out, they not only have the above-mentioned direct effects on students but also affect them in many indirect ways that they need on their path to the spiritual worlds. If we do these exercises enough, we will encounter many shortcomings and errors in our soul life and will discover the necessary means of strengthening and safeguarding the activity of our intellect, our feelings, and our character. Depending on our abilities, temperament, and character, we will certainly need many other exercises, but these will follow quite naturally from ample practice of the ones described above. In fact, we will notice that these exercises indirectly and gradually supply things that did not initially seem inherent in them. For example, after a certain time, people with too little self-confidence will notice that doing these exercises develops the self-confidence they need. The same is true of other soul qualities. (Specific and more detailed exercises can be found in my book *How to Know Higher Worlds*.)

It is significant that students of the spirit are able to advance to ever higher levels of the faculties indicated. They must develop their control of thoughts and feelings to the point where their souls have the power to establish times of complete inner tranquillity. During these times, students must keep their hearts and minds free of everything outer daily life brings with it in the way of joy and sorrow, satisfactions and concerns, and even tasks and demands. The only things that are allowed to enter the soul in this state of meditation are what the soul itself chooses to admit. It is easy for a certain prejudice to become apparent with regard to this. People might think that we would estrange ourselves from daily life and its tasks if we withdrew our heart and mind from them for certain periods during the day. In reality, however, this is not the case at all. If we give ourselves up to periods of inner stillness and peace, this engenders many powerful forces that are applicable even to our duties in daily life. As a result, we will not only not be worse at fulfilling our daily obligations but will certainly be better at it than we were before.

It is extremely valuable when people are able to detach themselves completely during these periods from thoughts about their personal concerns and rise to concerns that are shared by all. If they are able to fill their souls with communications from the higher spiritual worlds, and if this information is able to capture their interest to the same extent as their personal cares or concerns, this will prove especially fruitful for their souls.

If we make an effort to intercede in our soul life and regulate it in this way, we will also find it possible to observe ourselves and our own concerns with the same composure we apply to the concerns of others. Being able to look at our own experiences, joys, and sorrows as if they belonged to someone else is a good preparation for spiritual training. We can gradually acquire this ability to the necessary extent by taking time after our day's work is done to allow our experiences of the day to pass in front of us in the spirit. We should see ourselves in the images of these experiences; that is, we must look in on ourselves in our daily lives as if from outside. We acquire a certain facility in self-observation of this sort by beginning with visualizations of small isolated portions of our daily life. With practice, we become increasingly skillful in doing this retrospective view, so that after considerable practice we are able to form a complete picture in a short time. Looking at our experiences in reverse order is especially valuable for spiritual training because it forces us to free our visualizations from our normal habit of merely tracing the course of sense-perceptible events with our thinking. In this reversed thinking, we visualize things correctly but are not bound by their sense-perceptible sequence. This is something we need in order to find our way into the spiritual world. It makes our visualizing stronger in a healthy way. That's why it is also good, in addition to visualizing our daily life in reverse, to do the same with other things such as the sequence of a drama, a narrative, a melody, and so on.

For students of the spirit, the ideal increasingly becomes to relate to the events they encounter in life with inner certainty and tranquillity of soul and to judge them according to their own inherent significance and value rather than on the basis of a personal state of mind. With this ideal in view, students are able to create a foundation in their own souls for devoting effort to the above-mentioned meditation exercises on symbolic ideas or other thoughts and feelings.

The prerequisites described here must be met, because we build up our supersensible experience on the basis of our standing in ordinary soul life before entering the spiritual world. In two different ways, everything we experience supersensibly is dependent on the soul's point of departure for entering this world. If we are not concerned from the very beginning with making a healthy faculty of judgment the basis of our spiritual training, we will develop supersensible faculties that perceive the spiritual world inexactly and incorrectly. Our spiritual organs of perception will not develop properly, so to speak. Just as we cannot see properly in the world of the senses if our eyes are defective or diseased, we also cannot perceive properly with spiritual organs that have not been developed on the basis of a healthy faculty of judgment.

And if we take an immoral attitude as our point of departure, the way we ascend into the spiritual worlds will make our spiritual view seem clouded or dazed. We will confront supersensible worlds like someone observing the sensory world in a daze. Although in the sensory world, such a person will surely not be capable of saying anything significant about that world, even dazed spiritual observers are more awake than people in a normal state of consciousness, so their statements become errors with regard to the spiritual world.

The Members of the Human Being

The texts below aim to summarize essential aspects of the members of the human being. Every sentence or statement would need to be underpinned and expanded further. They are offered here to serve as starting points for more extensive documentation and argumentation, and as openings for discussion. They could also serve as reference points in daily practice with patients.

The physical; the solid state; dead nature

Together with the world which surrounds us, we as human beings belong to the *visible* world. We can become aware of this visible world because all visible things have a *surface*. Light reflects from these surfaces and makes things visible. All visible things have their own surface which always has an individual form. This individual form becomes visible as the *boundary* of things. All material objects live and exist next to one another therefore and cannot interpenetrate. Surfaces form impenetrable boundaries within which things have their own content. Everything physical is positioned in space and hence it is oriented in the various spatial directions and in relation to gravity.

The content of rocks, plants, animals and human beings is always filled with matter. On the material level forces of adhesion, cohesion and impenetrability reign. We cannot really enter matter. When we try, we create new surfaces. It seems as if the physical, sense perceptible world can be *subdivided* endlessly, and every division will create a new border surface. In this sense the physical world has *no inside,* but only an outside, and this is the only thing it can show us. All techniques of enlargement show us evermore surfaces hiding new contents. By means of the analytical approach we always end up with a *corpuscular worldview:* every single thing in turn consists of things. And even if we could get inside the physical things, we could not get to know it by means of analysis.

From the Practice Manual, used at the Louis Bolk Instituut, Driebergen, Netherlands.

Non-organic nature is *dead*. This means that things are changed *from the outside by forces* such as erosion, destruction by fire, dissolution, or by forces of the order of electricity, radioactivity and the like. These forces are controlled by *natural laws,* which must be viewed as *timeless,* at least to a certain degree. Physics and chemistry explore and use these natural laws. These forces working in from the outside are different from those at work in organisms which are capable of inner change. This kind of change manifests in growth and changes of shape (see section on the ether body).

The physical world can be *experienced* through the senses. Of all the senses, the sense of touch is most involved here. For it is through the sense of touch that we have the experience that what we touch is something with a surface and contour which takes up space. We also picture 'energy-particles' or 'photons' in a corpuscular sense. The physical world can only be *known,* however, by forming thoughts about data which were first acquired through *division, analysis, weighing, measuring and counting.* A paradox presents itself here with regards to our ability to actually know the physical or corpuscular world: these means of research only give us surface knowledge. Therefore it is impossible to give an answer to the question what the physical world actually *is*.

All natural things visible in space have their own physical manifestation. We denote this in physical nature with the word body, which is in the word corpuscular. In the physical, sense-perceptible world we are therefore always dealing with spatial bodies, with boundaries and content. Inasmuch as the human being is a 'natural object,' he or she therefore also has a physical body. It can be known through all current analytical means of research. During life physical forces do not dominate the human physical body as in a dead body, but interact with the other forces at work.

> *The physical body consists of space filled with matter; it has*
> *boundary and content, within which natural laws apply. Natural*
> *laws determine the shape in which the object manifests. Change*
> *comes about under the influence of natural laws, which affect the*
> *object from the outside. Left to itself, the physical body can only*
> *maintain the status quo and has no ability to change itself, by*
> *virtue of which it belongs to the dimension of timelessness.*

The etheric body

We commonly experience dead and living nature as two distinct realms. We experience all mountain chains and deserts which form the crust of the earth, including fossil remains, as dead nature. In the meantime, human beings have produced immeasurable amounts of dead matter beyond what was there to begin with. From the bronze age onward, human beings have either created and produced new materials or used existing ones. Examples are brick, glass, ceramics, metal alloys and, especially in this century, petroleum derivates. Ecological problems have shocked us into an awareness of what it means when substance is non-recyclable. Anything which cannot be reintegrated has the potential to destroy the life-cycle. Thereby the contrast between life and death has come sharply into focus in a new way; we now have direct experience of how whole sections of our flora and fauna have vanished for good. The independent character of the different life cycles, coupled with the impressive degree of interdependence of these cycles, have brought home to us the strong sense that 'life complexes' exist on several levels. Apparently matter can be part of a life complex either permanently or temporarily. This principle is applied in the preparation of fertilizer consisting of compost or manure.

Next to the physical world, a world of life cycles is in existence. These cycles are interdependent and can absorb matter and secrete it. Every life-cycle has its own character.

Walking through a meadow, we will usually find a variety of plants. Different grasses and flowers grow side-by-side and even intertwine. All the plant organisms share the same soil, breathe the same air and share the same light. Yet their life cycles are different and they form plants in completely different shapes. Furthermore, they will absorb different substances from the soil in different quantities. *The life-cycle* of the specific plant organism will determine when and how the plant will absorb or secrete, and how long it will live. One organism will blossom in the spring, another more towards the fall.

The individual character of a life-cycle manifests in a specific organism. Therefore one organism will form oneness of life within the totality of the living world. Thus understood, living cells are not the building blocks of life. It would be more apt to say that an organism differentiates into different cells. One individual cell is incapable of living outside the organism to which it belongs.

The astral body; awareness

We see animals moving around us in nature and we hear their sounds. Animal movements are usually clearly prompted by something felt or perceived. Such an experience can originate from outside and through sense perception call forth a reaction, as is the case when a gazelle flees from a lion. The sensory experience can also be based in physiological processes arising from within, as is the case when a creature feels hunger. This feeling of hunger causes a lion to go hunting. In both cases we are dealing with an *inner experience* which gives rise to a reaction which can lead to movement. We have the same inner experiences ourselves, and therefore we can recognize such behaviour in animals. It becomes even clearer that we are dealing with inwardly sensed experiences here when we see an animal reacting out of fear, fright or pain. From the reaction, we immediately recognize the whole process of perception, emotion and the reaction. These are all conscious experiences taking place inside of us, and therefore we also ascribe *consciousness* to the animal. That consciousness can be sharp and awake as is the case with eagles, but it can also be dull and undirected in animals like the worm or the jellyfish.

> *We recognize the presence of an astral body within an organism, and with that of inner life, when we see expressions of conscious experience of the world and reaction in the form of behaviour or movement. Consciousness, inner experience, reaction and behaviour are key words.*

Animals can be said to be 'programmed' to a certain degree; with regard to the way they sense things and their patterns of behaviour. For this we use the word instinct. Instinct determines what the animal will perceive and what it will react to. Our hunting techniques are based on knowledge of the animal's instinct, because we do not only know to what the animal will react, but also how it will react. Therefore one could speak of a *structure* in the way the animals experience the world, and of the structure in their reaction patterns. And just as we could use the word structure when we described the etheric, and use the term body for it, we can do the same for consciousness. Hence the word astral *body.*

Instincts are intimately connected to the organism. This connection with the organism comes into being because the astral body also shapes the organism. Viewed phenomenologically, both performance and action of the organism are a picture of the instinct (or astral body) of the animal under consideration. The animal's body has a form which fits the instinct. So the astral body has a formative effect both on the organism and the instinct. The astral body is the higher principle which is at work, and it manifests on different levels of reality.

> *Next to manifesting on the level of behaviour, the astral body also manifests on the level of organic processes. It affects both*

*morphology and physiology, and directs formative processes and
life processes.*

Striking physiological signs of the presence of an astral body are the
occurrence of tonus, as seen in the formation of blood pressure, the action
potential of the nerve, and the ability to build up considerable concentration gradients of salts such as those that occur in the kidneys.

Striking morphological signs are the existence of a nervous system,
muscles (being organs having tone), and senses.

The I; consciousness of self

We will treat three levels on which the I manifests. Consciousness of self
is a manifestation of the ego purely on a spiritual level; a picture of it
emerges in the biography, and it appears at the bodily level as an organism with physical functions.

Awareness of self

When we consider the human being, cultural phenomena and moral questions emerge in addition to biological phenomena. Cultural evolution has
a tempo all of its own and brings an impressive array of manifestations, in
contrast to the much slower principle of biological evolution. A central
aspect in this is human awareness and consciousness of self. Animals
manifest no signs of being aware of themselves in any form of ego consciousness or self reflection. We do see manifestations of a certain form of
reflection on their surroundings in animals. Higher animals exhibit behaviour which shows abilities to sort and combine separate things in order to
solve problems, yet they exhibit no signs of ever reflecting on themselves.

The human being strives to change from within, which comes out in
our efforts at self-education, self-development, and self-realization. The
experience that these possibilities are present in the human being can only
arise because we sense ourselves in the inner chambers of our souls. At
this point exploring what it means to be a human being becomes *intro-
spective* in its purest form. Having recognized and compared human and
animal behaviour, a deep sense of the essential difference between *all* animals and the human being gradually arises, and it is felt as something self-
evident. In using the concept of individuality for the human being, we
point to a sense of self deep within, which we call I. For this I the body is
just as much 'outer world' as other phenomena in nature. The I is a point
of consciousness in the moment; it denotes the present. The I derives a
sense of continuity from memory and anticipation of the future. For the
past works on within us and we anticipate the future coming towards us,

and these two flow together in the way the ego experiences itself in the moment. And even though the human I develops in time, it is itself not of a temporal nature.

> *The human being is able to reflect on and become aware of his or her individuality; thus the kernel of the personality, the I, is experienced deep within the psyche. The working of this I makes self-development and introspection possible. The I experiences itself in the present, on the cutting edge between past and future. The I develops in the course of time, but does not experience itself as a temporal being. It carries the principle of development as an inner potential. In structure and physiology, the human body is tailored to the presence of the I.*

Biography

The biography gives a picture of the development of the individual human being. Next to the constancy of the I, a biography shows continuous metamorphosis of bodily development to begin with, and later of psychological development. The human being takes exceptionally long to mature. It takes an extremely long time, comparatively speaking, before the human being is physically mature and grown-up. Then comes psychological development which again takes many years. And after this more or less 'natural psychological' development is completed, purely spiritual growth, brought about by self-development, can follow. The *patterns of development* originate in the I, which permeates and works on the levels of body, soul and spirit. Here, too, the law holds true that the lower is determined by the higher.

The human capacity to develop is in fact never exhausted. It is interesting to notice the uniqueness of each biography, the joys and sorrows of life, and to see what is gained and accomplished thereby. And it often turns out that a decline in bodily forces by no means implies a decline in spiritual forces. On the contrary, many people go through their greatest inner growth as their biological functions decline with age.

> *The biography of the human being is a picture of the development of the individual and carries the signature of the I.*

The human body

Evolutionary theory usually stresses the similarities between the higher primates and the human being, so that the impression is created that it is only a very small step from ape to human being. When we focus on just the physical differences between an ape and a human being alone, these differences turn out to be so numerous that it is actually a big leap instead of a small step.

To begin with, there is the capacity to walk upright and also to stand in quiet balance for long periods of time. From head to toe, this requires a body which differs in build from *all* apes. The human spinal column alone is biologically totally unique. The totality of the skeleton expresses the uniqueness of the human shape as if it were a symbol. Different apes show great similarity to each other in the structures of their bodies; in this respect the human being is in a separate category.

Another striking difference can be found in the way the whole *skin* is built, specifically in the way the capillary structure is built up below the skin, the fact that we are practically hairless, and hence have the ability to blush or turn pale. It is partly due to the blood supply to the skin that the human being has a warmth regulation which is biologically unique.

Another unique feature of the human being is the structure and function of the larynx and the way it is positioned in the neck.

In terms of biological development, the human being is a case apart when we look at the proportional development of for example the extremities, the teeth, sexual maturity and processes of aging in general.

This list of differences could be expanded at will. It seems important to still mention that the whole process of *health and illness* seems to be beyond evolutionary logic in the case of the human being. We have 'childhood illnesses,' which all have their characteristic course, then there are 'cultural illnesses,' such as a high blood pressure, and we should also mention the existence of illnesses with a psychosomatic component (asthma, stomach ulcer). The existence of these indicate that the human body takes up a special position in relationship to the animal kingdom.

> *In structure and function, the human body cannot be rightly placed within the framework of animal anatomy, physiology and pathology. Strong kinship exists in these categories among primates and higher apes themselves, but are missing when it comes to the human being. Biologically, therefore, the human being falls into a separate category.*
>
> *In human beings, biological processes are organized in such a way, in both form and function, that they form a basis for the human faculty of cultural expression.*

Freedom

Inner freedom is a uniquely human capacity. Only a human being can act out of freely gained insight. It *is* possible to transcend the compulsive effect of drives and instincts. The human I manifests more strongly to the degree in which the biography shows more of those 'free moments.'

The human being exhibits physiological, psychological and spiritual manifestations which are connected to the degree of freedom achieved.

The dynamics between the four members

The four members of the human being function in such a way that the relationships between them change continually. This goes both for rhythmical alternations of day and night and also for all changes related to growth and development of the human being. The relationship between the members is different in a baby and an elderly person and also differs between man and woman. In every individual the relationship differs from morning to evening.

Circadian rhythms, physiological processes of maturing and changing, and physiological differences between man and woman bear witness to this.

The dynamics between the I and the astral body

We have seen that the I is the carrier of the moral forces in the human being and that it determines the individual human character in both a bodily and a psychological sense. The I shapes the organism and the psyche in a way specific to each individual human being. Expressions of this are the slow physical development of the body and the long maturation time of the psyche. This bodily working of the I is an *unconscious* activity.

This implies that it directs the lower members in a hierarchical sense, as will be elaborated.

Human soul life (the astral body) can be influenced. This happens when we learn to think, or refine our feelings (developing them for example in learning to play music), and in all instances when we practice self-control. In all such situations, when we act out of careful consideration rather than out of impulse, the I dominates and shapes the soul. Words like 'self-education,' 'self-control' and the existence of 'scruples' and 'inner conflicts' all describe inner experiences belonging to the dynamic tension between the I and the soul. Everyone can experience how this I-activity is a *conscious* one. When the soul dominates the I we have situations in which the person reacts 'impulsively,' 'gets carried away' by emotions or even 'loses control.' The relationship between the astral body and the animal kingdom comes to expression in many sayings, and makes clear why 'bestial' behaviour is 'inhuman.' The dynamic tension between the I and the astral body on a conscious level lies between self-education on one side and losing control on the other.

The dynamics between astral body and ether body

Our emotional life is tied in with physiological phenomena. Heart palpitations, perspiration, goose bumps, turning red or pale, and intestinal cramps all indicate 'psychosomatic tendencies' of our physiology. The body is known to secrete many substances sparked by psychological reactions (adrenaline and neurotransmitters are two examples). This means that the ether body, as the carrier of biological processes, is influenced by the astral body 'from above' as it were. A number of specific bodily functions can be activated through this, for which specific organs exist which are closely related to the astral body. Examples are: the nervous system, the gonads, the adrenal glands, the thyroid gland and the heart. This activity of the astral body is conscious to begin with (thoughts and feelings), but extends into the unconsciousness of the body. The origin of the specific organs precedes their functioning, of course. During the embryological phase the astral body has already had a formative influence in building up these organs. This is the second way in which the astral body influences the etheric body: it directs and shapes the organs and their functions from the onset. This task of the astral body in forming the organs is an *unconscious* activity taking place deep inside the organism.

This unconscious activity comes first in the course of development, only to be followed later by conscious astral activity.

Next to this 'psychosomatic' direction there also is a reverse direction: from body to soul, in cases where etheric processes influence the astral body, which can result in abnormal states of consciousness. Here we find the origin of psychiatric phenomena and for that reason they can often be corrected chemically. Everyday life shows this influence, in mood swings during the course of the day, and also in the effect of coffee, nicotine and alcohol. All stimulants take effect this way, working from the body on the soul.

It may be clear from the examples given here that the etheric body can also influence the conscious astral body of the human being, without itself coming to consciousness. School readiness is a classic example of this. Head and brain must first be formed through the *unconscious* powers of the ether body. Once this process has been completed these ether forces can be used by the I and the astral body in order to learn to think independently and exactly. These can be called *freed* etheric forces. The ones which work to form the body, by contrast, are called *bound* etheric forces.

The dynamics between etheric and physical body

The ether body constantly attempts to keep the mineral substances of the physical body within the bounds of the biological processes. In edema the water descends out of the biological processes, and into the physical laws.

The etheric body orders, synthesizes and analyses bodily substances. As such it is at work in anabolic and catabolic processes. When the physical principle works on its own, substance will take on a contoured form, as we can see in gallstones, kidney stones, atheromatous plaques, lipid deposits and forms of osteoarthritis with calcium deposits. These are instances where the physical body *hampers* the function of the etheric body, which thereby deteriorates even more, sometimes causing compensatory life-processes.

Through these examples the reader can experience the flexible range of interrelationships of the members. They are some of the more obvious examples. The whole differentiation into organs and tissues within the human organism stems from all manner of different mixtures of the members. The skeleton is highly mineralized, the liver is strongly imbued with the etheric, the kidneys are 'astralized' and the heart is permeated by the I. It would go too far to describe all phenomena pertaining to this differentiation here.

In addition, it would be possible to describe even more interactions, for example between the I and the etheric body or between the I and the physical body. A conscious choice was made not to enter into this further here.

Endnotes

NT = Not available in English translation

Chapter 2

1 Report *Alternatieve Behandelwijzen en Wetenschappelijk Onderzoek (Alternative Medicine and Scientific Research),* August of 1993, p. 76ff.
2 Steiner, *Philosophy of Freedom.*
3 Steiner, R., *The Redemption of Thinking: A Study in the Philosophy of Thomas Aquinas.*

Chapter 4

1 From J.W. von Goethe, *Goethe's Theory of Colour.*
2 Bolk, L., *Hersenen en Cultuur,* 1917, p. 25. [Brains and Culture, p.25] (Dutch. NT)
3 R. Sheldrake, *A New Science of Life.*
4 J.H. van den, Berg, *Het menselijk lichaam,* Vol. 3, p. 100, Callenbach, Nijkerk 1961 [The human body] (Dutch. NT).
5 Karl Heinz Flau, *Urbild und Wandlung,* Ottiniberg 1980 [Archetype and change] (German. NT).
6 Rudolf Steiner, *Goethe's World View.*
7 Rudolf Steiner, *Goethe's World View.*
8 J.W. von Goethe, *Faust.* Full quote: 'Who for living knowledge thirsts seeks to drive out the spirit first. In the palm of his hand he holds all the sections, Lacks nothing, except the spirit's connections.'
9 O.J. Hartmann, *Die Gestaltungsstufen der Naturreiche.*

Chapter 6

1 Quoted lines are from Walter Kaufmann's translation. Original:
Dann steh' ich nur, ich armer Tor,
Und bin so klug als wie zuvor.
...
Dann hat er die Teile in der Hand,
Fehlt leider nur das geistige Band.

Chapter 8

1 R. Dawkins, *The Blind Watchmaker.* 'The difference [between physical and biological systems] lies in the complexity of the design.'

2 According to the second law of thermodynamics processes within a closed system, left to their own devices, will approach a state of equilibrium. As this happens, initial discrepancies in temperature, pressure etc between the different parts of that system will gradually disappear. In technical terms: the entropy of a closed macroscopic system remains the same or increases.
3 H.P. Fischer, 'Langzeitbeobachtungen über den Zusammenhang von Samenkeimung und Sonnenfleckentätigkeit,' *Berichte der Deutschen Botanischen Gesellschaft,* 1982, 95.457–64. [Long term observation regarding the relationship between seed germnination and sun spot activity] (German. NT).
4 J. Schwemmle, H.P. Fischer, 'Wodurch sind die großen Schwankungen bei der Keimung von Oenotheren-Samen bedingt?' *Berichte der Deutschen Botanischen Gesellschaft,* 1963, 76.147–53. [What determines the great variations in the germination of oenotherae-seeds?] (German. NT).
5 F.A. Brown Jr., C.S. Chow, 'Lunar-Correlated Variations in Water Uptake by Seen Seeds,' *Biol. Bull.,* 1973, 143.265–78.
6 Michael Endres, Wolfgang Schad, *Moon Rhythms in Nature.*
7 W. Reichel, 'The Biology of Aging,' *Journal of the American Geriatric Society* 1966, 14.431.
8 L. Hayflick, 'Human Cells and Aging,' *Scientific American* 1968, 218.32.

Chapter 10

1 Laura Barlow (Ed.) *The Autobiography of Charles Darwin,* Harcourt, Brace, New York 1959, pp. 138f.

Appendix 1

1 Baron Karl von Rokitansky (1804–1878), professor of pathological anatomy, author of *Handbuch der pathologischen Anatomie* ('Handbook of Pathological Anatomy'), 3 vols., Vienna 1842–1846.

2 Claudius Galenus (*ca.* AD 129–199), Greek physician to the gladiators in Parganum and at the court of Marcus Aurelius. Considered the founder of experimental physiology, he demonstrated the function of arteries. He is responsible for about 100 treatises on physiology and medicine.

3 Phillippus Aureolus Paracelsus Theophrastus Bombastus von (1493–1541), Swiss physician and alchemist. He investigated problems and diseases related to mining. He was forced out of mainstream medical practice because of his unorthodox ideas and methods. He emphasized a phenomenological approach to medicine and helped to establish chemistry as a part of medical practice. Johann Baptist van Helmont (1579–1644), Flemish physician and chemist who coined the term *gas* (suggested by the Latin and Greek *chaos*) to designate aeriform fluids. He was the first to distinguish gasses from air, such as carbon dioxide, and considered water a 'pure chemical.' He also suggested the use of alkalies to balance acidity in the stomach.

4 Georg Ernst Stahl (1660–1734), an advocate of animism.

5 Johannes Peter Müller (1801–1858), German physiologist and comparative anatomist. Ernst Heinrich Philipp August Haeckel (1834–1919) became professor of zoology at the University of Jena. He was a prolific writer and, by the age of sixty, had published 42 works.

6 Giovanni Battista Morgagni (1682–1771), Italian physician and considered the founder of padiological anatomy.

7 Christian Friedrich Samuel Hahnemann (1755–1843), founder of homeopathy. His chief work, *Organon der rationellen Heilkunde (Organon of Medicine)*, Dresden, 1810.

8 Theodor Schwann (1810–1882), professor of anatomy and physiology in Liege and Louvain. His chief work was *Mikroskopische Untersuchungen über die Übereinstimmung in der Struktur und dem Wachstum der Tiere und der Pflanzen* ('Microscopic Investigation of the Agreement between Structure and Growth in Animals and Plants'), Berlin 1839.

9 Rudolf Virchow (1821–1902), professor of pathological anatomy in Würzburg and Berlin; co-founded the Archive for Pathological Anatomy and Physiology and Clinical Medicine; explained cellular pathology in his *Vorlesungen über Zellularpathologie in ihrer Begründung auf physiologischer und pathologischer Gewebelehre* ('Lectures on Cellular Pathology: Its Basis in Tissue Physiology and Pathology'), Berlin, 1859.

10 Ignaz Paul Vital Troxler (1780–1866). Published works: *Blicke in das Wesen des Menschen* ('Glimpses into the Essential Nature of the Human Being'), Aarau 1812; *Naturlehre des menschlichen Erkennens oder Metaphysik* ('Natural History of Human Knowledge, or Metaphysics'), Aarau 1812; *Vorlesungen uber Philosophie, uber Inhalt, Bildungsgrenze, Zweck und Anwendung derselben aufs Leben* ('Lectures on Philosophy: Its Content, Delineation, Purpose, and Applicability to Life'), Bern 1835.

Appendix 5

1 Goethe, *Faust*, Part Two, Act 2.

2 Goethe. *Verses in Prose.*

3 A story attributed to the Persian poet Nizami (1141–1203), and adapted by Goethe for inclusion in his *West-östlicher Divan*. It is translated into English as 'Agraphon' in *Selected Poems*, Angelos Sikelianos, Princeton University Press, Princeton, 1979, pp. 137–139.

Bibliography

Compiled by Dr Frank Mulder

This list includes medical books and lectures by Rudolf Steiner, and material by other authors, selected on what some fifteen anthroposophical doctors worldwide said were the ten titles that had been most formative and helpful for them. Not all books listed are currently in print.

NT = Not available in English translation

Fundamental books and lectures by Rudolf Steiner
(The GA number refers to the volume of the German *Gesamtausgabe,* complete works.)

Steiner, R. & Wegman, I., *Fundamentals of Therapy* (bilingual study-edition, tr. C. van Tellingen) Mercury, New York 1999; or: *Extending Practical Medicine: Fundamental Principles based on the Science of the Spirit* (tr. A.R. Meuss) Steiner Press, London 1996 (GA 27).

Steiner, R. *Anthroposophical Spiritual Science and Medical Therapy,* Mercury, New York 1991 (GA 313).

—, *Course for Young Doctors,* Mercury, New York 1994 (GA 316).

—, *Curative Eurythmy,* Steiner Press, London 1983 (GA 315).

—, *Education for Special Needs. The Curative Education Course,* Steiner Press, Forest Row 1998 (GA 317).

—, *Fundamentals of Anthroposophical Medicine,* Mercury, New York 1998 (from GA 314),

—, *The Healing Process,* Steiner Press, Forest Row 2000 (GA 319).

—, *Introducing Anthroposophic Medicine,* Anthroposophic, New York 1999 (Also known as *Spiritual Science and Medicine)* (GA 312).

—, *The Invisible Man within us. Pathology Underlying Therapy,* Mercury, New York 2002 (from GA 221).

—, *An Occult Physiology,* Steiner Press, London 1983 (GA 128).

—, *Pastoral Medicine,* Anthroposophic, New York 1987 (GA 318).

—, *Physiology and Therapeutics,* Mercury, New York 1996, (from GA 314).

Workmen's Lectures. Steiner's lectures held to the workmen involved in building the first Goetheanum, extend over 8 volumes. They are not strictly medical, but nevertheless are a treasure trove for doctors.

—, *From Beetroot to Buddhism,* Steiner Press, Forest Row 1999 (GA 353).

—, *From Comets to Cocaine,* Steiner Press, Forest Row 2000 (GA 348).

—, *From Crystals to Crocodiles,* Steiner Press, Forest Row 2002 (GA 347).

—, *From Elephants to Einstein,* Steiner Press, Forest Row 1998 (GA 352).

—, *From Limestone to Lucifer,* Steiner Press, Forest Row 2000 (GA 349).

—, *From Mammoths to Mediums,* Steiner Press, Forest Row 2000 (GA 350).
—, *From Sunspots to Strawberries,* Steiner Press, Forest Row 2002 (GA 354).
—, *Health and Illness,* 2 vols. Anthroposophic, New York 1981, 1983 (GA 348).

Fundamental books by other authors

Bott, Victor, *Spiritual Science and the Art of Healing,* Healing Arts, 1982.
Drake, Stanley, *Though You Die,* Floris, Edinburgh 2002.
Dunselman, Robert, *In Place of Self — How Drugs Work,* Hawthorn, Stroud 1995.
Evans, Michael & Rodger, Iain, *Healing for Body, Soul and Spirit — An Introduction to Anthroposophical Medicine,* Floris, Edinburgh & Anthroposophic, New York, 2000.
Goebel, Wolfgang, & Glöckler, Michaela, *A Guide to Child Health,* Floris, Edinburgh 2003.
Hauschka, Rudolf, *The Nature of Substance,* Steiner Press, Forest Row 2002.
Hauschka-Stavenhagen, Margarethe, *Rhythmical Massage as indicated by Dr Ita Wegman,* Mercury, New York 1991.
Heiligtag, Hans-Richard (ed.), *Anthroposophical Medicine and Therapies for Cancer,* Mercury, New York 1995.
Holtzapfel, Walter, *Children with a Difference,* Lanthorne Press, East Grinstead.
—, *Children's Destinies,* Mercury, New York 1984.
—, *Children's Illnesses,* Mercury, New York 1985.
—, *The Four Organs,* Lanthorne Press, 1993.
Husemann, Armin, *The Harmony of the Human Body. Musical Principles in Human Physiology,* Floris, Edinburgh 2002.
Husemann, Friedrich & Wolff, Otto et al., *The Anthroposophical Approach to Medicine,* 3 vols. Anthroposophic, New York 1982, 1987.
Kirchner-Bockholt, Margarete, *Fundamental Principles of Curative Eurythmy,* Steiner Press, London 1977.
König, Karl, *In Need of Special Understanding,* Camphill Press 1999.
—, *A Living Physiology,* Camphill Press 1999.
Leroi, Rita, *Illness and Healing in the Context of Cosmic Evolution,* Temple Lodge, London 1988.
Lievegoed, Bernard, *Man on The Threshold,* Hawthorn, Stroud 1985.
—, *Phases: The Spiritual Rhythms of Adult Life,* Steiner Press, London 1979.
Marti, Ernst, *The Four Ethers,* Schaumberg, Illinois 1984.
Pelikan, Wilhelm, *Healing Plants: Insights Through Spiritual Science,* Mercury, New York 1997.
—, *The Secrets of Metals,* Anthroposophic, New York 1973.
Treichler, Rudolf, *Soulways,* Hawthorn, Stroud 1989.
Twentyman, Ralph, *The Science and Art of Healing,* Floris, Edinburgh 1992.
Vogel, Heinz-Hartmut, *Finding Remedies; Spiritual Knowledge of Man and Nature,* Medizin Verlags 2000.
Wolff, Otto, *Remedies for the Typical Diseases,* Mercury, New York 1996.

Chapter 1: Modern books on the history of medicine:

Conrad, L.I. et al., *The Western Medical Tradition,* Cambridge University Press 1995
Lindeboom, G.A, *Inleiding tot de geschiedenis van de geneeskunst,* Erasmus, Rotterdam 1993. [Introduction to the history of medicine] (Dutch. NT).
Temkin, O, *Hippocrates in a World of Pagans and Christians,* John Hopkins University Press, Baltimore 1991,

Primary sources:

There is a wide choice of readers of pre-Socratic texts on the market

Hahnemann, S., *Organon of Medicine*, various editions

Hippocrates, *The Nature of Man; Aphorisms*, Loeb, London 1984

Homer, *Iliad*, various editions

Homer, *Odyssey*, various editions. Only the Cotterill translation is in hexameters, Harrap, London 1911.

Hufeland, C.W., *Enchiridium medicum*. (German. NT).

Hufeland, C.W., *Makrobiotik*. Insel, Frankfurt 1984. (German. NT).

Lessing, G.E., *The Education of the Human Race*, London & New York 1927.

Paracelsus, Th., *Sämtliche Werke*, Vol.1 (Ed B. Aschner), Fischer, Jena 1926 [Collected works] (German. Various readers and selections in print).

Paracelsus, Th., *Werke: medizinische Schriften*, Vol. 2, (Ed. W.E. Peuckert), Schwabe, Basel/Stuttgart 1981 [Works: medical writings] (German.Various readers and selections in print).

Plutarch, *Socrates' Daimon*: in *Selected Essays and Dialogues*, Oxford University Press 1993.

About the consciousness of the ancient Greeks:

Dietz, K.M., *Metamorhposen des Geistes*, Vol. 1, Freies Geistesleben, Stuttgart 1989 [Metamorphoses of the spirit] (German. NT).

Stein, W.J., Die Mysterien des Asklepios, *Natura* 10/11, Dornach 1927 [The mysteries of Asclepios] (German. NT).

Steiner, R., *Riddles of Philosophy*, Anthroposophic Press, New York 1974 (from German GA 18).

About ancient mystery streams

Muijres, B. (Ed), *Mysteriën en inwijdingen in het oude Europa en de nieuwe mysteriën*, Pentagon, Amsterdam 1989 [Mysteries and Initiations in ancient Europe and the new mysteries] (Dutch. NT).

Steiner, R, *Christianity as Mystical Fact*, Anthroposophic Press, New York 1997 (from German GA 8).

Wegman, I., *The Mysteries*, Temple Lodge, London 1995.

Others

König, K., Hahnemann und seine Zeit, in *Beiträge zu einer Erweiterung der Heilkunst*, 1955.1 [Hahnemann and his time] (German. NT).

Steiner, R., *An Occult Physiology*, Rudolf Steiner Press, London 1983 (from German GA 128).

Steiner, R., *Introducing Anthroposophic Medicine*, Anthroposophic, New York 1999. (Another translation *Spiritual Science and Medicine*) (from German GA 312).

Chapter 2

Rapport van de Gezondheidsraad: Alternatieve Behandelwijzen en Wetenschappelijk Onderzoek, W.V.C. 1993 [Health Council Report: Alternative approaches to treatment and scientific research, 1993] (Dutch. NT).

Bor, J. & Teppema, S., *Vijfentwintig Eeuwen Filosofie*, Boom, Meppel & Amsterdam 1992 [Twenty-five centuries of philosophy] (Dutch. NT).

Bortoft, H., *The Wholeness of Nature*, Lindisfarne, New York & Floris, Edinburgh 1996.

Brakel, J. & Brink, J.T. van de, *Filosofie van de wetenschappen*, Coutinho 1988 [Philosophy of the Sciences] (Dutch. NT).

Dietz, K., Rudolf Steiners 'Grundlinien' im Zusammenhang der Bewusstseinsgeschichte; in *Tycho de Brahe Jahrbuch*, 1986 [Rudolf Steiner's 'Goethean Science' in the Context of the History of Consciousness] (German. NT).

Ephraim, M., *De goetheanistische fenomenologie als additieve onderzoeksmethode bij en als verruiming van het gangbare (medische) natuurwetenschappelijke onderzoek*, privately published 1988 [Goetheanistic phenomenology as a method of research in addition to and as an extension of conventional (medical) scientific research] (Dutch. NT).

Kiene, H., *Grundlinien einer essentialen Wissenschaftstheorie*, Urachhaus, Stuttgart 1984 [Outline of an essential theory of science] (German. NT).

—, *Schulmedizin-Komplementärmedizin*, Schattauer, Stuttgart 1994 [Orthodox medicine — complementary medicine] (German. NT).

Kracht, T. (Ed.), *Erfahrung des Denkens*, 1996 [The experience of thinking] (German. NT).

Kuhn,T., *The structure of scientific revolutions*, University of Chicago Press, 1962.

Schaik, J., van (Ed.), *Van Aristoteles tot Steiner. De metamorfose van het denken*, 1995 [From Aristotle to Steiner. The metamorphosis of thinking] (Dutch. NT).

Steiner, R., *The Philosophy of Freedom: The Basis for a Modern World Conception*, Rudolf Steiner Press, London 1999 (Alternative translation: *Intuitive Thinking as a Spiritual Paath*, Anthroposophic, New York 1995) (from German GA 4).

Steiner, R., *The Redemption of Thinking: A Study in the Philosophy of Thomas Aquinas* Anthroposophic, New York 1983. (from German GA 74).

Steiner, R., *The Boundaries of Natural Science*, Anthroposophic, New York 1988 (from German GA 322).

Steiner, R., *Truth and Knowledge: Introduction to the Philosophy of Spiritual Activity* Steinerbooks, New York 1981 (from German GA 3).

Steiner, R., *Theory of Knowledge Implicit in Goethe's World Conception*, Anthroposophic, New York 1988 (from German GA 2).

Verbrugh, H., *Op de huid van de tijd*, De Toorts, Haarlem [Under time's skin] (Dutch. NT).

Chapter 3

Steiner, R., *Goethe the Scientist*, Anthroposophic, New York 1950 *(Goethes naturwissenschaftliche Schriften*. Freies Geistesleben, Stuttgart 1962.)

Bockemühl, J. (Ed.), *Toward a Phenomenology of the Etheric World*, Rudolf Steiner Press, London. *(Erscheinungsformen des Ätherischen*, Freies Geistesleben, Stuttgart 1977.)

Husemann, A.J., *Der Zahnwechsel des Kindes, ein Spiegel seiner seelisches Entwicklung*, Freies Geistesleben, Stuttgart 1996. [The change of teeth in children, a reflection of their soul development] (German. NT).

Chapter 4

Poppelbaum, H., *Man and Animal*, Anthroposophical Publishing Co., London n.d.

Poppelbaum, H., *A New Zoology*, Philosophic-Anthroposophic Press, Dornach 1961.

Hartmann, O.J., *Die Gestaltstufen der Naturreiche*, Die Kommenden, Freiburg 1967 [The stages of form in the natural kingdoms] (German. NT).

Hartmann, O.J., *Dynamische Morphologie*, Klostermann, Frankfurt a.M. 1959 [Dynamic morphology] (German. NT.).

Verhulst, J., *De eerstgeborene*, Cahier Vrije School, Antwerp 1990 [The Firstborn] Dutch. NT).

Mees, L.F.C., *Dieren zijn wat mensen hebben,* Vrij Geestesleven, Zeist 1984 [Animals are what humans have] (Dutch. NT).

Naydler, J., (Ed.) *Goethe on Science,* Floris, Edinburgh 1996.

Steiner, R., *Goethe's World View,* Mercury, New York 1985 (from German GA 6).

Chapter 5

Most of the drawings presented here are from George Adams & Olive Whicher, *The Plant between Sun and Earth,* Rudolf Steiner Press, London 1980. There is a treasure trove of exercise material in this book specially aimed at fathoming the processes of form in the plant world. The study of this book is warmly recommended.

Whicher, Olive, *The Idea of Counterspace,* Rudolf Steiner Press, London 1996.

Whicher, Olive, *Sunspace,* Rudolf Steiner Press, London 1989.

Whicher, Olive, *Projective Geometry: Creative Polarities in Space and Time,* Rudolf Steiner Press, London, 1985.

Adams Kaufmann, George, *Strahlende Weltgestaltung, synthetische Geometrie in geisteswissenschaftlicher Beleuchtung* Philosophisch-Anthroposophischer, Dornach 1965 [Radiant world formation] (German. NT).

Locher-Ernst, L., *Urphänomene der Geometrie,* Philosophisch-Anthroposophischer, Dornach 1980 [Archetypal phenomena in geometry] (German. NT).

Edward, L., *Projective Geometry,* Floris, Edinburgh 2003.

Chapter 6

Bockemühl, J. (Ed.) *Toward a Phenomenology of the Etheric World,* Rudolf Steiner Press, London. *(Erscheinungsformen des Ätherischen,* Freies Geistesleben, Stuttgart 1977.)

Goethe, J.W. von, *Goethe's Botanical Writings,* various editions (e.g. Ox Bow Press 1989).

Grohmann, G., *The Plant, a Guide to Understanding its Nature,* Rudolf Steiner Press, London 1974 *(Die Pflanze,* Verlag Freies Geistesleben, 1991, Stuttgart).

Pelikan, W., *Healing Plants, Insights Through Spiritual Science,* Vol 1. Mercury Press, New York 1997 *(Heilpflanzenkunde,* Philosophisch-Anthroposophischer, Dornach 1958).

Colquhoun, M., and Ewald, A., *New Eyes for Plants,* Hawthorn Press, Stroud 1996.

Chapter 7

Husemann, F. and Wolff, O. (Ed.) *The Anthroposophical Approach to Medicine,* 3 vols. Anthroposophic Press, New York 1982–2003 *(Das Bild des Menschen,* Freies Geistesleben, Stuttgart 1993).

Marti, Ernst, *Das Ätherische,* Basel 1989. (German. NT).

Marti, Ernst, *The Four Ethers,* Schaumberg, Illinois 1984.

Chapter 8

Evans, M., and Rodger, I, *Healing for Body, Soul and Spirit — An Introduction to Anthroposophical Medicine,* Floris Books, Edinburgh and Anthropsophic, New York 2000.

Hauschka, M., *Fundamentals of Artistic Therapy Based on Spiritual Science,* Rudolf Steiner Press, London 1992.

Hauschka, M., *Rhythmical Massage,* Rudolf Steiner Press, London 1979.

Husemann, F. and Wolff, O. (Ed.) *The Anthroposophical Approach to Medicine,* 3 vols.

Anthroposophic Press, New York 1982–2003 *(Das Bild des Menschen,* Freies Geistesleben, Stuttgart 1993).

Pelikan, W., *Healing Plants – Insights Through Spiritual Science,* Mercury New York 1997.

Schoorel, E., *De eerste zeven jaar,* Christofoor, Zeist 1998 [The first seven years] (Dutch. NT).

Sheldrake, R., *A New Science of Life,* Blond & Briggs, London 1981.

Wijnbergh, F., *De twee stromen,* Cicero, Schoorl 1995 [The two streams] (Dutch. NT).

Chapter 9

Lindenau, C., Life Organisation and Thought Organisation. In: Bockemühl, J. (Ed.) *Toward a Phenomenology of the Etheric World,* Rudolf Steiner Press, London. (Erscheinungsformen des Ätherischen, Freies Geistesleben, Stuttgart 1977.)

Steiner, R., *The Education of the Child in Light of Anthroposophy,* Rudolf Steiner Press, London 1989 (from German GA 34 and 36).

Steiner, R., *Theosophy,* Anthroposophic Press, New York 1989 (from German GA 9).

Chapter 10

General Path:

Lipson, Michael, *Stairway of Surprise, Six Steps to a Creative Life,* Anthropsophic, New York 2002.

Smit, J., *How to Transform Thinking, Feeling and Willing,* Hawthorn Press, Stroud.

Steiner, R., *Guidance in Esoteric Training,* Steiner Press, Forest Row 1998 (GA 245).

—, *How to Know Higher Worlds,* Anthroposophic Press, New York 2003 (Other translations *Knowledge of Higher Worlds, and how to Attain it)* (from German GA 10).

—, *Theosophy,* Anthroposophic Press, New York 1989 (from German GA 9).

—, *True and False Paths in Spiritual Investigation,* Anthroposophic, New York 1969 (GA 243).

Profession-specific Path:

Steiner, R., *Course for Young Doctors.*

Steiner, R. & Wegman, I., *Fundamentals of Therapy.*

Van de Weg, J., *Lof der hindernissen; inwijdingsmotieven in het dagelijks leven,* Vrij Geestesleven, Zeist 1996. [The challenge of setbacks; initiation in daily life] (Dutch. NT).

Addresses

If you have difficulty ordering from your local (anthroposophical) bookshop, or for up-to-date information, contact the publisher.

Steinerbooks (Anthroposophic Press), www.steinerbooks.org
PO Box 960, Herndon, VA 20172-0960
Tel. 800-856-8664 Fax 800-277-7947 E-mail: service@anthropress.org
Steinerbooks distribute all book of Steiner Press, Floris Books, Temple Lodge and Hawthorn Books in USA.

BookSource, 32 Finlas Street, Glasgow G22 5DU, UK.
Tel. 0141-558 1366, Fax: 0141-557 0189, Email: orders@booksource.net
BookSource distributes all book of Steiner Press, Floris Books, Temple Lodge and Hawthorn Books.

Floris Books, www.florisbooks.co.uk, order from BookSource
Hawthorn Press, www.hawthornpress.com, order from BookSource
Mercury Press, 241 Hungry Hollow Road, Spring Valley, NY 10977, USA.
Rudolf Steiner Press, www.rudolfsteinerpress.com, order from BookSource
Temple Lodge Publishing, www.templelodge.com, order from BookSource
Healing Arts, via Steinerbooks
Camphill Press, Botton Village, Danby, Whitby YO21 2NJ, UK.
Natur Mensch Medizin Verlag, www.nmm-verlag.de/index.htm (German only)
Louis Bolk Instituut, Hoofdstraat 24, 3972 LA Driebergen, Netherlands.

Index